THE NURSING MOTHER'S COMPANION

THE BREASTFEEDING BOOK MOTHERS TRUST, FROM PREGNANCY THROUGH WEANING

KATHLEEN HUGGINS, R.N., M.S., I.B.C.L.C.

Foreword by Jessica Martin-Weber
Preface by Kelly Bonyata
Appendix on Drug Safety by Philip O. Anderson

HARVARD
COMMON
PRESS

TO THE NURSING MOTHERS OF SAN LUIS OBISPO, WHO HAVE BEEN MY TEACHERS

Inspiring | Educating | Creating | Entertaining

Brimming with creative inspiration, how-to projects, and useful information to enrich your everyday life, Quarto Knows is a favorite destination for those pursuing their interests and passions. Visit our site and dig deeper with our books into your area of interest: Quarto Creates, Quarto Cooks, Quarto Homes, Quarto Lives, Quarto Drives, Quarto Explores, Quarto Gifts, or Quarto Kids.

© 2017 Quarto Publishing Group USA Inc.
Text © 2015 Kathleen Huggins

First Published in 2017 by The Harvard Common Press, an imprint of The Quarto Group, 100 Cummings Center, Suite 265-D, Beverly, MA 01915, USA.
T (978) 282-9590 F (978) 283-2742 QuartoKnows.com

The Harvard Common Press titles are also available at discount for retail, wholesale, promotional, and bulk purchase. For details, contact the Special Sales Manager by email at specialsales@quarto.com or by mail at The Quarto Group, Attn: Special Sales Manager, 100 Cummings Center, Suite 265-D, Beverly, MA 01915, USA.

21 20 19   5

ISBN: 978-1-55832-882-2

Originally found under the following *Library of Congress Cataloging-in-Publication Data*
Huggins, Kathleen.
  The nursing mother's companion : the breastfeeding book mothers trust, from pregnancy through weaning / Kathleen Huggins, R.N., M.S., I.B.C.L.C. ; foreword by Jessica Martin-Weber ; preface by Kelly Bonyata ; appendix on Drug Safety by Philip O. Anderson. — 7th edition.
    pages cm
  Includes bibliographical references and index.
  ISBN 978-1-55832-849-5 (paperback : acid-free paper)
  1. Breastfeeding—Popular works. I. Title.
  RJ216.H845 2015
  649'.33--dc23
                                                                    2014041988

Cover illustration by Susie So
Cover and Text design by Laura H. Couallier, Laura Herrmann Design
Illustrations by Susan Aldridge and Arden Vincent

Contents

Foreword

N EARLY 16 YEARS AGO I WAS BREASTFEEDING my first newborn in the middle of the night and in agonizing pain. Both my baby and I were frustrated and in tears. Having already asked for help from various sources, including my mother, a local breastfeeding support group, and health-care professionals, I was ready to quit. A friend had given me a few breastfeeding books, but the one I had started just left me feeling even more overwhelmed. I needed answers that were easy to find in my sleep-deprived and emotionally spent state. That night I looked at the basket of books and selected another one to try, *The Nursing Mother's Companion*. After reading the introduction, I flipped to the index and found a title that looked like what I was dealing with. Ten minutes later I carefully broke the painful latch of my daughter and, following the suggestions I had just read, readjusted my hold, positioning her differently and paying attention to her chin, lips, and tongue, and latched her again. There was still pain, but I could tell it was different. Within a day

I was healing and my baby was more satisfied. Just like that, a woman I had never met saved my breastfeeding relationship. Throughout my personal breastfeeding journey with six babies, Kathleen Huggins, through her manual, has been my guide and support. More than a dry textbook on human lactation, *The Nursing Mother's Companion* not only put information I could easily understand and apply right at my fingertips at all hours, it also showed me I wasn't alone. Kathleen's voice of experience blends clinical support with the relatable presence of a friend.

Today, my original copy of *The Nursing Mother's Companion* looks well loved. This is the only book I give to breastfeeding mothers as a gift—I trust it like a good friend to support moms and help them tap into their own strength and power in mothering their children. It is such a pleasure and an honor to share this revised edition with thousands of other mothers on their breastfeeding journeys and to call Kathleen my personal friend. I wish all the best to you along your own breastfeeding journey and assure you that you couldn't have a better companion.

—Jessica Martin-Weber
Creator, *The Leaky Boob*, www.theleakyboob.com

Preface

AT SOME POINT, EVERY MOTHER IS GOING TO HAVE QUESTIONS about breastfeeding—this is a new experience, after all, and it changes from week to week and from child to child! More than 75 percent of mothers begin breastfeeding when their child is born, but one-third of them stop within six months, often because of problems they encounter along the way. As a lactation consultant, one of my goals is to help connect mothers with the information they need to combat these problems and have a successful breastfeeding experience.

Our babies and our breasts are biologically hardwired to breastfeed, but that doesn't mean that it always comes easily. If you had been born into an earlier generation when breastfeeding was the norm, you would have seen babies breastfeeding and heard mothers talking about breastfeeding since you were very young; if you had questions, you would be able to look to the women around you for answers. Despite the increase in breastfeeding rates over the last 30 years, many new mothers still have never seen a breastfeeding baby and have never known another woman who had a successful breastfeeding relationship.

The good news is that in our modern information culture, many good sources of breastfeeding information are available to mothers. This book, written by a board-certified lactation consultant and registered nurse who breastfed her own children, has been a trusted source of breastfeeding information for more than 30 years. It has been newly updated to provide mothers with the most current information on many topics, including

- latching on and positioning;
- safety of medications, tattoos, and milk sharing;
- breastfeeding problems and their treatments, including sore or injured nipples, plugged ducts, insufficient glandular tissue, mastitis and MRSA, and low milk supply;
- infant issues such as biting and teething, tongue or lip tie, breast refusal and torticollis, high palate, laryngomalacia, and colic;
- insurance coverage of pumps and lactation consultant visits;
- employer support for breastfeeding mothers under the Fair Labor Standards Act; and
- breast pumps, "hands-on pumping," and paced bottle-feeding.

This easy-to-use guide has a simple format that can be read a little at a time as your baby grows. Chapters on pregnancy planning, the first week after birth, and breastfeeding your baby at different ages also contain information on self-care and baby care, in addition to breastfeeding. Each chapter on what to expect at each age ends with a useful "Survival Guide" that describes common problems and possible solutions. Other chapters feature advice on special medical situations, expressing milk, traveling with baby, separations from baby, and breastfeeding after you go back to work. The appendices include a comprehensive list of additional breastfeeding resources, growth standards, and medication safety guidelines.

The information in this book will help you build confidence in yourself as a breastfeeding mother so you can more quickly become an expert on your own baby.

—Kelly Bonyata, B.S., I.B.C.L.C.
Founder and author, www.kellymom.com

Acknowledgments

MORE THAN 30 YEARS AGO, a first-time nursing mother came to me about a difficulty she was having breastfeeding her baby. After we successfully resolved it, she suggested I write a book on breastfeeding that included problem-solving techniques. Although I was flattered, such a project seemed monumental. But later, as I recalled her enthusiasm, I began to consider the insights I had gained over years of assisting so many mothers, first as a maternity and newborn nurse and later after founding a breastfeeding clinic (one of the first in the United States) and telephone counseling service. Certainly, I was more than familiar with the common concerns of mothers who are learning to breastfeed, as well as with the occasional problems that can interfere with the development of a successful nursing relationship. The next day I wrote my rough outline. Without that mother's words to me, this book would never have been written.

During the year I spent writing this book, I received a great deal of encouragement and guidance. I am tremendously indebted to Lynn Moen for her support along the way. I also wish to thank Penny Simkin, R.P.T.

For their thoughtful review of the text I thank Marian Tompson; Andrea Herron, R.N., M.S., C.L.C.; Kathleen Rodriquez Michaelson, B.A., C.L.C.; Vicki McDonald, R.D.; Judith La Vigna; Julie Merrill, R.N.; Tom Robinson; and Kathleen Auerbach, Ph.D.

Jim Litzenburger; Vicki Gadberry, R.N., C.N.M.; Marilynn Schuster, R.N.; Kathleen Long, M.D.; and Dawn Edwards, R.N.C., are most appreciated for their encouragement as well as their friendship.

I am grateful to Donna Janetski for her commitment to this project in preparing the manuscript. My thanks also to Mike Sims for his generosity, and to Susan and Kirk Graves for their efforts.

This book would never have been possible without my husband, Brad, whose love, patience, and faith sustained me. Kate, my beautiful daughter and former nursing companion, was my inspiration throughout.

Note to the Second Edition: For help in preparing this edition I would like to thank Trina Vosti, I.B.C.L.C., and Andrea VanOutryve, I.B.C.L.C. And thanks to John, my current nursing companion.

Note to the Third Edition: For their extensive review of the text I wish to thank Olga Mireles, R.N., C.L.C., and Ellen "Binky" Petok, I.B.C.L.C.

Note to the Fourth Edition: For their generous assistance with revisions, I thank the following women: Dayna Ravalin, R.D.; Sue Petracek, B.S. Ed.; Paula Meier, D.N.Sc., R.N., F.A.A.N.; Lois D. W. Arnold, M.P.H., I.B.C.L.C.; Jan Barger, R.N., I.B.C.L.C.; Darillyn Starr; and Rachel Vireday.

Note to the Fifth Edition: Several years ago, on a parenting website, I was lucky enough to meet "Honeysucklemama," who was nursing her first child. Rarely have I encountered such a thoughtful and supportive counselor assisting other mothers with her insightful writing. Thank you, Tricia Bulger Zack, for your fresh look at this book, as well as your support during my year of recovery from breast cancer.

ACKNOWLEDGMENTS

I would also like to thank perinatal health educator Patricia Donohue-Carey, L.C.C.E., C.L.E.; Nancy Wight, M.D.; Jack Newman, M.D.; Lenore Goldfarb, I.B.C.L.C.; Thomas Hale, Ph.D.; James McKenna, Ph.D.; Cynthia Good Mojab, M.S., I.B.C.L.C., R.L.C.; and Darillyn Starr for reviewing portions of this new edition. My friends Binky Petok, I.B.C.L.C.; Gretta Blythe, R.N., I.B.C.L.C.; and Jan Ellen Brown, I.B.C.L.C., I thank you for your love and support.

Note to the Sixth Edition: Two physicians who specialize in lactation have been particularly helpful with this edition. Dr. Jane Morton has devoted herself to assisting nursing mothers and has shared her experience and research with mothers as well as health-care providers. Dr. Jack Newman, a Canadian pediatrician, has also graciously shared his vast breastfeeding knowledge with mothers and lactation professionals.

In this edition I have included information about the impact of hospital maternity care on breastfeeding. My friend and co-worker Claudia Goff, R.N., was kind enough to assist me with this.

Penny Simkin, P.T., was helpful in sharing information on mothers who have been sexually abused and the effects of the abuse on breastfeeding.

This edition contains more information on expressing milk, including in-depth reviews of breast pumps. For this, I must thank Catherine Watson Genna and Richard Weston.

There is now a new approach to feeding solid foods to babies. Dawn Wilt, R.D., C.L.E., assisted me greatly to incorporate this information, as did Gill Rapley and Stefan Kleintjes, European experts on breastfeeding.

A surprising resource for me during this past year was my daughter, Kate Gulbransen. After years of working in banking, Kate became a lactation educator. She helped me a great deal with this edition.

Note to the Seventh Edition: First, I thank my husband, Brad, who for the past 30 years has encouraged and supported me. Without him, there never would have been *The Nursing Mother's Companion*.

Although Philip O. Anderson, Pharm.D., is now retired, he kindly agreed to update the drug information in Appendix D for this edition.

I must also thank Maria Lynch, I.B.C.L.C., who was helpful in my understanding of the Affordable Care Act. I appreciate Barbara Wilson-Clay, I.B.C.L.C., and Catherine Watson-Genna, I.B.C.L.C., for their reviews of portions of the text.

Lastly, I must acknowledge Linda Ziedrich, my editor extraordinaire, who has held my hand and polished my words for the past three decades.

Introduction

Is Breastfeeding Really Better?

•

What's in It for Mom?

•

Breastfeeding Isn't Always Easy

SINCE THE BEGINNING OF HUMANKIND, women have put their infants to breast. Extending the physical bond that begins at conception, they have nourished and protected their young with their bodies. These tender moments, in return, have brought pleasure and fulfillment to the task of mothering. If you are now pregnant, you are probably looking forward to the time in which you will nourish, comfort, and protect your child in the same way as others before you—at the breast.

Perhaps you already feel committed to the idea of nursing. For you, there is no question that you'll breastfeed your baby. Or perhaps, like many women, you have some uncertainties but still feel it's worth a try. Your outlook depends on many things—the value you place on breast-feeding, how your partner feels about it, how your friends have fed their babies, your lifestyle, and your feelings about yourself and your body.

You probably also have some notions about what nursing will be like. Perhaps you think it will be easy and convenient. Maybe you worry that it might not fit in with your activities and plans. You may have concerns about your ability to nurse. Probably you know of other women who tried to nurse but soon gave up. Whatever your attitudes, expectations, and concerns about breastfeeding, these may become powerful deter-minants in your ultimate success or failure to nurse your baby happily.

Is Breastfeeding Really Better?

You may be under the impression that the decision to breastfeed or bottle-feed is simply a matter of personal preference. Don't let anyone fool you into believing that breast milk and formula are equally good— they are not. Without a doubt, mother's milk alone promotes optimum health and development for babies. It is uniquely designed to meet the complete nutritional needs of the growing human infant. It also protects the infant against illness throughout the entire first year and beyond, as long as nursing continues. Artificial human milk, whether made from cow's milk or soybeans, will never be able to duplicate nature's formula.

Although they do grow on processed infant formulas, babies, like all young mammals, do best with milk from their own species. Human milk contains proteins that promote brain development. In contrast, cow's milk contains proteins that favor muscular growth. Thenutritional prop-erties of breast milk are designed for babies' specific growth and devel-opmental needs. Formula manufacturers are continually challenged to include all of the nutrients in breast milk that scientists are gradually identifying as important to infant growth and development.

If a multinational company developed a product that was a nutritionally balanced and delicious food, a wonder drug that both prevented and treated disease, cost almost nothing to produce, and could be delivered in quantities controlled by the consumers' needs, the very announcement of their find would send their shares rocketing to the top of the stock market. The scientists who developed the product would win prizes and the wealth and influence of everyone involved would increase dramatically. Women have been producing such a miraculous substance, breast milk, since the beginning of human existence.

—Gabrielle Palmer, *The Politics of Breastfeeding*

In recent years, for example, formula manufacturers have acknowledged that the fatty acids in breast milk are necessary to babies' intellectual, motor, and visual development. Now 90 percent of formula in the United States includes ARA and DHA (arachidonic acid and docosahexaenoic acid) made from fermented microalgae and soil fungus. These lab-produced chemicals are meant to substitute for the omega-3 and omega-6 fatty acids that are naturally found in breast milk. When formula manufacturers started adding ARA and DHA to their products, says Marsha Walker, executive director of the National Alliance for Breastfeeding Advocacy, the price of formula immediately rose by 30 percent. Research has shown little evidence for the companies' claims of beneficial effects on brain and eye development, but we do know that some infants suffer from diarrhea and other side effects after drinking these formulas.

Human milk differs from formula, too, in that it contains specific immunities against human illness. In contrast, cow's milk contains specific immunities against bovine disease. For this and other reasons, babies on a formula diet are at greater risk for illness and hospitalization. Diarrheal infections and respiratory illnesses, including respiratory syncytial virus (RSV), are more frequent and serious among these babies. (RSV is the most common cause of pneumonia and bronchiolitis—inflammation of the small airways in the lung—in children younger than one year of age in the United States.) Formula-fed babies develop many more ear infections, which may lead to later speech and reading problems. Urinary tract infections and bacterial meningitis are also more common among artificially fed infants.

Although most parents don't know this, powdered formula is not sterile. Besides lacking the anti-infective components of breast milk, powdered formula may be contaminated with bacteria (*Cronobacter spp.,* formerly known as *Enterobacter sakazakii*) that can make infants sick. For this reason, both the World Health Organization and the Food and Agriculture Organization of the United Nations recommend that infants at greatest risk of infection—those younger than two months old, born at a low birth weight, or born prematurely—receive liquid rather than powdered formula. Yet most hospitals routinely give mothers powdered formula samples in gift bags when their newborns are discharged.

Recently, formula companies have added probiotics, live intestinal bacteria, to their powdered infant formulas to help prevent diarrheal infections. This poses a dilemma for parents, as the instructions say to mix the powdered formula with cool water so these beneficial bacteria will not be destroyed. But the World Health Organization advises always mixing powdered formula with boiling water, to kill any dangerous bacteria that may be present in the formula.

Infant formula may contain other toxins besides bacteria. High levels of aluminum have been identified in most formulas. In 2008 some formulas were found to contain another toxic chemical as well. After Chinese manufacturers poisoned thousands of infants in China by adding melamine to formula to fake higher protein levels, the U.S. Food and Drug Administration (FDA) announced that it could not establish any safe level of melamine in formula. The FDA then tested the most popular brands of formula sold in the United States to be sure they were free of melamine. Apparently because the chemical is used in some plastic food packaging and in a cleaning solution used on food processing equipment, some of the U.S. formulas were found to have trace amounts of melamine. The agency then changed its view, and declared that the amounts of melamine found in U.S. formulas were acceptable.

From time to time, manufacturing errors in the production of infant formula have had serious consequences. More commonly, though, contaminants are introduced at home. Babies have suffered lead poisoning when their formulas have been mixed with tap water high in lead content. Water pollution is a potential problem even if water is purchased in a sealed bottle. And older feeding bottles can contain toxins that can leach into the baby's formula (see page 251).

Formula-feeding has other risks for babies:

- Formula-fed infants have higher incidences of colic, constipation, and allergic disorders. In fact, a significant number of babies are allergic to formulas, both those based on cow's milk and those based on soy.

- Formula-feeding appears to be one of several factors implicated in sudden infant death syndrome (SIDS). Babies who have received formula, in any amount, have a doubled risk of SIDS at one month of age compared with babies who are exclusively breastfed. (The reason for this is unknown. Perhaps it's that. breastfed infants are generally healthier than formula-fed babies and therefore resistant to whatever causes SIDS.)

- Tooth decay, malocclusion (improper meeting of the upper and lower teeth), and distortion of the facial muscles may also directly result from sucking on bottles.

Some studies suggest that the benefits of breastfeeding extend into later childhood, adolescence, and adulthood. Breastfed babies have lower cholesterol levels and less coronary artery disease, on average, when they become adults. Breastfeeding is protective against chronic digestive disorders, such as Crohn's disease and ulcerative colitis. Although asthma rates are not significantly different between breastfed and non-breastfed babies, adults who were breastfed have a lower rate of asthma. Breastfed babies have a smaller chance of developing obesity, which can start with overfeeding in infancy, and both type 1 (juvenile-onset insulin-dependent) and type 2 (late-onset) diabetes. Cancers, including leukemia and cancer of the lymph glands, are also less common in children who were breastfed.

There is mounting evidence that artificially fed infants more often develop learning disorders and generally experience lower levels of intellectual functioning. Recent large-scale, international studies confirm previous studies' findings that children who were breastfed have higher IQs and perform better in reading, writing, mathematics, and other school subjects. Studies also reveal that it is breast milk, not the act of breastfeeding, that is responsible for this superior cognitive development.

Breastfeeding helps, of course, in establishing a close bond and meeting the emotional needs of a child. Nursing women produce hormones that promote a physiologic bonding between mother and child. And in what better way can a baby be nurtured, comforted, and made to feel secure than snuggled within his mother's loving arms, against the warmth of her breast?

Although some rationalize that bottle-feeding mothers can capture a similar warm feeding relationship, in reality they do not. This is partly because bottle-feeding doesn't require much human contact. The bottle-fed baby generally receives less stroking, caressing, and rocking than the breastfed baby. He is talked to less often, and he spends more time in his crib away from his parents. Although no one knows how prevalent the practice of propping bottles for young infants is, probably the overwhelming majority of babies who are able to hold their own bottles become almost entirely responsible for feeding themselves.

For all of these reasons, the American Academy of Pediatrics recommends that infants be offered only breast milk for the first six months after birth, and that breastfeeding continue throughout the first year and then as long as mutually desired.

What's in It for Mom?

Although the health of an infant and the emotional benefits of breastfeeding are reasons enough to nurse, women frequently have other motives. Experienced nursing mothers boast about the ease and convenience of breastfeeding. They are often quick to add that information, guidance, support, and reassurance were essential at the start. After the first few weeks, however, nursing a baby simplifies life considerably.

Nursing saves money. Feeding your baby on 8-ounce cans of ready-to-feed formula would cost about $4,000 for the first year of life. Using 32-ounce cans instead would cut the cost to about $1,800. Concentrated formula, which must be reconstituted with water, would cost about $1,500 for the year, and using powdered formula would cut the price a little more, to about $1,200.

Most experienced nursing mothers are glad not only that they don't have to buy formula but that they don't have to prepare bottles. Instead up getting up at night to fix a bottle, you can simply pull the baby to your breast and doze off again. You can go on outings with your baby without carting around formula, bottles, and nipples. (But just because the breastfed baby is easy to take along doesn't mean she can't be left behind. When you and your infant must be apart, you can leave your own milk for her. See Chapter 6 for more information.) Many mothers have been grateful that they could nurse their babies through natural disasters such as storms, flooding, and fires when formula and clean feeding supplies were unavailable.

Many women worry about how they will look after they have had a baby. The fat you accumulate during pregnancy is intended for caloric reserves while nursing. Rigorous dieting is not a good idea during the nursing period, but it isn't necessary, either; most mothers find that they gradually lose weight while they are breastfeeding so long as they are not overeating. Women who formula-feed their babies may have a much harder time losing the fat they gained during pregnancy. Furthermore, two separate studies confirm that breastfeeding mothers who nursed for three months or longer after each birth had less belly fat than mothers who did not breastfeed, and no more belly fat than women who had never been pregnant.

Breastfeeding has other beneficial effects on a woman's body. Recent studies have found that women reduce their risk of type 2 diabetes by as much as 12 percent for each year they breastfeed. Swedish researchers

Needless Fears about Breastfeeding

Breastfeeding will be inconvenient. In fact, experienced nursing mothers boast about the ease and convenience of breastfeeding.

Breastfeeding will be painful. Normally, women find nursing comfortable and pleasurable. Some women develop sore nipples during the early days of nursing, but most soreness can be avoided by correctly positioning the baby at the breast (see "Positioning at the Breast," page 44). You may have heard that babies sometimes bite their mothers while nursing. When a baby is sucking, his tongue covers his lower gums and teeth so he cannot bite. Still, some babies do occasionally bite at the end of feeding, usually during a period of teething. Most babies learn very quickly not to do this.

Breastfeeding will be embarrassing. Although we all know that making milk is the natural function of our breasts, many of us feel embarrassed about exposing them. At first you may be more comfortable nursing in private, but most women find that, with a little time and experience, nursing in the presence of others can be discreet and comfortable.

Breastfeeding will tie you down. In fact, you can take your nursing baby anywhere with as little equipment as a spare diaper.

You'll have to stop breastfeeding when you go back to work. Today, a growing number of women are combining motherhood, nursing, and working,

have determined that mothers who nurse for at least 13 months cut their risk of developing rheumatoid arthritis in half. Many studies report lower rates of ovarian cancer and breast cancer among women who have breast-fed, and it appears that the risk of cancer decreases the longer a woman nurses. New studies also reveal that breastfeeding has a significant impact on reducing the risk of developing heart problems in women. While it is well known that obesity, high cholesterol, and diabetes all lead to heart disease, it is less known that breastfeeding reduces the risk of all these. There is some evidence, too, that nursing offers protection against devel-

and doing it quite successfully, thanks to recent advances in milk collection and storage equipment. Having a healthy baby is especially important to a working mother, and breastfed babies are sick less often.

Breastfeeding will ruin the shape of your breasts. Pregnancy typically causes the breasts to enlarge and sometimes to develop stretch marks. During the first few months of nursing, women whose breasts are normally small or medium-sized generally find them to be bigger. As the baby gets older and begins nursing less often, most women notice their breasts reduce in size. At weaning, the breasts typically appear smaller still and somewhat droopy, but within six months they often resume their usual size and shape. A recent U.S. study found that increased maternal age, more pregnancies, higher body-mass index, larger pre-pregnancy bra size, and smoking were all independent risk factors for sagging breasts. But women who nursed generally had no more sagging than women who bottle-fed.

Your milk may be inadequate for your baby. Some mothers wonder if their diet, breast size, or temperament will keep their milk from being rich or abundant enough. None of these factors affect the amount of breast milk produced, which depends on the frequency of feedings and the baby's effectiveness at the breast. And the quality of a mother's milk is rarely an issue.

oping osteoporosis (brittle bones) later in life. And breastfeeding generally lengthens the time before menstrual periods resume after childbirth; most nursing women have no menstrual cycle for several months to two years after delivery, so long as they are nursing frequently. Recent studies comparing breastfeeding and bottle-feeding mothers suggest a lower rate of postpartum depression among nursing mothers as well.

Some mothers are repelled by the smell and taste of many formula preparations, not to mention the unpleasant odor of the bowel movements and spit-up milk of the formula-fed baby and the stains formula may leave on clothing. Breast milk smells sweet, if it smells at all, and as long as a baby is exclusively breastfed, her spit-up and bowel movements smell mild and inoffensive.

Breastfeeding Isn't Always Easy

If breastfeeding is natural, it must be easy, right? Sometimes it isn't. Today, close to half of all mothers who start out nursing their babies give it up within the first six weeks. The reason for this failure is rarely that the mother is unable to produce enough milk. Typically, it is because she is alone in her efforts to nurse. All too many new mothers know little about the nursing process and the breastfed infant, have little or no guidance, and lack support while they are learning. Although breastfeeding is natural, it is not instinctive—it must be learned. The chapters that follow will tell you what you need to know.

Many excellent books have already been written on the benefits of nursing over artificial feeding methods. I set out, however, to provide mothers with a practical guide for easy reference throughout the nursing period. The first part of the book provides basic information about

There's no pleasure to equal watching your baby grow from the nourishment of your own body.

the breast, preparation for nursing, and nursing during the first week; the remainder of the book is intended for reading as the baby and the nursing relationship grow and develop. There are chapters on each of the three later phases of nursing—from the first week through the second month, from the second month through the sixth, and after the sixth month. Following each of these chapters is a Survival Guide—a quick yet thorough reference for almost any problem you or your baby may encounter during the phase covered. Although you may rarely need to consult the Survival Guides, I have included them to ensure that, when you do, you will be able to identify and resolve your problem as quickly as possible. Because many nursing women occasionally find themselves in need of medication, Dr. Philip O. Anderson has provided an appendix on drugs and their safety for the breastfed baby.

Mothers who nurse do so not only because they want the very best nourishment and protection for their babies and because they personally derive many practical benefits from breastfeeding, but simply because they enjoy the experience. The loving relationship established between mother and infant at the breast is emotionally fulfilling and pleasurable. You'll know no greater reward as a mother than witnessing your child grow from your body—first in the womb, and then at the breast.

CHAPTER

one

LOOKING FORWARD: PREPARATIONS DURING PREGNANCY

- Learning about Breastfeeding
- Your Breasts
- Ensuring the Purest Milk

- Planning for a Normal Birth
- Planning for the First Days
- Planning for the First Weeks

12

Y OU MAY HAVE DECIDED TO NURSE your baby long before you became pregnant. Or perhaps you have just begun to consider breastfeeding. Although nourishing a baby at the breast is natural, many new mothers are surprised to find it is a learned skill—one that usually takes several weeks to master.

Success at nursing often depends upon a woman's confidence and commitment. You can develop your confidence by learning as much as possible about breastfeeding ahead of time. You can strengthen your commitment to nurse by developing a strong support system for yourself.

Learning about Breastfeeding

Generations ago, most new mothers turned to their own mothers for support and guidance on breastfeeding. Happily, many women today can do so, too. But many can't.

If your mother didn't breastfeed, or if she gave it up quickly, there are several ways you can learn about nursing ahead of time. Reading about it is certainly beneficial. In some communities, breastfeeding classes are offered. Expectant mothers are also most welcome to attend La Leche League meetings, which are held monthly in most areas. La Leche League is the organization of nursing mothers whose purpose is to support breastfeeding worldwide. In some areas, other groups, such as the Nursing Mothers Counsel, provide classes and telephone counseling for pregnant and nursing women. These groups are listed in Appendix A (see page 357). In addition, hospitals, county health departments, and WIC (the Special Supplemental Nutrition Program for Women, Infants, and Children) programs may sponsor prenatal breastfeeding classes. See Appendix A, page 359, for more information about WIC.

Another excellent way to learn about breastfeeding is to spend time with women who are nursing their babies. It may be that you have never seen, close-up, a mother and baby breastfeeding. Most nursing mothers will delight in your interest, and one or two may become good sources of information and support for you in the days to come. Be sure to ask them about their first weeks of nursing. Most likely you will hear of a variety of experiences, and perhaps you will develop a sense of what the early period of breastfeeding can be like.

Your Breasts

During pregnancy, many changes occur in your breasts in preparation for nourishing your baby. In early pregnancy, you probably noticed they were more full and tender than usual. Their increasing size during the first few months of pregnancy is caused by the development of the milk-making structures within them. Most women prefer to wear a supportive bra throughout pregnancy, although a few women are just as comfortable without one. From early or mid-pregnancy on, your rib cage expands. You will probably find that your bra band feels tighter, and this may require you to purchase new bras or bra extenders.

As your breasts grow in size, the blood flow to them increases, and veins in the breasts may become clearly visible. Some women develop stretch marks on their breasts, like the ones that can occur on the abdomen during pregnancy.

The nipple and the area around the nipple, the areola, may double in size and deepen in color; this darkening may serve as a visual cue to the newborn. Also during this time, small glands located in the areola, known as Montgomery's tubercles, become pronounced. Their function is to secrete an antibacterial lubricant that keeps the nipple moist and protected during pregnancy and breastfeeding. This is why soaps and special creams are unnecessary in caring for your breasts, and may even be harmful: soaps remove the breast's natural lubricant, and creams may interfere with its antibacterial action.

The nipples often become more sensitive during pregnancy. Some women find that their nipples even hurt when touched. This sensitivity diminishes as pregnancy advances; it should not make breastfeeding uncomfortable. Other women enjoy the sensitivity and feel great pleasure when their breasts are fondled during lovemaking.

By the fifth or sixth month of pregnancy, the breasts are fully capable of producing milk. Some women begin to notice drops of fluid on the nipple at this time. This fluid, known as colostrum, comes from several tiny openings in the nipple and is the food your baby will receive during the first few days after birth. Some women do not leak colostrum, but it is there in the breasts just the same.

As women, we all receive messages about our bodies and what they "ought" to look like. These messages affect our self-image, including our feelings about our breasts and how they look. You can probably remember how you felt about your breasts as they developed in early adolescence. You may have felt proud as they grew larger and you began wearing a bra. Perhaps you were embarrassed if they developed earlier or grew larger than the other girls'. You may have felt anxious if they took a long time to grow or self-conscious if they were small.

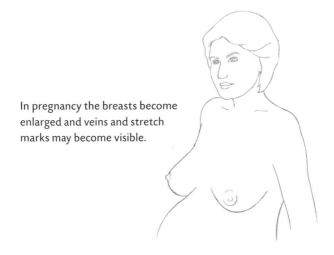

In pregnancy the breasts become enlarged and veins and stretch marks may become visible.

Caring for Your Breasts

During the last months of pregnancy, avoid soaping your breasts; just rinse them during your bath or shower. Soaps tend to dry the nipples and the areola. If your breasts are dry or itchy, a mild cream or lotion may feel soothing, but avoid getting it on the nipple or areola.

Even now you may wish that your breasts were smaller or larger, fuller or less droopy. You may not resemble the women with "perfect" breasts portrayed in photographs of nursing mothers. Women with large breasts, especially, often feel insecure about nursing, fearing that their breasts will grow much larger still or leak milk excessively. Actually, large breasts seldom grow bigger after delivery, and they tend to leak less than small breasts.

Each woman's breasts are different from all others, but most breasts, regardless of size, are perfectly designed for their ultimate purpose—to nourish and nurture our children. The breasts not only provide an infant with superb nutrients for growth and development but offer the warmth, the comfort, and the security that every growing baby needs. In this respect, they are most beautiful.

Breasts come in all shapes and sizes.

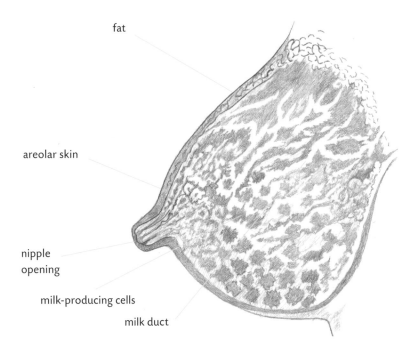

fat

areolar skin

nipple opening

milk-producing cells

milk duct

Cross-section of a lactating breast

The Making and Giving of Milk

After the birth of your baby, colostrum is readily available for her first nursings. Colostrum is the ideal food for her first days; it is both perfect nutritionally and important for protection against infection. Mature milk generally appears by the second or third day, but occasionally not until the fourth or fifth day or even later. The late onset of milk production, which is becoming a common problem, may be related to events that occur during birth (see "Planning for a Normal Birth," page 20).

A woman's body is signaled to initiate milk production with the delivery of the placenta. This causes the hormone prolactin to activate the milk-producing cells of the breast. The initial manufacture of milk occurs whether the baby nurses or not. Continued milk production is another matter. This depends on frequent and regular stimulation of the breast and the drainage of milk. The baby's sucking stimulates the nerve endings in the breast, which in turn trigger the release of the two hormones essential to milk production and release—prolactin and oxytocin.

Prolactin, as mentioned previously, activates the milk-producing cells in the breast to manufacture milk. Oxytocin is responsible for the release of the milk from the tiny sacs where the milk is made. This release is referred to as the ejection or let-down reflex. As the baby nurses, the milk is propelled forward toward the nipple. It is the baby's job to get the milk out by compressing the areola with her tongue and gums as she nurses. During the early months of her life, your baby will receive plenty of milk as long as you nurse her frequently (at least eight times in 24 hours), she latches on and sucks properly, and you allow her a sufficient amount of time to complete each feeding. This is because breastfeeding works by supply and demand. The more your breasts are stimulated and emptied by the baby's sucking, the more milk you will produce.

Ensuring the Purest Milk

A mother may occasionally wonder if her milk is entirely safe for her child. Most frequently, this concern arises because she needs to take medication. Although most medications pass into the breast milk, the vast majority pass in only small amounts and are considered safe for the nursing infant. A comprehensive guide to drugs in breast milk, by Dr. Philip O. Anderson, can be found in Appendix D (see page 374). Another source of such information is LactMed, an online database developed by Dr. Anderson for the National Library of Medicine. You can find LactMed in the list of databases at www.toxnet.nlm.nih.gov.

More and more questions have arisen about the environmental pollutants we are exposed to, such as insecticides and other toxic chemicals. Many of these substances are stored in fatty tissues of the body; as a result, small amounts may be detected in breast milk. Experts on the subject, however, have been unable to identify any risks to the baby from such amounts, and most believe that the nutritional and immunological benefits of breast milk far outweigh the possible risks of environmental pollutants. Sadly, our children receive even greater exposure to some of these chemicals in the womb than they do at the breast.

If you want to minimize your baby's exposure to toxic chemicals, follow these guidelines during pregnancy and as long as you are breastfeeding:

- Stop using pesticides in the home, in the garden, and on pets.

- Avoid exposure to organic solvents, which are in paints, furniture strippers, gasoline fumes, non-water-based glues, nail polish, and dry-cleaning fluids. Air dry-cleaned and mothballed clothes outdoors before wearing them, and avoid permanently moth-proofed garments.

- Avoid eating fish species that have been found to have high levels of mercury and PCB, including shark, swordfish (also known as *kajiki*), king mackerel (which is among the species known as *saba* in Japanese restaurants), tilefish (also known as golden or white snapper), and fish caught in contaminated waters, especially the Great Lakes.

- Adopt a diet low in animal fat by choosing lean meats and low-fat dairy products.

Seafood, Safe and Not

The U.S. Food and Drug Administration says that pregnant women should avoid eating shark, swordfish, king mackerel, and tilefish but can safely eat 12 ounces per week of any other types of cooked fish. The Environmental Working Group is even more conservative; this nonprofit organization suggests also avoiding fresh tuna (including varieties sold in sushi restaurants as *ahi, maguro, meji, shiro,* and *toro),* sea bass, Gulf Coast oysters, marlin *(makjiki),* halibut, pike, walleye, white croaker, and largemouth bass, and eating no more than 3 to 6 ounces per month of canned tuna, mahi-mahi, blue mussels, Eastern oysters, cod, pollock, Great Lakes salmon, Gulf Coast blue crab, wild channel catfish, yellowtail (known in sushi restaurants as *hamachi, kanpachi, inada,* or *buri),* bonito *(katsuo),* wild trout, and lake whitefish.

Safe fish and shellfish, with mercury levels lower than 0.2 parts per million, include farmed trout, farmed catfish, fish sticks, shrimp, pollock, wild Pacific salmon, haddock, summer-caught flounder, croaker, clams, flatfish, mid-Atlantic blue crab, freshwater sport fish, and scallops. Check with your state or local health department about the safety of local species.

Tattoos

Some nursing mothers consider getting a tattoo and wonder if it is safe. Many tattoo artists will not knowingly perform work on a pregnant or nursing mother, as it is recommended that women wait a year after giving birth before getting one. However, there is no evidence that getting a tattoo has any effect on breast milk.

It is very important to screen tattoo artists to verify that they follow adequate safety measures, as local or even systemic infections can occur otherwise. Some local health departments have specific laws and regulations in place, so you might begin your search there. The tattooist should follow universal precautions, such as sterilizing the tattoo machine with an autoclave, using single-use needles, ensuring that the inks are not contaminated, and wearing gloves. When these precautions are not followed, diseases such as hepatitis, tetanus, and even HIV can be transmitted.

If you do get a tattoo, be sure to guard against a local infection by washing the tattooed area with mild soap and water. Avoid picking at the scabs and keep the area covered when in the sun.

Laser removal of tattoos can safely be done while nursing. The laser causes the pigments of the tattoo to break up into small particles and then be filtered out by the body. There is no bleeding, and the procedure has minimal side effects.

- Avoid smoking and the company of those who smoke around you.
- Carefully wash or peel fresh fruit and vegetables. Avoid crash diets, which can increase the excretion of toxic substances into breast milk.
- If you work with chemicals, ask your doctor to refer you to a specialist who can advise you about their safety.

Planning for a Normal Birth

Over the past two decades, the numbers of mothers who have their labor induced, who have epidural anesthesia, and who deliver by cesarean section have skyrocketed. It is now known that these high-tech interventions often affect breastfeeding.

A complicated birth often ends with the separation of mother and baby. This may make the start of breastfeeding more difficult.

All too often, a complicated birth also means the late onset of milk production. Several factors may be responsible: a long labor, epidural anesthesia, the use of synthetic oxytocin (Pitocin) to augment or induce labor, and the administration of large volumes of intravenous fluids. When milk production is delayed beyond 72 hours after birth, the newborn may become jaundiced, lose too much weight, and require supplemental feedings. A mother in this situation becomes more likely to abandon nursing.

A complicated birth often doesn't begin naturally but is induced by the breaking of the bag of waters. A doctor may suggest doing this when a mother nears or passes her due date. Induced labor all too often makes other medical interventions necessary. The rupture of the membranes may or may not stimulate labor, but it certainly increases the risk of infection to mother and baby. Once the bag of waters is broken, the clock begins ticking. In most cases, the baby needs to be delivered within 24 hours to minimize the chance of infection.

Sometimes problems during pregnancy make induction a good choice. It may be risky for the baby to remain in the uterus when pregnancy has lasted 42 weeks, when the mother has high blood pressure or an infection of the uterus, or when she has another health problem such as diabetes. Induction may also be the best option if the baby stops growing or if the amount of amniotic fluid is very low. But many doctors schedule inductions for the convenience of mothers, physicians, and hospital staff. A doctor may persuade a mother by describing induction as a routine procedure to avoid a middle-of-the-night run to the hospital and to guarantee that certain family members can be in attendance, or by voicing concern about the baby's size. Some mothers may request induction simply because they are tired of being pregnant.

None of these are good reasons for induction. Studies of thousands of cases have shown that inductions increase the incidence of labor complications and surgical delivery without improving newborn outcomes.

Nature begins preparing for birth during the last weeks of pregnancy. The baby drops down into the pelvis; the cervix tilts forward and begins to soften. The baby's lungs mature, he receives maternal antibodies that will protect him against infection in the early weeks of life, and he puts on a layer of fat. His body stores more iron, and he develops a coordinated sucking and swallowing ability. When the baby is ready to be born, he releases a small amount of a hormone that in turn stimulates the mother's body to secrete the hormones that initiate labor. When the baby, maternal hormones, uterus, cervix, and placenta are ready, labor begins. When labor begins on its own in this way, the labor tends to be easier, and the baby is usually born ready to breastfeed.

A mother who has agreed to an induction usually finds herself admitted to the hospital before labor is well established or even begun. If her due date was incorrectly estimated, the baby may be born weeks early. A developmentally immature newborn is at increased risk for complications such as temperature instability, low blood sugar, respiratory problems, and jaundice. Babies born three weeks or more early often don't learn to nurse well until near the time that they were meant to be born.

If breaking the water bag fails to bring on effective contractions, artificial oxytocin (Pitocin) may be used to strengthen them. During a normal labor, the mother produces her own oxytocin, which leads her body to also manufacture endorphins, natural pain reducers. Artificial oxytocin, given intravenously, does not reach the brain and so does not stimulate the release of natural endorphins. Besides feeling more painful, Pitocin-induced contractions are often longer, and Pitocin may prevent the uterus from fully relaxing between contractions. Because Pitocin can increase the stress to both the uterine muscle and the baby, the mother will need continuous electronic monitoring. As a result, she may be confined to a bed instead of helping her labor along by moving freely, and she may be unable to take relaxing baths or showers to ease her labor pains.

A recent study of thousands of first-time mothers revealed that those whose labors were induced—by rupture of the membranes, Pitocin, or both—were four to ten times more likely to undergo cesarean surgery. Many of these women will deliver their future children by cesarean as well.

Whether or not their labors are induced, most women today choose to have epidurals. An epidural is an injection of a narcotic and an anesthetic into the space around the spinal cord. The drugs block the nerve impulses from the lower spinal segments, and this results in decreased sensation in the lower half of the body.

For 80 percent of laboring women, an epidural provides good pain relief. But it may also cause undesirable complications. Labor is usually longer. Contractions become weaker and less frequent, because an epidural lowers the mother's own production of oxytocin, the substance that causes the uterus to contract. This means that she is more likely to need artificial oxytocin. She will not experience the peak in oxytocin that produces the powerful final contractions that end in birth and that help the mother fall in love with her baby at first sight.

Epidurals have other side effects. Because the drugs block the nerves that regulate blood pressure, one-third of women who have epidurals experience low blood pressure, and in 12 percent of these cases the drop is low enough to seriously deprive the baby of oxygen. In an attempt to prevent a blood-pressure decrease, the mother may be given large amounts of intravenous fluids before the epidural. These fluids may be a factor in the delayed onset of milk production.

Having both an epidural and Pitocin can affect the baby's heart rate. A survey of first-time mothers who experienced both of these interventions found that half required cesarean births for fetal distress.

Epidural anesthesia also often causes relaxation of the pelvic-floor muscles, which can interfere with the normal flexion and rotation of the baby's head as it passes through the birth canal. This interference can lead to an abnormal presentation (that is, the baby descends facing the mother's front or side), which makes delivery difficult, or to the baby's failure to descend, an indication for a cesarean. An epidural also reduces a mother's ability to push (and occasionally makes it impossible for her to move her lower body at all), so delivery by forceps or vacuum extractor may be necessary. The incidence of cesarean section increases by three times when epidurals are given. Mothers having an epidural are also at greater risk for excessive bleeding after birth.

About 24 percent of women who have an epidural will develop a fever. Any elevation in temperature could mean that the mother has an infection, so the newborn will need to be checked. If the baby also has a fever, he will be further tested and treated with antibiotics. In one large-scale study, mothers who had fevers during delivery more often had babies with low Apgar scores, poor muscle tone, and seizures than did babies of mothers without fever. And a baby who is being tested and treated for fever is separated from his mother during the hours when breastfeeding ideally begins.

Not only do mothers whose labors are lengthened and complicated by medical interventions tend to get their milk in later, but their babies tend to be less able at the breast. In general, a baby's breast-feeding ability is highest when the mother has given birth with neither intravenous narcotics nor an epidural. The baby's breastfeeding ability is lowest when the mother has used both intravenous and epidural drugs during labor.

Despite high satisfaction with pain relief, many mothers who have undergone epidurals report low satisfaction with their birth experiences. If you're sure you need medication in labor, you might ask for patient-controlled epidural anesthesia, or PCEA. Available in many hospitals and birth centers, PCEA allows a mother to give herself a bolus of narcotic and anesthetic when she feels the need. The dose is low, so it blocks the pain sensors but allows more movement in bed. Once the cervix is totally dilated, the epidural is turned off so the mother can respond to her desire to push. The mother's recovery tends to be better after PCEA; she can walk about sooner, and walking may help prevent her bladder from becoming distended and may also prevent excessive bleeding. Because the baby has taken in less narcotic with PCEA, he tends to show a more normal interest in and ability at the breast.

If You Must Schedule a Cesarean Birth

As many surveys have shown, babies born more than seven days before their due date tend to have complications. Respiratory problems, infections, low blood sugar, and the need for intensive care are especially common in babies born at 37 weeks' gestation or earlier. These problems usually result in separation of mother and baby and a delay in the start of breastfeeding. In addition, babies born at 37 weeks or

Prepare For a Normal Birth

- Attend childbirth classes, preferably ones taught by certified Lamaze or Bradley instructors, to learn more about normal birth.
- Recognize that your due date is approximate. Let your caregiver know that you prefer to wait until labor begins on its own.
- If your caregiver is concerned about the well-being of the baby, ask to have a non-stress test (electronic fetal monitoring) every two to four days for reassurance that the baby is well.
- Stay at home during early labor until your water breaks or your contractions are coming every 3 to 4 minutes and are lasting for 1 minute.
- Consider hiring a doula to assist you in coping with the discomforts of labor and birth.
- When you begin to push, try to rest between contractions. Push only when the urge comes or when your caregiver or nurse directs. Short pushes, of no more than 4 to 6 seconds each, will help conserve your energy.
- Take advantage of a water tub or shower to lessen the intensity of contractions.
- Try to delay an epidural until after labor is well established and your cervix is dilated 5 centimeters.
- If you feel you need pain medication, ask about PCEA.
- Once your cervix is completely dilated, use upright positions to assist gravity and to increase the diameter of your pelvis, so as to help the baby descend through the birth canal.
- When you begin to push, try to rest between contractions. Push only when the urge comes or when your caregiver or nurse directs. Short pushes, of no more than 4 to 6 seconds each, will help conserve your energy.

earlier are often poor feeders (see "The Very Premature or Sick Baby," page 138).

In spite of these risks, one-third of cesareans are performed before 39 weeks' gestation. If you must have a cesarean, insist that it be scheduled for after 39 weeks or after tests show that the baby's lungs are mature.

For advice on breastfeeding after a cesarean birth, see page 51.

Planning for the First Days

Nipple preparation

Often mothers who plan to breastfeed are advised to prepare their nipples during pregnancy. In fact, studies have shown that nipple "toughening" maneuvers, such as brisk rubbing or twisting, do little to prevent soreness during early breastfeeding. Whether or not they have especially sensitive skin, blondes and redheads do not generally experience any more nipple soreness than other women. Sore nipples are usually prevented by correct attachment of the baby at the breast (see "Positioning at the Breast," page 44).

If you have had one or both nipples pierced, remove the jewelry before giving birth and leave it out as long as your baby is nursing. You'll probably be able to nurse without complication, but you may find that you leak milk from the site of the piercing.

One preparation is very important during pregnancy: You should make sure your nipples can extend outward. Your baby may have difficulty grasping the breast if the nipples do not protrude enough on their own or cannot be made to protrude. Even if you had a breast exam earlier in your pregnancy, your nipples may not have been fully checked. Take the time to perform your own assessment.

First, look at both your nipples. They may protrude, or one or both may be flat, dimpled, folded in the center, or inverted. Next, do the "pinch test": Gently squeeze just behind the nipple with your thumb and forefinger. This imitates the motion your baby will make while nursing. See how both nipples respond. If your nipples are flat, pull them outward to determine if they can lift away from the inner mass of the breast. The chart on page 27 will help you determine whether you need to take further steps to minimize initial nursing difficulties.

When nipples need correction. The flat nipple that cannot be pinched outward, or the nipple that moves inward or flattens when compressed, is said to be "tied" to the inner breast tissue by tiny adhesions. The physical changes of pregnancy help the nipples to stand out, but one or

USUAL NIPPLE APPEARANCE	APPEARANCE WHEN PINCHED	
	SATISFACTORY	NEEDS CORRECTION
Protruding	Nipple stays protruded	
Flat	Nipple can be pinched outward	Nipple moves inward or cannot be pinched outward
Dimpled or folded	Entire nipple extends outward	Nipple moves inward or flattens
Inverted	Entire nipple extends outward	Nipple extends out only slightly, remains inverted, or inverts further

Breast shells can improve nipple shape.

both may still need correction. In this case, special plastic breast shells may solve the problem before breastfeeding begins.

Worn inside the bra, breast shells exert a steady but gentle pressure on the areola and cause the nipple to extend outward through the opening in the shell. This may help to loosen adhesions beneath the nipple. Breast shells should be worn as soon as you have determined that improvement is needed, ideally from about mid-pregnancy on. They can be purchased in most maternity shops or ordered through Medela (see Appendix A, page 361). Gradually work up to wearing the shells most of the day, letting comfort be your guide.

The Postpartum Setting

Too few mothers realize ahead of time the tremendous effect the immediate postpartum experience—in a hospital, in a birth center, or at home—can have on their breastfeeding success. It is most worthwhile to evaluate the situation you will be in after delivery to make any necessary arrangements for early nursing.

The maternity unit's policies should encourage mothers and babies to remain together for the first few hours after birth, or at least assure that nursing takes place within the first two hours, when the baby is likely to be alert and eager to suck. Ideally, the baby isn't swaddled, weighed, bathed, and placed in a crib after birth but simply dried and placed naked against his mother's bare chest; then they are both covered. Newborns treated this way tend to have more respiratory stability and higher blood-sugar levels and to cry much less than other babies. If the birth was unmedicated, the baby will generally be quiet but alert and able to crawl to the breast and latch on unaided in 30 to 60 minutes (you can see a video of a newborn crawling to the breast at www.breastcrawl.org). Weighing, bathing, eye treatment, and other baby care procedures are best postponed until after the first feeding.

Breastfeeding goes best when nursing is frequent, every one to three hours, during both day and night. "Rooming in"

Studies show that mothers who nurse during the first two hours after giving birth are much more likely to be successfully nursing weeks and months later.

with the baby, at least during the day and evening, is conducive to frequent nursing and allows the mother and baby to become better acquainted before going home. Preferably, the nursing staff does not routinely give the babies water or formula supplements, as this lessens their interest in nursing and sometimes interferes with their ability to breastfeed. It can be an added bonus if the nurses enjoy assisting breastfeeding mothers or if one nurse is specifically responsible for breastfeeding counseling.

Some women have the opportunity to select among several hospitals or birth centers for their delivery. If you are making such a choice, be sure to get a recommendation from your childbirth educator or a local breastfeeding counselor. She will probably know which places are most supportive of nursing mothers and infants. Even if only one hospital is available to you—and many birth attendants practice at only one—it is well worth your time to ask about the policies of the maternity unit. This will help assure that your nursing gets off to the best possible start.

Take advantage of the maternity tours, teas, and classes that most hospitals and birth centers offer, or call the postpartum unit to learn about policies and routines. Be sure to inquire:

- How soon after delivery will I be able to nurse? What if I have a cesarean birth?
- Will I be able to hold the baby skin-to-skin right after the birth?
- How often is nursing encouraged during the day and at night?
- Can the baby stay in the room with me? If not, how often and for how long will we be together?
- What assistance with breastfeeding does the nursing staff offer?
- Does the staff avoid supplemental bottle-feeding?
- Is there a lactation professional on staff?

In 1990, the United Nations Children's Fund and the World Health Organization created an award of recognition for those hospitals worldwide that have enacted ten policies to support breastfeeding mothers and babies. Hospitals that have implemented the "Ten Steps" are awarded the designation "Baby-Friendly." As of this writing, 203 U.S. hospitals and birthing centers in 45 states and the District of Columbia are considered baby-friendly, while another 500 are working toward the designation. When inquiring about a hospital's breastfeeding policies, ask if it has earned or applied for the Baby-Friendly certificate. If it has, you can be assured that the nurses are committed to your breastfeeding success. If it hasn't, perhaps your inquiry will inspire the hospital to enact baby-friendly policies. You can find all "Baby-Friendly" hospitals in the United States listed at www.babyfriendlyusa.org.

If the nurse is friendly and receptive to your questions, you might also ask which pediatricians she feels are particularly knowledgeable about breastfeeding and supportive of it.

If you are planning an early discharge from a hospital or birth center, or will be delivering at home, you may also want to inquire about home visits by a nurse, lactation professional, or midwife during the first few days.

The Baby's Doctor

Your breastfeeding experience can be greatly influenced by your choice of physician for your child. You may want a pediatrician for your baby, or you may prefer to use a family practitioner, perhaps the one who may attend your baby's birth. In selecting a doctor, start by getting the names of some who are said to have a positive attitude about breastfeeding. Ask your obstetrician, midwife, childbirth educator, or a lactation professional for recommendations. You might also inquire about physicians in your area who work with nurse practitioners. These nurses have advanced education and training in well-baby care, and they usually provide mothers with extra attention and counseling on a variety of parental concerns, including breastfeeding.

Most doctors and nurse practitioners will set aside time for a preliminary visit with expectant parents. Usually this visit is free of charge. Be sure to visit at least two before making a final decision, even if the first one seems satisfactory. At each office, meet the nurse. She will often be the one who will answer your questions or concerns when you call during office hours. She can be a good resource for you, especially if she has breastfed successfully herself or has a special interest in breastfeeding.

Let the doctor or nurse practitioner know that you are going to breastfeed your baby. To gauge his or her overall support of nursing mothers, ask what the recommendations would be should you experience difficulty in breastfeeding. The best pediatric practitioners offer practical assistance with breastfeeding or referrals to lactation professionals. Other practitioners provide reassuring words about feeding infant formula. Take time to discuss your preferences for feeding the baby in the hospital. If the maternity unit's policies are not ideal, ask about written orders to allow early nursing and rooming-in and to prevent the feeding of supplements to your baby. A few pediatric practices have lactation consultants on their staff or can refer you to experienced lactation consultants in your area.

There may be other questions you will want to ask about the hospital or birth center, or about well-baby care. Bring a list with you so you don't forget any of them. Be sure to inquire about any necessary procedures for notifying the doctor or nurse practitioner when the baby is born. It is often said that the pediatrician takes care of the parents perhaps even more than the child. Trust your intuition when making your final choice about which pediatrician, family doctor, or nurse practitioner is right for you.

Nursing bras and pads

During the early weeks of breastfeeding, the average breast weighs three to four times as much as it did before pregnancy. Although a bra isn't an absolute necessity in this period, you'll probably be more comfortable

A nursing bra makes the breast available with only the motion of one hand.

in one, at least if it fits well. If you leak milk and want to use breast pads, you'll definitely need a bra to hold them in place. A stretch bra that can be pulled out of the way may work fine if you're small-breasted, but otherwise you may prefer a nursing bra with removable cup flaps.

After you give birth, both your cup size and band size will most likely change. If you buy a nursing bra in early pregnancy, it may not fit when milk production begins. A better time to shop for nursing bras is during the last couple of weeks of pregnancy or after your baby is born. To be on the safe side, limit your purchase to two or three bras; you'll be more sure of the size and style that suits you after a few weeks of nursing.

The salesperson in the maternity shop or department may be able to help you choose a bra that will fit well while you are nursing. If she doesn't know a lot about bras, though, you can figure out your size yourself by following these guidelines: While standing, wearing an unpadded bra and breathing normally, measure your chest just under your arms with a tape measure. Round up to an even number of inches; this number is your band size. Now measure around your body at the fullest part of your bust. As shown in the chart on page 33, the difference between the bust measurement and band size determines your cup size.

Since finding larger bra sizes can be difficult, you may have to use a mail-order supplier. To locate one, see Appendix A, page 360.

To check a bra for fit, fasten it on the outside row of hooks. Before raising the straps over your shoulders, bend forward, allowing your breasts to fill the cups. Now stand straight, and adjust the straps.

Check the cup fit. When the flaps of a nursing bra are hooked at their highest points, the cups should have just a little extra room at the top for when milk production begins. If the cups are roomier than this, try a smaller cup size. If your breasts are overflowing at the top, outsides, or center, you need a larger cup size.

Next check the bottom band. While fastened on the outside row of hooks, the band should be snug; an inner row of hooks will allow you to tighten the band as your rib cage contracts after birth. Check to see that the band is level all around or slightly lower in the back. If the bra rides up in the back, the shoulder straps may be too tight. Otherwise, try a larger cup size.

Aside from a good fit, other valuable features of a bra for breastfeeding include all-cotton or microfiber cups to absorb moisture, nonelastic straps for better support, and front-flap fasteners that are manageable with one hand.

A word about underwire bras: Poorly fitted ones are associated with plugged milk ducts and breast infections. If you want to wear an underwire bra while nursing, it is very important to get one that fits properly. The bend of the wire must be wide enough to fall where there are no milk ducts—that is, well behind the breast tissue. If you have a lot of breast tissue below the armpits, as many women do, a soft-cup bra is definitely preferable. If you do use an underwire bra while nursing, alternate it with a soft-cup bra, and never wear the underwire bra during sleep.

You may also wish to purchase breast pads before delivery, to keep your bra and clothing dry during the early weeks of nursing (not all women leak, so you may want to start with just one pack). Breast pads are sold in two varieties, disposable and reusable. Whichever you select, be sure the pads do not contain plastic or waterproof liners, as these can contribute to nipple soreness. If you prefer, you can use handkerchiefs or cut-up cloth diapers instead of commercially made pads.

Sometimes mothers consider using plastic breast shells instead of pads to keep dry. The primary purpose of these shells is to improve nipple shape. When they are routinely worn in place of pads, milk may leak excessively.

DIFFERENCE BETWEEN BUST MEASUREMENT AND BAND SIZE	CUP SIZE
Up to 1 inch	A
1 to 2 inches	B
2 to 3 inches	C
3 to 4 inches	D
4 to 5 inches	DD or E
5 to 6 inches	F
6 to 7 inches	G
7 to 8 inches	H

Other Purchases You May Be Considering

The arms of an adult are never a safe place for an infant or small child riding in an automobile. If you use a car, buy an infant restraining seat; every U.S. state now requires the use of one.

Although all infant car seats sold today must meet federal safety standards, the seats vary considerably in both features and price. The best car seats for infants are rear-facing, semi-reclined, and labeled for use with babies up to 30 or 35 pounds in weight or, depending on the seat, up to 32 inches in height. These seats cradle young infants more securely than do convertible infant-toddler seats. In choosing a model, look for latches you can operate easily. You may also prefer a washable cover.

Some parents use car seats both in and out of the car to carry their babies outside the home and to contain them within the home, whether the babies are awake or asleep. A baby who spends many hours each day in a car seat may experience delayed muscular and sensorimotor development because the lower brain is not stimulated by normal movement. In addition, many newborns have trouble keeping their airways open when they are placed in car seats because their chins rest on their chests. The Snuggin Go infant positioner, a product invented by a neonatal nurse practitioner, helps young infants keep their heads well positioned in car seats and strollers. It can be ordered at www.snuggingo.com or other online retailers for about $35.

Unless it's from a rental or loan program sponsored by a hospital or other agency, think twice about getting a used car seat. The seat may not meet current standards or may have been recalled, as many are. If you decide to use a secondhand seat, be certain that it is not more than two years old, that the model is still in production and has not been recalled, and that you have the instructions for installation and use. In addition, the National Highway Traffic Safety Administration recommends that you never use a car seat that has been involved in a moderate to severe car accident, as its integrity may have been compromised.

Infant car seats are often improperly installed. Install yours according to the manufacturer's directions, and then shake it hard. It should not move more than 1 inch in any direction. You might also have the installation checked by a child passenger safety technician. Your local health department or highway police department can help you find one for a free inspection. See page 63 for further information on car seat safety.

You'll want to either buy diapers or arrange for a diaper service for the first few weeks. Besides being more environmentally responsible than disposable diapers, cloth diapers are more economical as well, if you have access to a washer and dryer. A diaper service is usually no more expensive than disposable diapers and is a luxury all new parents deserve.

A comfortable armchair can make positioning your newborn at the breast much easier and provide more support for you while nursing. An upholstered living-room, dining-room, or office chair with arms, or a wooden rocking chair, may make a great place for nursing your baby. If your breasts are large, a recliner may be most comfortable. Consider borrowing an appropriate chair or buying one secondhand if you can't afford a new one.

You can get by without an armchair, of course. Most couches are too deep to sit up straight on, and propping yourself upright against the headboard of your bed makes it hard to position the baby and may contribute to poor posture and muscle fatigue. But either a couch or bed can work well if you lean far back and position your baby for latch-on using "biological nurturing," as described in Chapter 2 (see page 50).

Babies need to spend most of their time in a horizontal position, whether in someone's arms or on a safe, level surface. A bouncer seat, bassinet, or blanket on the floor is a better place than a plastic carrier to leave your baby for extended periods. Or carry your baby in a pouch or sling, keeping your arms free for other things. Holding, rocking, and carrying your baby against your body will stimulate his physical and mental development while strengthening the loving bond between you.

Although ordinary bed pillows can work well in helping to position a baby for nursing, a variety of pillows are marketed specifically for this purpose, and they are becoming very popular for the early weeks of nursing. If you'd like to try one of these pillows, choose one with flat surfaces rather than one that is shaped like a croissant. The latter type creates a gap between the pillow and the mother's body, and the baby tends to slip down in between. See Appendix A, page 364, for information about my favorite nursing pillow.

Many mothers have found that a footstool specially designed for nursing is very helpful in reducing the strain of holding the baby at the breast. The angled stool raises the mother's feet and legs, lifting her lap. This relaxes her abdomen and supports her lower back, preventing arm and shoulder strain. Nursing stools are available from some nursing |supply retailers; see Appendix A, page 364.

Some mothers buy breast pumps before delivery. Although a pump is not a necessity for everyone, you may at some time want to use one. Or you may prefer to learn the technique of hand expression, which is described on pages 225 to 227. If you decide to purchase or rent a pump ahead of time, see pages 258 to 283 for reviews of various models and information on obtaining them. Your insurance provider may be required to provide you with a breast pump, although the models that they offer may not be very effective, so check carefully. See Chapter 5, page 230, about ordering a pump through your insurance carrier, and be sure to ask about the window of time you have for ordering your pump. You might also speak with a lactation consultant, who will have experience with high-quality breast pumps and may even have them available for sale if your insurance carrier does not offer breastfeeding equipment to nursing mothers. Many mothers end up disappointed with pumps they buy at discount, baby, and big-box stores.

Some mothers need a clinical-grade electric pump in the first few days after delivery. Whether you buy another sort of pump or not, find out where you can rent a clinical-grade pump should the need arise. If your baby isn't nursing well upon leaving the hospital or is at risk of underfeeding for another reason (see page 57), you should go home with a clinical-grade electric pump, ideally with a double collection kit. You can locate a rental station by calling the toll-free numbers provided in Appendix A, page 361.

In the first weeks after giving birth, many mothers find it helpful to keep a log of their nursings and their babies' stools and urine output.

One study has suggested that women who keep such logs tend to breastfeed longer than those who don't. You might consider purchasing *The Nursing Mother's Companion Breastfeeding Diary* (see "Suggested Supplemental Reading," page 414) as a handy record book and keepsake for the early weeks.

Planning for the First Weeks

During your first few weeks of motherhood, caring for the baby and yourself will take just about all of your time and energy. Most new mothers find they are often tired and have emotional highs and lows. Planning ahead can make these important first weeks go much more smoothly for both you and your family.

If your partner can possibly manage to take time off from work, by all means encourage him to do so. Not only can he help in fixing meals, managing the household, and caring for any other children at home, but he also needs and deserves time to get to know the baby. And he can be a great source of support and encouragement while you are learning to breastfeed.

Other family members can also make these weeks easier, but invite them to stay with you only if you feel they will make a positive contribution and be supportive of your nursing.

Perhaps some of your friends in the area have already offered to help when the baby arrives. There are many things they can do, like fixing a meal, washing a load or two of laundry, running errands, minding any older children, or spending an hour or so straightening up your house.

It's also a good idea to stock up on groceries before the birth. Include foods that are easy to prepare and plenty of things to drink. You may also want to plan some simple menus or freeze a few dinners ahead of time.

Your Support System

About half of American women who start out breastfeeding give up and begin bottle-feeding within the first three months after birth. As Dana Raphael wrote more than 35 years ago, "The odds in our culture today are stacked heavily against successful breastfeeding, and the emotional price for failure is high." Although more breastfeeding help is available now, those words still hold true. Mothers frequently give up breastfeeding in the learning stage because they have too little information, guidance, and support.

When a nursing mother is encouraged and cared for by others, her motivation can carry her through almost any difficult situation. When she feels alone and unsupported, however, the nursing relationship seems to fall apart at the slightest provocation.

As enthusiastic as you may feel now, you probably have difficulty imagining that during the early weeks you may sometimes doubt your ability to nurse. In fact, many new mothers experience periods of anxiety while they are learning to breastfeed. If you are lucky, you can turn to your own mother for advice and reassurance about nursing. Many of today's grandmothers, however, nursed for only a few weeks. You may hear them say, "The baby was never able to take the breast" or "I just didn't make enough milk" or "Nursing hurt too much." Comments such as these reflect an era when women received little encouragement and support in their efforts to nurse, and the lactation consulting profession was in its infancy. Consider for a moment the idea of giving birth all alone. Awful, right? It is probably important to you that someone you love and trust will be with you, encouraging you each step of the way. During your early weeks of breastfeeding you need the same kind of upport—the presence of someone who provides reassurance, guidance, and encouragement.

You may be fortunate enough to have friends who have nursed—or are nursing—their babies, and a partner who believes with you that breastfeeding is healthy and natural. Even so, you may discover in time that not everyone in your life shares your feelings about breastfeeding. In fact, many people feel indifferent, and some downright opposed, to this way of feeding and nurturing a baby. Your partner, mother, or best friend may not be entirely enthusiastic about your decision. Some people may even try to discourage you along the way. Perhaps

You can find the names of International Board Certified Lactation Consultants in your area by going to www.ILCA.org and clicking on "Find a Lactation Consultant."

they feel a bit threatened, fearful, or even jealous of the intimate relationship you will be establishing with the baby. The sad fact of the matter is that despite the renewed enthusiasm of young women today toward breastfeeding, many new mothers still get too little support —from family, friends, health professionals, and society in general.

Develop a support system for yourself ahead of time. Let your partner and other family members know how much breastfeeding means to you and how important they will be to your success. If they have concerns or fears about nursing, find out what they are and provide them with the information they need to correct any misconceptions. If you have older children, talk with them about nursing so they know what to expect.

Be sure to identify sources of guidance. Perhaps you are close to women who have successfully nursed their babies. Many WIC (the Special Supplemental Nutrition Program for Women, Infants, and Children) offices provide breastfeeding support and guidance (see Appendix A, page 359). Take time to find the names of lactation professionals in your community. Your childbirth educator, your hospital's maternity unit, or your obstetrician's or pediatrician's nurse may know of some. In addition, your insurance carrier may be required under the Affordable Care Act to cover the cost of consulting a lactation professional with no cost sharing. When you have gathered these supports, you will have stacked the odds in your favor.

OFF TO A GOOD START: THE FIRST WEEK

- In the Beginning
- Ensuring Your Milk Supply
- The First Week of Nursing

Y OU MIGHT EXPECT THAT AFTER THE WORK of labor and birth a mother and her newborn infant would be too exhausted to greet each other. But no matter how fatigued birth may have left her, the mother usually brightens with renewed energy to explore her baby. Some mothers seem to meet their infants for the first time with puzzlement, as if searching for some sign of familiarity. Others react as if they have always known this tiny being and are overjoyed to meet him at long last.

After several minutes of adjustment to breathing, the temperature change, and lights and sounds, the unmedicated infant likewise becomes alert, opening his eyes and moving his mouth. The newborn who is placed skin-to-skin with his mother is soon crawling toward the breast and is actively rooting about. With his fists to his mouth, or perhaps his lips against his father's arm, he seeks out the comfort of the breast. Ideally, the mother and baby should be left skin-to-skin until the first nursing takes place.

In the Beginning

Colostrum

Throughout the first two hours after birth, the infant is usually alert and eager to suck. At this time he is most ready for his first nursing.

It is not unusual to hear a first-time mother tell a nurse, "I don't think I have anything yet to feed the baby." Although small in amount, colostrum is available in the breast in quantities close to the stomach capacity of the newborn. This "liquid gold," which is often yellow but may be colorless, is more like blood than milk in that it contains protective white blood cells capable of attacking harmful bacteria. Colostrum also acts to "seal" the inside of the baby's intestines, preventing the invasion of bacteria, and provides the baby with high levels of antibodies from the mother. Not only does colostrum thus offer protection from sickness, it is also the ideal food for the newborn's first few days of life. It is high in protein and low in sugar and fat, making it easy to digest. Colostrum is also beneficial in stimulating the baby's early bowel movements. The black, tarry first stools, called meconium, contain bilirubin, the substance that causes newborn jaundice. Colostrum in frequent doses helps eliminate bilirubin from the body and may lessen the incidence and severity of jaundice.

In the hospital the first nursing may take place in the delivery room, the birthing room, or the recovery area. With minimal assistance from your nurse or partner, the baby will probably seek out your breasts and suck within the first hour or so. It is ideal for the baby to be naked against your bare chest (see page 28).

Many specialists believe that when the first nursing is delayed much beyond the first two hours, the infant may be somewhat reluctant to take the breast thereafter. Most babies fall asleep about two hours after birth, and they become more difficult to rouse over the next few hours. Nursing without delay also boosts the confidence of the mother and stimulates the action of hormones that cause the uterus to contract and remain firm after delivery. These contractions may help speed delivery of the placenta and minimize blood loss afterward (breastfeeding alone is insufficient, however, in the case of postpartum hemorrhage, when prompt intervention by the medical staff is essential). During the first few days after birth, some mothers feel these contractions, or "afterpains," while nursing. Mothers who have had other children may be quite uncomfortable with afterpains. If you experience these contractions during breastfeeding, you can ask for a mild pain reliever like acetaminophen (Tylenol) or ibuprofen (Motrin, Advil) an hour or so before nursing.

Should you not have the opportunity to nurse right after delivery, or if you can't persuade your baby to take the breast, don't get discouraged. Many mothers have established successful nursing hours or even days after giving birth.

Just the Breast

When you have finished your first nursing in the hospital, let the nurses know (if you have not done so previously) that you prefer your baby be given no supplementary bottles of water or formula and no pacifiers. Water or formula is unnecessary, and artificial nipples may cause your baby to have difficulty recognizing your nipple while she is learning to breastfeed. A recent study reveals that mothers whose babies received supplements or pacifiers in the hospital were far less likely to achieve exclusive breastfeeding.

Newborns do not normally require any fluids other than colostrum (the exception is the baby who has low blood sugar—because her mother is diabetic, her birth weight was low, or she underwent unusual stress during labor or delivery). Supplemental feedings, moreover, can be harmful: They may cause the baby to lose interest in the breast and to nurse less frequently than needed. This is because bottle nipples may lessen the baby's instinctive efforts to open her mouth wide, as she needs to do to grasp the breast, and condition her to wait to suck until she feels the firm bottle nipple in her mouth. The baby who has sucked on bottle nipples may also become frustrated while nursing, since milk does not flow as rapidly from the breast as it does from the bottle.

Giving newborns large amounts of water can be dangerous. Because young babies can't excrete water quickly, large amounts can lower sodium levels in their bodies, causing complications that include low body temperature and, sometimes, seizures.

A newborn trained to take a pacifier may fail to recognize her mother's soft, short nipple and therefore have trouble latching on to the breast. Introducing a pacifier now could lead to later problems, too. Recent studies associate the use of pacifiers with early weaning, and older babies who use pacifiers are more likely than others to have frequent ear infections.

Some hospitals now have policies against giving bottles and pacifiers to nursing newborns, but not all do. To be sure all the nurses know of your preference, ask them to place a sign on the baby's crib like this one:

To all my nurses:

While I'm here and learning to breastfeed, PLEASE, NO BOTTLES OR PACIFIERS. My mom will be happy to nurse me whenever I fuss.

Thanks!! Baby Reynolds

Time at The Breast

Many doctors and nurses tell mothers that to prevent sore nipples they should limit their nursing time during the first several days. Probably nothing else about breastfeeding is as poorly understood as the causes of sore nipples. It may be explained that keeping feedings short will prevent soreness and will help "toughen" the nipples. Actually, sore nipples usually result from improper positioning of the baby on the breast, not from long nursings. Another myth often heard by new mothers is that the breast "empties" in a prescribed number of minutes. Most newborns require 10 to 40 minutes to complete a feeding. As long as your positioning is correct and nursing is comfortable, there is no need to restrict your nursing time. Besides being unnecessary, limiting nursing time may frustrate the baby and lead to increased engorgement when milk production begins.

Positioning at the Breast

A baby is correctly positioned at the breast when he has latched on to it with a wide-open mouth so that his lower gum is well below the base of the nipple on the areola, the dark area around the nipples. In this off-center or "asymmetrical" position he will compress the sinuses located

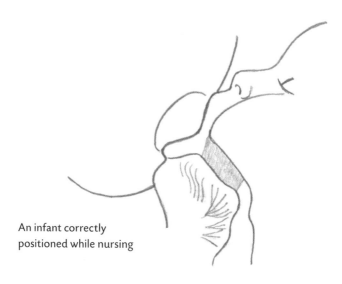

An infant correctly
positioned while nursing

It's hard to control a newborn's head using the cradle hold.

beneath the areola to draw out milk. If he instead latches on to the nipple only, or latches on with the nipple centered in his mouth, and starts sucking, the nipple will probably become sore and cracked and may even bleed. The baby will also be unable to compress the sinuses beneath the areola well and may therefore get too little milk.

Probably the most important skill for you to master, initially, is that of getting the baby on the breast correctly. Some mothers can do this easily, but many need practice.

The cradle hold, or cuddle hold, in which the baby's head is held in the crook of the mother's arm, is considered the classic breastfeeding position. I have come to believe that for most new mothers and babies, this position is neither the easiest nor the most effective for getting a baby well latched on to the breast. In the first few weeks after birth, a baby hasn't developed enough muscular coordination of the head and neck to easily latch on without help; she needs a good deal of direction from her mother. But it is difficult to direct a newborn's head accurately with the inside of one's forearm. Also, it is usually not possible to get an off-center latch using this position. Although most mothers sooner or later begin using the cradle hold for most of their daytime nursings, in the early days of breastfeeding the crossover and football holds are generally more useful.

The crossover hold. Take time to position yourself comfortably. If you are nursing in a hospital bed, sit up as straight as possible with a pillow behind you. As soon as you are able, sit in a chair with arms (most couches are too deep). Unwrap your baby; this will encourage his interest in latching on and make it easier for you to check his position. Place one or two pillows on your lap so that the baby is at the level of your breast. Lay him on his side with his chest and abdomen against your body.

Instead of placing the baby's head in the bend of your elbow, as in the cradle hold, hold him with the opposite arm so that your hand rests between his shoulder blades and supports the back of his neck and head. Place your thumb behind and below one ear and your other fingers behind and below the other ear. Tip his head back slightly so that when you pull him onto the breast, his chin will reach it first. Now shift the baby, if necessary, so that the area just above the upper lip—not his mouth—is right in front of your nipple. In this position he is most likely to latch on asymmetrically, with his lower jaw far below the base of the nipple.

If you're starting on the left breast, hold it with your left hand so that your thumb is positioned at the margin of the areola, about 1½ inches from the nipple, at the spot where the baby's upper lip will touch the breast (or at about two o'clock, if you imagine a clock face printed on your breast). Place your index finger the same distance from the nipple at the spot where the baby's chin will touch the breast (or at about eight

Crossover hold   Hand position for the crossover hold

o'clock). Gently compress the breast to match the shape of your baby's open mouth.

Before you bring the baby onto the breast, you must stimulate him to "root." With the baby's forehead tipped back, touch the baby just under the nose with your nipple, and wait until he opens his mouth wide. When his lower jaw is dropped all the way down, quickly bring his shoulders and head together to the breast. With his head tipped slightly back, his chin should reach the breast first. Don't lean into the baby or move your breast. Keep the areola compressed until he begins sucking. You'll know that he is well latched on if his lips are far apart and flared, if he has more of the bottom of the areola in his mouth than the top, and if you feel comfortable.

You may need to repeat this process a few times before the baby latches on correctly. Common mistakes include lining up the baby's mouth rather than the upper lip area with the nipple, pulling the baby on before his mouth is wide open, not pulling him on quickly enough or far enough, and letting go of the breast before he is well latched on.

When you're first learning to get a baby latched on, it helps to see someone else do it. Dr. Jane Morton, a pediatrician in general practice,

Just before latch-on: Tip the baby's head back a bit, and aim your nipple at his upper lip.

Just before latch-on, from your point of view

a clinical professor at Stanford University, an executive board member of the American Academy of Pediatrics' Section on Breastfeeding, and a fellow of the American Academy of Breastfeeding Medicine, has produced wonderful videos about breastfeeding (see Appendix A, page 359). "A Perfect Latch" is intended for physicians but is also helpful for mothers who are learning to get a baby latched on. This video is available for viewing online at http://newborns.stanford.edu/Breastfeeding/FifteenMinuteHelper.html.

Once the baby is actively nursing, you'll probably need to support the breast for him by gently pressing your fingers against the underside. If your breasts are small, though, you may be able to let go of the breast or even switch arms and continue nursing using the cradle hold.

Football hold. The football hold is a great position to use in the following circumstances:

- You have had a cesarean birth and want to avoid placing the baby against your abdomen.
- You need more visibility while getting the baby to latch on.
- Your breasts are large.
- You are nursing a small baby, especially if he is premature.
- You are nursing twins.

Football hold

Hand position for the
football hold

Sit in a comfortable armchair with a pillow at your side to help support your arm and lift the baby. Support the baby in a semi-sitting position facing you, with her bottom at the back of the chair. Your arm closest to your baby should support her back, with your hand holding her neck and head. Place your thumb behind and below one ear and your other fingers behind the other ear. Position the baby with her head just below the breast and her nose in front of the nipple. This way she'll latch on to the areola off-center, with her lower jaw well below the base of the nipple.

Support your breast with your free hand so that your thumb is about 1½ inches above the nipple, at twelve o'clock, and your index finger is the same distance below the nipple, at six o'clock. Compress the areola with your thumb and index finger so that your hand forms a C-shape. This will more closely match your breast to the shape of your baby's mouth so she can take in more of the breast. As with the crossover hold, stimulate the baby to open her mouth wide, and bring her up onto the breast.

Side-lying position. The side-lying position is an especially good choice for nursing in these cases:

- You must lie flat after a cesarean birth.
- You are uncomfortable sitting up.

Side-lying position

- You need help from someone else to get the baby latched on.

- The baby is sleepy and reluctant to begin nursing or stay awake very long.

- You are nursing during the night.

You and your baby lie on your sides, tummy to tummy as with the cuddle hold. Place your fingers beneath the breast and lift upward, wait for the baby to root with a wide-open mouth, and then pull him in close.

The side-lying position becomes much easier after four to six weeks, when the baby has better head control and can come onto the breast without much assistance.

Biological Nurturing

Recently, a new approach to getting a newborn latched on to the breast has been described by Dr. Suzanne Colson, a nurse-midwife from England. "Biological nurturing" employs the normal reflexes of newborn infants, which, Dr. Colson teaches, are present in part to assist the baby to latch on to the breast by himself. The technique uses a very comfortable position for mothers and may be especially helpful with newborns who are struggling to achieve a good latch.

With this technique, the mother leans back against pillows, and the baby is placed vertically or obliquely on top of her. The baby, wearing no more than a diaper, lies against the mother's bare skin with his face on top of her breast and his feet touching her thighs so he can use his crawling reflex to reach the nipple area. The feel and smell of the breast stimulate the baby to open his mouth very wide and bob his head up and down and from side to side as he searches for the nipple. Because the mother is leaning back, the baby is able to use gravity to his advantage and so takes the nipple deeply into his mouth. The mother can support the baby's bottom with one hand and help present the breast with the other. On his website (www.breastfeedinginc.ca), Canadian pediatrician Dr. Jack Newman offers a video of a baby latching on, for the first time, with this technique—click on "Videos/Info Sheets" and then choose "Baby-Led Mother-Guided Started Upright Left Breast, Latches."

To learn more about biological nurturing, visit Dr. Colson's website, www.biologicalnurturing.com.

Ending the Feeding

Waiting until your baby lets go of the nipple is the ideal way to end a feeding. If the baby does not come off the breast by himself after 20 to 25 minutes on a side, and you want to switch breasts or rest awhile, you can take him off by first breaking the suction. Even if he is not actively sucking, his hold on the nipple is tremendously strong. To release the suction, place your finger at the corner of the baby's mouth, pulling the skin gently toward his ear, until you hear or feel the release.

After taking the baby off the breast, leave your bra flaps down so that the air can dry your nipples. If your nipples are tender or damaged and you want to soothe them, you may be offered a modified lanolin preparation or a gel pad. However, recent studies suggest that using gel pads may lead to higher rates of breast infections when used by nursing mothers. If your nipples are tender or injured and you are using a nipple ointment, be sure to wash your hands frequently and especially right before nursing. I also suggest some other products for treating tender or injured nipples in "Survival Guide: The First Week," page 67.

After a Cesarean Birth

If you are awake for your delivery, let the staff and the baby's physician know that you wish to nurse as soon as possible. While some hospitals allow the mother to hold the baby against her skin in the operating room while she is being sutured, many do not, and, frankly, some mothers do not feel well enough to enjoy this experience. Also, surgical suites are kept cool for the doctors' comfort, and the low room temperature can cause a mother's body temperature to drop so low that she may not be able to keep the baby warm enough.

As long as neither you nor the baby is having difficulties, however, there is no reason to delay nursing for long. One option is to have a nurse or your partner bring your baby to you in the recovery room. If you were not fully conscious during the delivery, or if the doctor orders that the baby be kept in the nursery, you can still begin nursing after your initial separation.

When the baby arrives, place him against your skin, and cover him. Enjoy his attempts to crawl to the breast and nurse. If he doesn't latch on even with your help, have your partner or the nurse help you feed him in the side-lying position. Leave the side rails of the bed up so that turning will be easier. A pillow behind your back and one between your legs may be helpful.

Because you will be recovering from surgery, you will face some discomfort and possibly some difficulty in maneuvering the baby to your breast. The pain medication you'll receive, probably a narcotic, is important for your comfort during the first few days, and it will not hurt the baby. If you take the medication right after you nurse, moreover, only a minimal amount will be in your milk at the next feeding. After the first couple of days, a non-narcotic pain reliever, like acetaminophen (Tylenol) or ibuprofen (Motrin, Advil), may be adequate to control your pain most of the time.

When you begin sitting up to nurse, a pillow or two on your lap will make you more comfortable. The football hold may work well if you want to keep the baby off your abdomen, but some mothers may not get a good off-centered latch and may find that they get sore nipples using this hold.

After a couple of days you may want to keep the baby in the room with you. Remember to ask for help whenever you need it. Sometimes the staff may forget you gave birth by cesarean.

Whether or not your cesarean was planned, your milk should come in just as if you had delivered vaginally, although it may be delayed if you had a long or complicated labor and received large amounts of intravenous fluids (see page 70).

Ensuring Your Milk Supply

Frequent nursing

Most babies nurse infrequently during the first 24 hours of life. But thereafter your baby should be nursing often, at least eight times in 24 hours. Studies show that the numbers of daily nursings on the second, third, and fourth days of life are directly related to how much milk is produced on days 5 and 14. Until your milk comes in, your baby needs frequent feedings of colostrum. After your milk comes in, probably about 72 hours after the birth, a good feeding every few hours will help ensure a plentiful milk supply.

During the first few days after birth, many babies are sleepy. If your newborn has not nursed after three hours (counted from the start of the last feeding), unwrap her from her blankets. Rub her back and talk to her, or place her, dressed in only her diaper, against your bare chest. She will probably then become interested in nursing.

In the hospital, keeping the baby with you in your room helps ensure frequent nursing. If you are not sharing a room with your baby, ask the nurses to bring her to you at least every three hours (more often if she fusses), including whenever she wakens in the night.

Encourage the baby to have a good feeding each time you nurse her. Until your milk is in, you can probably persuade her to take both breasts at each feeding. Listen for the sound of your baby swallowing; when you hear it, you will know that she is taking colostrum or milk.

Dr. Jack Newman, of the Newman Breastfeeding Clinic and Institute in Canada, has produced some excellent videos that show both babies who are latched on and swallowing well and others who are taking very little milk. You can find links to these videos at www.breastfeedinginc.ca. The clip entitled "Really Good Drinking" shows a baby who is a few days old. The mother's milk has come in, and the baby is vigorously sucking and swallowing. Not only can you see the baby drinking and occasionally hear him swallowing milk, but you can see that he has taken the breast deeply into his wide-open mouth. (Before the milk has come in, a baby may not swallow as much.) For contrast, you can see a baby who is only nibbling at the breast, with little if any swallowing, in the video clip entitled "Nibbling."

In the video entitled "Baby 28 Hours Old, Baby-Led Mother-Guided Latching," a lactation consultant and Dr. Newman show a mother how to compress her breast to stimulate milk flow to the baby. With the help of breast compression, this one-day-old baby begins swallowing colostrum. Breast compression is easy to do: When the baby is sucking but is not

You can burp the baby by sitting her up, one hand under her jaw. Firmly pat her lower back with the other hand.

swallowing, gently squeeze the breast until the baby begins taking long sucks with pauses for swallowing.

When your baby has released the nipple, or when you have nursed her for 20 to 25 minutes and she is no longer swallowing, burp her. Hold her up over your shoulder and pat her back, or sit her upright, bent slightly forward with your hand supporting her lower jaw, and firmly pat her lower back. After burping, she will probably regain interest in nursing and take the second breast. If she doesn't burp within a few minutes, just switch sides. If she refuses to nurse on the second breast or nurses for only a short time, be sure to start her on that side at the next feeding.

The first days of milk production are the critical period for determining whether a mother ends up with a generous milk supply or an inadequate one. If little milk is removed from the breast, the resulting pressure causes the breast to slow down production. If no milk is removed, milk production stops entirely (this is how women who don't nurse stop producing milk). So ensuring a good milk supply depends on having a vigorous nursing baby, or an effective breast pump, that drains at least one breast every few hours around the clock.

Avoiding Supplements

Another way to help ensure your milk supply is to avoid supplemental feedings. Some babies develop a strong preference for an artificial nipple when a bottle is introduced during the first few days (see "Just the Breast," page 42). Glucose (sugar) water offers few calories and may discourage the baby's interest in nursing. Also, babies fed glucose water more frequently develop jaundice in the first few days after birth. After taking formula, a baby frequently will not want to nurse for four hours or longer, since formula takes longer to digest than breast milk. The decrease in breast stimulation may decrease milk production.

Putting Your Fears to Rest

In the early days of breastfeeding, you may be surprised at how often your baby wants to nurse. He may be especially fussy on the second night following birth, before milk production begins; most babies want to nurse nearly hourly during this period. Even after your milk comes in, your newborn may seem fussy and hungry much of the time. This may make you wonder if you have enough milk, and if you should pump your milk and feed it by bottle to see how much the baby is getting. Well-meaning friends and family members may even suggest you supplement your milk with formula.

Most newborns want to nurse 8 to 12 times in each 24-hour period after the first day or two of life. This frequent nursing is normal; it seldom reflects a poor milk supply, and it never reflects "weak milk." Unless you or your baby falls into one of the categories described under "Babies Who May Not Get Enough" (see page 57), your baby is probably getting plenty of milk.

Without introducing a bottle, though, how can you know your baby is getting enough? You can look for these signs of adequate milk intake:

- *Your milk has come in by the third day after birth.* When milk production begins, the breasts become firmer and heavier. The firmness may be less apparent with large breasts, but the breasts should still feel heavier.

- *Your baby is nursing at least eight times in a 24-hour period after the first 24 hours.* This means your baby is nursing every two to three hours (measured from the start of one feeding to the start of the next) during the day, with a sleep stretch of up to five hours at night. If your baby isn't nursing this often, you may have to wake her for feedings.

- **Your baby is nursing for 10 to 45 minutes at each feeding and seems content after feedings.** Babies vary in the length of time they nurse, but they typically need 10 to 45 minutes to complete a feeding. Although babies don't always fall asleep after nursing, they should usually seem satisfied after feedings.

- **Your baby has several periods of swallowing during each feeding.** When babies are getting milk, they take long, drawing sucks and can be heard swallowing or gulping (see page 59).

- **Your breasts feel softer or lighter after the baby has nursed.** Once milk production has begun, you should be able to feel a decrease in fullness or heaviness after feeding your baby.

- **Your baby is having bowel movements every day, and by the fifth day they have turned yellow.** This is the clearest sign that a baby is getting enough colostrum at first, and then later enough breast milk. Most newborns have at least two to three bowel movements each day during the first month. Only after the first month is it normal for breastfed babies to go several days without a bowel movement.

- **Your baby is wetting more diapers by the fifth day after birth.** Before your milk comes in, your baby will urinate infrequently, but by the fifth day you should notice more frequent and wetter diapers. Be aware that most disposable diapers today are so absorbent that they can make wetness difficult to detect.

If not all of the points just listed hold true for you and your baby, you should have him weighed and examined. In the first four to five days after birth, a baby loses weight. After the fifth day, a baby should gain an ounce every day. An initial loss of 10 percent or more of a baby's birth weight suggests the baby is underfed (see Appendix B, page 369). Even if your baby has lost less than 10 percent of his birth weight, have him weighed again in a couple of days to see if he has started gaining an ounce per day.

Babies Who May Not Get Enough

Some mothers and babies at risk for underfeeding can be identified even before the milk comes in. This group includes

- babies who are born at 37 weeks' gestation or earlier (see "The Near-Term Baby," page 136);
- babies weighing less than 6 pounds at birth (see "The Near-Term Baby," page 136);
- babies who may have poor muscle tone, such as those with Down syndrome (see "Developmental and Neurological Problems," page 151);
- babies who have unusual conformations in their mouths, such as a short frenulum (the string of tissue on the underside of the tongue) near the tongue's tip, a high palate (see page 98), or a cleft lip or palate (see "The Baby Who Has Not Yet Nursed," page 97, and "Cleft Lip and Palate," page 150);
- babies who aren't yet latching on or sustaining sucking 24 hours after birth (see "Sucking Problems," page 102);
- mothers with nipples as large as or larger in diameter than a quarter (see "Sucking Problems," page 102);
- mothers who have very soft breasts with no noticeable change in fullness and no other signs of milk production at 72 hours following birth (see "Late Onset of Milk Production," page 70);
- mothers who have had previous breast surgery involving an incision around the nipple or areola, such as in some breast augmentation and reduction procedures (see "Nursing after Breast Surgery," page 119);
- mothers who have polycystic ovary syndrome, or PCOS (see page 119);
- mothers who have widely spaced, long, thin breasts that did not get larger in pregnancy and that may differ markedly from each other in size (see page 116); and
- mothers who have placental fragments still in their uterus (see "Late Onset of Milk Production," page 70).

If you or your baby falls into one of these risk groups, a few days of sluggish nursing and limited milk removal could have a devastating effect on your milk production, even if breastfeeding seems to be getting off to a good start. Consider renting a clinical-grade breast pump, preferably with a double collection kit, which may be more reliable than your baby in stimulating continued milk production. Starting on the third day after birth, pump for 5 to 10 minutes with a double collection kit right after each daytime and evening nursing. If you don't have a double collection kit, pump each side twice, for a total pumping time of 10 to 15 minutes. If your baby isn't able to latch on or clearly isn't sucking effectively, start pumping earlier than the third day, and pump for 10 to 20 minutes with a double collection kit or 10 to 15 minutes per side without one. This should assure that you'll have an abundant milk supply even if your baby's sucking is sluggish. You can freeze the pumped milk for later use.

If your baby is latching on and sucking, watch her closely for the reassuring signs of adequate milk intake listed on pages 55 and 56. Weigh her at three to four days of age and approximately every two days thereafter until she is clearly gaining an ounce a day. If she loses 10 percent or more of her birth weight or does not gain an ounce a day after five days of age, she needs your pumped breast milk or formula as a supplement. If she has regained her birth weight, you can gradually stop pumping over a few days. Before returning the pump, though, make sure the baby has gained an ounce a day since the last weighing. See "Treatment Measures for Underfeeding," page 108.

The First Week of Nursing

Although most unmedicated babies are alert and eager to nurse during the first two hours after birth, during the next few days they may sleep much of the time. The average baby, after the first couple of days, begins to wake up to nurse about every one to three hours. At night, he will sleep from one to five hours at a stretch. If your baby is not waking on his own to nurse at least eight times in each 24-hour period, including at least once in the night, awaken him for feedings.

The typical length of a feeding varies greatly from baby to baby. A baby who is "all business"—who sucks and swallows with few pauses —may complete a feeding in as little as 10 minutes. At the other extreme is the baby who sucks and swallows five or six times and then pauses. This pattern of frequent pausing may extend a feeding beyond 40 minutes. Most babies' feedings fall between these extremes; the average is 20 to 30 minutes. Although your baby may not fall asleep after feeding, he should seem content.

A baby who takes longer than 45 minutes to complete most of his feedings may not be getting sufficient amounts of milk and should be weighed to make sure that he has not lost too much weight or, after the fifth day of life, that he is gaining weight.

After your milk comes in, you should hear a lot of swallowing while nursing the baby. Swallowing sounds something like "eh, eh, eh." Some babies gulp noisily, whereas others swallow more quietly. Between swallows, babies take long, drawing sucks. (They take short, choppy sucks when they are not swallowing milk.) These long, drawing sucks usually occur in bursts, that is, five to ten continuous sucks followed by a resting pause. Babies who are taking enough milk usually have several bursts of continuous sucking and swallowing during a feeding.

You should not hear clicking noises while your baby nurses. Clicking often means that the baby is not sucking adequately and therefore may not be receiving enough milk. Some babies make clicking sounds if they have a very high palate (roof of the mouth). The baby may not be able to press the nipple up against it if it is very high, deeper than the underside of a teaspoon. Some babies have such high palates that you will need to place your cheek on their chest to be able to see the top of it. The baby should have such a strong hold on the breast that the nipple does not easily slip from his mouth when you pull him slightly away. His cheeks should remain smooth with each suck; dimples on the cheek while nursing are a sign of inadequate suction and faulty sucking (see "Sucking Problems," page 102, if your baby's cheeks are dimpling or if you don't hear much swallowing). One exception to clicking being abnormal can occur when a baby is getting so much milk and is swallowing so much that she momentarily unlatches without coming off the breast, which also causes a clicking sound.

During the first day after birth, babies sometimes spit up mucus they have swallowed during delivery. Occasionally a baby will gag on this mucus. After the first 24 hours, this is usually no longer a problem.

Some babies also spit up colostrum or milk. The amounts are usually smaller than they seem, though you may wonder if your baby is keeping anything down. Spitting up a teaspoon or two after feedings is normal for some babies in the first week.

Babies also get hiccups, often after a feeding. Hiccups are the result of the baby's full tummy. You may remember the baby hiccuping in utero after drinking amniotic fluid. If the baby starts hiccuping after nursing at the first breast, it may be difficult to interest him in the other. You don't need to give him water or anything else. The hiccups are painless for him; just wait until they go away.

The baby's first stools, called meconium, are black and sticky. Having bowel movements every day and yellow stools by the fifth day usually indicates an adequate intake of colostrum, first, and then breast milk. Frequent yellow stools are one of the surest signs that a newborn is getting enough to eat. Most newborns have at least two bowel movements each day during the first month.

The yellow stools of a breastfed baby are soft, loose, or even watery, and sometimes they look seedy. Babies normally strain and grunt when passing their stools. This does not mean they are constipated.

Wet diapers are usually infrequent in the first few days, but they should be more frequent and wetter by the fifth day. Eight or more diapers wet with pale urine each day, along with daily yellow stools, are usually a sign of sufficient milk intake. (This rule may not hold true if the baby is receiving water or formula supplements.)

All newborns lose weight after birth. Expect your baby to lose 5 to 9 percent of his birth weight. He should begin gaining weight by the fifth day, about an ounce a day.

Caring For Your Breasts

Your daily bath or shower is sufficient for cleaning your breasts. Avoid getting soap or shampoo on the nipple and areola; this would counteract the naturally occurring oils that cleanse this area. Antiseptic applications to the nipples are also unnecessary, but do take care to wash your hands before nursing.

You will probably want to wear a nursing bra for convenience and comfort, especially after your milk comes in. Again, bras with cotton or microfiber rather than synthetic cups allow for better air circulation to the nipples.

If the baby does not come off the breast by herself when the nursing session is over, take care to release the suction by pulling with your finger at the corner of the baby's mouth, toward her ear. Leave your breasts exposed to the air for 5 to 10 minutes before covering up.

In the past, nursing mothers were discouraged from using nipple creams, since some women develop sore nipples in reaction to preparations containing lanolin, vitamin E, or cocoa butter. Some lanolin preparations were also discovered to be contaminated with pesticide residues. However, a purified form of lanolin has been developed; it rarely causes allergic reactions. Another aid for sore nipples are gel pads, but while they are soothing to sore nipples, they have been associated with breast infections. Other options for soothing tender or injured nipples are discussed in "Survival Guide: The First Week," page 67.

If you are using plastic breast shells to improve the shape of your nipples, you may find during the first few weeks that they cause your milk to leak excessively and keep your nipples damp. You might try placing the shells in your bra just 10 to 20 minutes before the feeding (milk collected this way should be discarded if it has been in the cups longer than a half hour or so). Don't routinely use breast shells in place of nursing pads; this usually causes more leakage. Breast shells should be washed after each nursing in hot soapy water and rinsed thoroughly.

When Your Mature Milk Comes In

Mature milk production generally begins on the second or third day after birth, but occasionally not until the fourth day or later (if your milk hasn't come in by the third day, see "Late Onset of Milk Production," page 70). At first the milk will be mixed with colostrum, and so will be pale orange in color. After a few days the milk will become whiter. This mature milk will look more watery than cow's milk; it may resemble skim milk.

Most women notice that their breasts become larger, fuller, and more tender as the mature milk comes in. Large-breasted women may notice only a change in heaviness. This change, known as engorgement, is caused by increased blood flow to the breasts as well as beginning milk production. Fullness may be more apparent if your breasts are normally small or medium-sized. They may feel lumpy, and the lumpiness may extend all the way to your armpits, since milk glands are also located there. After nursing, your breasts should feel softer or lighter.

Engorgement normally lasts 24 to 72 hours. During this time a nursing bra will provide support and comfort. Frequent nursing, at least every two to three hours, is the best treatment. Heat treatments such as warm showers, hot packs, and heating pads may worsen the swelling. You may get relief, though, with cool applications to the breast and by gentle massaging or compressing the breast while the baby is nursing. This will encourage more milk to let down. It is important to pay careful attention to the way the baby latches on while the breast is engorged. When latch-on is incorrect, because the baby isn't positioned well or the areola is overly full, soreness often follows. If the areola is hard, you can express some milk, by hand or with a pump. (For further advice on managing engorgement, see "Engorged Breasts," page 68.)

When you put your baby to breast, you may feel any of these normal sensations: warmth, relaxation, sleepiness, thirst, and even hunger.

It is normal for milk to leak from the breasts. When the baby nurses at one breast, milk may drip or even spray from the other. This leaking may continue for several weeks, or it may never happen at all.

For women who leak milk, nursing pads are usually necessary to prevent wet or spotted clothing. You can buy the pads in two varieties: reusable and disposable. A new type that helps lessen leaking is called LilyPadz. Made of gas-permeable silicone, these pads apply a gentle pressure on the nipple to stop milk leakage (see Appendix A, page 361, for ordering information).

From Hospital to Home

In many hospitals, it is customary at the time of discharge to give new mothers an array of sample products that manufacturers would like them to try. You might conclude that the staff endorses these products, but this is not necessarily so. One of the gifts is usually something that may be labeled a "breastfeeding kit"—infant formula (often powdered, although powdered formula isn't safe for newborns—see page 4), bottle nipples, and a pamphlet on breastfeeding, which may contain misleading information. Since you have chosen to breastfeed, it is best to leave the kit behind. You won't be needing it.

Well worth taking home, however, are the names and telephone numbers of people who have a good reputation for helping nursing mothers and infants. Ask any nurse who has been encouraging or helpful with your early breastfeeding for this information. She may know of volunteers in La Leche League or the Nursing Mothers Counsel, or experienced lactation professionals in your community.

When you're getting ready to leave the hospital by car, have ready some small blankets to support your baby in her car seat, even if you'll have a short drive home. Because a newborn can't control her head well, she needs special support to allow her to breathe freely while riding in a car seat. A study of car seat models (Tonkin et al., 2006) found that all newborns need blanket rolls at either side of the body and another across the top of the head. Many also require a blanket roll between the crotch belt and the legs to keep from sliding down in the seat. This is particularly important for infants born early. The Snuggin Go infant positioner is a soft insert that helps preterm and term infants stay well positioned in their car seat (see page 34).

If a baby has been born before 37 weeks' gestation, the American Academy of Pediatrics recommends that the hospital staff observe her while she reclines in a car seat to be sure her breathing, heart rate, and oxygen levels remain normal. Nurseries that care mainly for full-term babies may not be aware of this recommendation, so you may need to ask for your baby to be monitored before she is discharged.

At home. As any experienced nursing mother can tell you, the first few days at home with a baby are exhausting and, at times, emotional. These days are best spent caring for only yourself and the baby. Besides recovering from the birth, you are doing the important work of getting to know your baby and learning to breastfeed. Rest and a quiet, pleasant environment are important in preventing anxiety and "baby blues." Try to eat well, but don't worry if your appetite has lessened; this can be normal during the first couple of weeks after delivery. Do be sure to drink enough water in order to stay hydrated. Ideally, you should spend the first several days nursing and resting with the baby, while a supportive partner or helper (or both) manages your home, meals, and callers.

Because all newborns are susceptible to declining oxygen levels when they remain seated for a long time, researchers recommend minimizing car travel and avoiding the use of car seats as carriers and other seating devices, such as swings, in the early months of life.

If you have another child or children, you'll want help with them, too. Otherwise you may find yourself feeling suddenly, unexpectedly impatient or irritable with a beloved older child. When my second child was born, I found myself wishing someone could take away my nine-year-old for a while. Such feelings may arise from a natural protective urge that allows a mother to focus her total attention on the vulnerable newborn; shifting hormones and lack of sleep may contribute, too. Other species also defend their babies aggressively. For instance, picking up the new babies of a household pet may make the new mama growl, though in a few weeks she may not care at all when someone handles them.

In women, as in cats and dogs, such feelings usually lessen over time. In the meantime, they present a fine opportunity for your older child to strengthen a relationship with Dad, Grandma or Grandpa, or another adult. This is also a great chance for your older child to learn patience and responsibility. You can encourage him to accept the big-kid role by saying outright that "the baby comes first." Your child may feel proud to help by fetching a diaper or glass of water, and he may later be able to apply the baby-comes-first principle with other helpless creatures, such as pets.

Some parents find it helpful to keep a log of the baby's feedings and urine and stool output during the early days of breastfeeding. This information may reassure them that the feedings are going well and help a doctor or lactation professional analyze any problem that may arise. If you don't have a copy of *The Nursing Mother's Companion Breastfeeding Diary* (see "Suggested Supplemental Reading," page 414), your caregiver may give you a blank log, you can find one on the Internet (for example, at www.kellymom.com), or you can create your own. For each 24-hour period, include the number of nursings, the number and color of stools, and, perhaps, the number of wet diapers. There is seldom any reason to keep such a log after the baby has regained his birth weight, which usually happens between 10 and 14 days of age. There are also now smartphone apps to keep track of infant feedings.

Regardless of how you gave birth, you may continue to require pain medication for the first week or so at home. Use over-the-counter pain relievers such as acetaminophen (Tylenol) or ibuprofen (Motrin, Advil) as often as you need for afterpains or pain from an episiotomy or cesarean incision. Use narcotic pain relievers only when the over-the-counter medications are not enough.

Taking narcotic pain relievers often and for more than one week after birth can, in some instances, make a baby sleepy and in rare cases lead mothers to experience withdrawal symptoms when the medication is stopped. Withdrawal symptoms may include depression, anxiety, crying, difficulty sleeping, nausea, vomiting, diarrhea, excessive sweating, and dilated pupils. Some of these symptoms mimic a normal postpartum emotional upset, but others do not.

It is not uncommon for things to suddenly "fall apart" shortly after a new mother comes home from the hospital. Suddenly responsible for a new baby, you may feel shaky, and at times your confidence may vanish. The dramatic hormonal shift that begins immediately after birth may also affect your emotional state for a while. You may find yourself exhausted and upset—especially if you've been taking responsibility for more than the baby and yourself.

Many new mothers have times when they feel that nursing "isn't working" and think about giving it up. Combined with the mood swings that follow birth, fears that the baby may not be getting enough milk, struggles with getting the baby to latch on, or problems like sore nipples, nursing can be overwhelming. A father may become very concerned when he is witness to these struggles and emotional episodes, and he may become anxious to find a solution. If your partner can't "fix" your breastfeeding problems, he may encourage you to give up on nursing.

Your partner will be more supportive if he feels he plays an important role in helping the family adjust after childbirth. So encourage him to help—even if he puts the diaper on backward! He might hold the baby while you nap, put meals together, tidy the house, care for other children, and even track down a lactation consultant for you (see Appendix A, page 358).

Despite tearful moments, rest assured that most early nursing difficulties can be overcome with patience and help. Don't hesitate to seek assistance. Just a phone conversation with a knowledgeable person may be enough to get you and your baby back on track.

The postpartum period is a time of physical and emotional adjustment. As with most of life's great transitions, this one is usually accompanied by some turmoil. It will take several weeks, and most of your time and energy, to get to know your baby and learn how to care for her. So don't do more than you must, and accept offers for help. Adjusting to motherhood is always easier when you are supported and cared for by others.

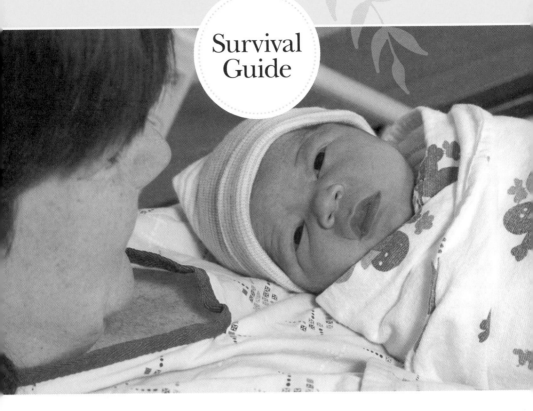

THE FIRST WEEK

Concerns about Yourself

- Engorged Breasts
- Late Onset of Milk Production
- Sore Nipples
- Breast Pain
- Leaking Milk
- Let-Down Difficulty
- Milk Appearance
- Difficult Latch-on: Flat, Dimpled, or Inverted Nipples
- Fatigue and Depression

Concerns about the Baby

- Sleepy Baby
- Bowel Movements
- Jaundice
- Difficult Latch-on: Refusal to Nurse
- Sucking Problems
- Fussiness and Excessive Night Waking
- Underfeeding and Weight Loss

Concerns about Yourself

Engorged Breasts

Two to three days after a woman gives birth, her breasts usually become engorged, or temporarily swollen. The breasts typically feel fuller, although large-breasted women may notice only more heaviness. Engorgement is caused by the increased flow of blood to the breasts and the start of milk production. For some women the breasts become only slightly full, but for others they feel very swollen, tender, throbbing, and lumpy. Sometimes the swelling extends all the way to the armpit.

Engorgement may cause the nipples to flatten, making it difficult for the baby to latch on. The problem usually lessens within 24 to 72 hours, but the swelling and discomfort may worsen if nursing is too brief or infrequent or if the baby sucks ineffectively. If engorgement is unrelieved by nursing or pumping, milk production declines and ultimately stops altogether.

Although many health-care providers recommend applying direct heat (warm washcloths, heating pads, hot water bottles, or hot showers) to engorged breasts, this may actually aggravate engorgement.

Treatment Measures for Engorged Breasts

1. Wear a supportive nursing bra, even during the night. Be sure your bra is not too tight.

2. Nurse frequently, every one and a half to three hours. This may mean waking the baby (see "Sleepy Baby," page 88).

3. Avoid having the baby latch on when the areola is very firm. To help keep the baby's mouth from sliding down onto the nipple and injuring it, use a technique developed by Jean Cotterman (2004): Just before nursing, soften the areola by placing two or three fingers at the base of the nipple and pressing firmly against the areola. Hold this position for at least 1 minute, and then move your fingers to a different spot at the base of the nipple and repeat the pressure. Or soften the areola and extend the nipple

by manually expressing or pumping a little milk (see Chapter 5, page 225). Wearing plastic breast shells for half an hour before nursing may also help to soften the areola.

4. Encourage the baby to nurse for at least 10 minutes or longer. It is preferable to nurse on just one side until the breast is soft, even if the baby goes to sleep, than to limit the baby's nursing time on the first side so you can nurse from both sides in one feeding.

5. Gently massage or compress the breast by squeezing it gently as the baby nurses. This will encourage the milk to flow and will help relieve some of the tightness and discomfort you feel (see Chapter 2, page 53).

6. To relieve the pain and swelling, apply a cold pack to the breast for a short period after nursing. You can use ice in a plastic bag or, better, soak a disposable diaper in water, shape it, and then freeze it. Lay a thin cloth over your breast before applying the cold pack or diaper.

The breasts may grow astonishingly big and hard as milk production begins.

7. If you need to, take a mild pain reliever such as acetaminophen (Tylenol) or ibuprofen (Motrin, Advil).

8. If, 48 hours after your milk has come in, you still find yourself overly full right after nursing, use a pump to drain both breasts as completely as possible. In this first week, habitual pumping along with nursing can lead to more engorgement and chronic overproduction, but pumping after nursing once every 24 hours or so should relieve your engorgement, not prolong it.

9. If the baby is not nursing well enough to soften at least one breast every few hours, use a clinical-grade pump as necessary (see Chapter 5, page 232).

Late Onset of Milk Production

Occasionally milk production is delayed beyond 72 hours; sometimes it begins days later. In the meantime, the breasts remain soft, and the baby sucks but gets little milk. In these circumstances, some babies seem sleepy and content, but most act dissatisfied. They may spend a long time sucking at the breast only to act hungry when they stop. They have infrequent bowel movements, many become jaundiced, and they lose more weight than normally expected.

Events during labor and birth can delay the onset of milk production. Overhydration with intravenous fluids during labor is a frequent cause of delayed milk production (see Chapter 1, page 21). Retained placental fragments are another possible, although uncommon, cause. It is thought that the hormones secreted by even small placental parts still attached to the uterine wall can keep the milk from coming in. Suspect retained placental fragments if you experienced postpartum hemorrhage or if, since the birth, you've had some of these symptoms: cramping, heavy bleeding, passing of tissue, foul-smelling lochia, and fever. Even some women who have delivered by cesarean have had retained placental fragments. When a doctor removes the fragments, milk production usually begins.

Most newborns lose weight following birth. While some professionals believe that a weight loss of up to 8 percent is normal, others are comfortable with a weight loss of up to 10 percent. Loosing 10 percent or more of birth weight may be a red flag that the baby has lost too much weight, which can lead to dehydration, jaundice, and poor feeding (see the "Ten-Percent Weight Loss" chart in Appendix B, page 369).

If your milk is late coming in, you may need to supplement with whatever colostrum you can express and/or formula until it does. But you should continue to nurse frequently in the meantime.

Treatment Measures for Late Onset of Milk Production

1. If, 72 hours after the birth, you suspect that your milk is not in, have your baby weighed. If he has lost 10 percent or more of his birth weight (see the chart in Appendix B, page 369), nurse frequently, every two to two and a half hours during the day or evening, or more often if the baby seems hungry, and every three hours in the night, or more often if the baby wakes sooner.

2. Check the baby's weight every day or two.

3. Seek advice from a lactation professional, if possible.

4. While the baby is at the breast, listen for swallowing. When he drifts off to sleep and is no longer swallowing, massage or compress your breast (see Chapter 2, page 53). You can also switch breasts as the swallowing slows, to help the baby wake and begin swallowing again. Massaging, compressing, and switching back and forth for 20 to 30 minutes will help stimulate the breast and maximize the amount that the baby takes.

   After each nursing, hand express your colostrum or breast milk and/or use a clinical-grade electric breast pump with a double collection kit. You can read about manual expression and pumping in Chapter 5, pages 225 to 229. You can also learn the technique of hand expression from a lactation consultant or by viewing a help-ful video made by Dr. Jane Morton of Stanford University at http://newborns.stanford.edu/Breastfeeding/HandExpression.html.

5. Express or pump your breasts for 5 to 10 minutes, and then feed your baby the colostrum you collect along with any necessary formula (see Appendix B, page 370, to determine how much milk

Herbs for More Milk

Various herbs are known to stimulate milk production. One of the most effective may be fenugreek, whose fragrant seed is used as the flavoring ingredient in artificial maple syrup. You can make a tea from the seeds, but more convenient and effective is the capsule form, available in most health-food stores. Mothers who take three 580- or 610-milligram capsules three times a day typically notice an increase in the milk supply within one to three days. Although fenugreek capsules are usually taken for just a few days, some mothers continue to use them for weeks or months without any difficulties. Fenugreek capsules cost about $10 for a bottle of 100.

Fenugreek is generally harmless, although your sweat and urine will probably take on a distinct odor of maple. Rarely, mothers taking fenugreek report having diarrhea, but it quickly subsides when the fenugreek is stopped. There have also been reports of asthmatic women developing symptoms while taking fenugreek.

Blessed thistle (*Cnicus benedictus*) is also helpful in stimulating milk production. Like fenugreek, this herb is available in most health-food stores in capsule form. The typical dosage is three 390-milligram capsules three times a day. Consider using fenugreek and blessed thistle together to stimulate greater milk production.

Two other herbal preparations I recommend are More Milk Plus and More Milk Special Blend, both manufactured by Motherlove Herbal Company. More Milk Plus contains fenugreek, blessed thistle, nettle, and fennel, and is designed to increase milk production quickly. More Milk Special Blend, with the same herbs plus goat's rue, is designed to stimulate the development of breast tissue as well as increase the milk supply in women who have polycystic ovary syndrome (PCOS), who have a history of breast surgery involving an incision around the areola, or who have underdeveloped breasts (see "Insufficient Glandular Tissue," page 116). It is often used by mothers who are adopting. Both preparations are offered in capsule and tincture form. Tinctures are stronger and faster acting than capsules. For information on sources and ordering, see Appendix A, page 362.

Another herbal preparation is Go-Lacta. Go-Lacta is made from the leaves of the Malunggay tree and has been shown to increase milk pro- duction in one study. It can be taken with other herbal supplements, like More Milk Plus or More Milk Special Blend. See Appendix A, page 363.

or formula your baby needs). If you want to avoid using a bottle, you can offer your colostrum or milk using a spoon. Some mothers may be given or sold a supplementer by a lactation consultant for feeding the baby additional milk with a small tube while the baby nurses at the breast (see Appendix A, page 362).

6. Consider using herbs known to stimulate milk production (see box on facing page).

7. If you have possible symptoms of retained placenta (see page 70), call your doctor or midwife.

8. When your milk comes in, refer to "Underfeeding and Weight Loss," page 107, for guidance in estimating your production and weaning your baby off expressed milk or formula. Have the baby weighed often as you gradually stop using formula and pumping. After the fifth day of life, all babies should be gaining an ounce per day.

Sore Nipples

There is no doubt about it: Sore nipples can make a trial of what ought to be a joyous experience. For a few days after giving birth, you may feel slight tenderness during the first minute of nursing, when the baby latches on and the nipple stretches into her mouth. Such tenderness is normal at this time.

If your nipples become really sore, however, they are probably injured or irritated and require treatment beyond simple comfort measures. It is important for you to identify the cause of the problem so that you can help your nipples heal. At any time that you are unable to tolerate the pain and the position changes recommended do not help, consult a lactation professional. If none is available, you may want to temporarily stop nursing; pump your milk with a clinical-grade rental pump using a double collection kit for 24 to 72 hours, or until the nipples heal (see Chapter 5, page 225, for information on expressing milk).

There are two basic types of sore nipples: the traumatized nipple and the irritated nipple. The traumatized nipple may be blistered, scabbed, or cracked. The irritated nipple is very pink and often burns. Occasionally a mother may have both types of soreness at once.

In addition to the specific treatments listed for each category of sore nipples, the tips below will help speed healing and provide comfort.

General Comfort Measures for Sore Nipples

1. A half hour before nursing, take acetaminophen (Tylenol), ibuprofen (Motrin, Advil), or a pain reliever prescribed by your doctor.

2. Avoid nipple shields (see page 85) for nursing, unless you are under the care of a lactation consultant. These thin, soft silicone nipple covers are designed to help infants who are having difficulty latching on to the breast. Nipple shields can make the soreness worse, and they can decrease your milk supply. Nipple shields come in different sizes; a wrong fit may not allow adequate breast compression and can cause the baby to get too little milk.

3. Do not delay nursings. Shorter, more frequent nursings (every one and a half to two hours) are easier on the nipples than longer, infrequent nursings.

4. While nursing, massage or compress your breasts (see page 53) to encourage the milk to flow and to speed emptying.

5. If you are sore during the entire feeding, restrict nursing to one breast only or restrict the time to 10 to 15 minutes per side. This will probably mean nursing more often, every hour or two. If nursing is still too painful, rent a clinical-grade pump with a double collection kit. You may find that Medela's Symphony pump feels gentler on your nipples (see Chapter 5, page 260).

6. Release the baby's suction carefully (see page 61) before removing him from the breast.

7. After nursing, wash your hands and then apply a thin coating of modified lanolin (see page 61) or other ointment to your nipples to soothe them and promote healing.

8. Another soothing ointment is Motherlove Nipple Cream, which contains three herbal remedies for healing sore or injured nipples. Medical-grade Manuka honey is well known for its healing and antibacterial properties; see Appendix A, page 365, for help locating a local distributor.

9. Between nursings, you might wear vented, hard plastic breast shells to keep your bra off your sensitive nipples. If you use plastic breast shells, wash them daily.

10. Avoid wearing hydrogel dressings. These cool, soothing pads may feel good but are associated with the development of breast infection.

11. Change disposable or cloth nursing pads after each nursing and when they become wet.

12. Wear cotton or microfiber bras. Other fabrics do not allow adequate air circulation.

13. Suds and rinse your nipples in your daily shower and rinse them in warm water after each nursing. Take care to wash your hands before handling your breasts.

14. If you are using a breast pump instead of nursing during a period of soreness, pump your milk often—at least eight times a day—to keep up your supply. Again, anything other than a clinical-grade rental pump with a double collection kit may not be effective enough to maintain your milk supply. (See Chapter 5 for more information on expressing milk.)

Traumatized nipples. Cracks, blisters, and abrasions usually result because a baby is improperly positioned for nursing; her gums close on the nipple instead of the areola. This often occurs when a baby fails to open her mouth wide enough or when her gums slide off the areola onto the nipple, commonly because the breast is engorged or unsupported.

Babies who have a faulty suck or who are "tongue-tied" (see page 98) can also cause cracks, blisters, and abrasions. Cracking may also occur with irritated nipples (see page 77) and thrush nipples (see page 78).

Treatment Measures for Traumatized Nipples

1. Carefully review "Positioning at the Breast," page 44, so that you clearly understand the details of correct latch-on technique. The crossover or football hold is highly recommended. Review the video recommended on page 48. You might also try "biological nurturing" (see page 50).

2. If your breast is so full that the areola cannot be easily compressed, soften it by pressing with your finger, as described on page 69, or by manually expressing or pumping a little milk. This will allow the baby to get more of the areola into her mouth and help stimulate the milk to let down.

3. If your baby is reluctant to open her mouth wide, don't let her chew her way onto the breast. Patiently wait until she opens her mouth wide. Letting the baby suck on your finger for a few seconds may stimulate her sucking reflex and encourage her to open wider.

4. Do not hesitate to take the baby off the breast as soon as you realize that she is not in the right position. You may need to help her latch on a couple of times before you succeed at getting her far enough onto the breast. Ask your partner or a lactation consultant to observe your latch-on technique. A helper can also guide your arm when the baby opens wide so that she is pulled in as quickly and as close as possible.

5. Don't turn to a nipple shield when dealing with traumatized nipples. You may not find the correct size shield, which can make nipple pain worse or may not allow the baby to empty the breast well.

6. Apply a thin coating of modified lanolin (see page 61) or Mother-love Nipple Cream (see Appendix A, page 364) with clean hands right after nursings.

7. Consider trying medical-grade Manuka honey, which has been irradiated to destroy any botulism spores and therefore is safe to use while nursing a newborn. This honey protects against the damage caused by bacteria and has anti-inflammatory properties that can quickly reduce pain and inflammation. You can use a nursing pad to keep your nipple from sticking to your bra. See Appendix A, page 361, for ordering information.

8. Ask your midwife or physician about trying APNO (all-purpose nipple ointment), Dr. Jack Newman's ointment recipe for healing sore nipples. It was developed to treat nipple soreness or injury stemming from any number of underlying causes including bacteria, yeast, and inflammation. This ointment needs to be ordered by a doctor or midwife and mixed by a pharmacist, usually in a compounding pharmacy. It is well absorbed into the skin and the baby will not take in very much at all. The mixture is to be used sparingly after each feeding and not wiped or washed off prior to nursings, although rinsing both nipples after nursing and before applying the ointment is still recommended by lactation consultants. (See the entire prescription written out for your doctor on page 185.)

9. Bacteria in an open wound from the surrounding skin and hands can delay healing, and one study found that 75 percent of mothers with injured nipples at five days postpartum or beyond, usually from a faulty latch, develop mastitis in the coming weeks (Livingstone and Stringer, 1999). Because so many mothers develop wounded nipples during the early days of nursing, I often recommend oral antibiotics to help the wound heal and prevent getting a breast infection later. If you have injured nipples at or after five days post partum, call your midwife or obstetrician for a prescription of antibiotics.

Irritated nipples. Irritated nipples are reddened and sometimes slightly swollen, and generally they burn. Some mothers may feel burning

Thrush often appears as white, cheesy patches on the insides of the cheeks and lips.

between, as well as during, feedings. In severe cases, the nipples may be cracked, peeling, or oozing. Nipple irritation may be caused by yeast (thrush), bacteria, a chemical sensitivity or allergy, or a skin condition such as eczema or impetigo.

Thrush nipples. When a mother's nipples become sore after weeks or months of comfortable nursing, thrush (see page 182) is the usual cause. But a thrush infection can also occur in the early weeks after delivery, and when it does, it may be overlooked as the cause of the nipple soreness. A newborn with thrush may have picked up a yeast infection in the birth canal during delivery; this often happens if the mother is diabetic. A thrush infection may also result if a mother or her baby is given antibiotics (after a cesarean, antibiotics are often given in intravenous fluids).

If you suspect a case of thrush, carefully inspect the baby's mouth. You may see white patches on the inside of the cheeks, inside the lips, and possibly on the tongue. Sometimes a baby will have no symptoms in the mouth but will have a diaper rash caused by yeast. This rash, usually in the genital area, will be very defined, very red, and a bit raised. It may also appear in the folds of the baby's diaper area. There may be "satellite" areas apart from the main rash, and the rash may appear scaly. Another difference is that a yeast rash will not respond to typical remedies like frequent cleaning and the usual diaper rash creams. For treatment, see page 182.

Nipple dermatitis. A slight reddening and a burning feeling in the nipples, in the absence of thrush or another underlying skin condition, usually indicate dermatitis. Nipple dermatitis can result from bacterial growth on the nipples or an allergy or sensitivity to a nipple cream or oil, laundry detergent, or fabric softener.

Common offenders are vitamin E preparations—oils, creams, or capsules. Mothers allergic to chocolate may develop an allergic reaction to preparations with cocoa butter, such as Balm Barr. Unmodified lanolin can also cause an allergic response, usually in a mother who is allergic to wool (from which lanolin comes) or very sensitive to it. Lanolin is found in pure hydrous and anhydrous forms and in many commercial creams, such as Massé breast cream, Mammol ointment, Eucerin, and A+D ointment. Modified lanolin, which has had the allergenic component removed, seldom causes allergic reactions.

Simply discontinuing use of the cream or oil, or switching to hypoallergenic detergents (free of perfumes and dyes), may bring relief, but usually additional measures are necessary.

Treatment Measures for Nipple Dermatitis

1. You might try using Dr. Jack Newman's APNO on your nipples for a few days. See page 185.

2. Consult a doctor, preferably a dermatologist. Usually, a moderate- or high-strength anti-inflammatory cream and an antibiotic cream are prescribed.

3. Apply the medication to the irritated areas after every other nursing with clean hands, making sure your nipples are completely dry first. Apply the cream sparingly so that all of it is absorbed. If you see traces on your nipples when you are ready to nurse again, you are using too much. Dab the area with a tissue to absorb the excess.

4. Use the medication for as long as advised by your doctor. Although the pain may be gone in a day or two, the dermatitis may take from one to two weeks to completely heal.

5. Should you find that the medication aggravates your soreness, stop using it immediately. This may indicate that yeast is present and should be treated (see "Thrush Nipples," page 78).

6. Place cool, wet compresses on the nipples after nursing.

7. Review "General Comfort Measures for Sore Nipples," page 74.

Eczema and impetigo. Eczema can appear on the nipple and areola, making the area burn, itch, flake, ooze, or crust. Women with a history or current outbreak of eczema elsewhere on the body are most often affected. If you suspect eczema, seek treatment from a dermatologist.

Impetigo is a severe infection that causes continual sloughing off of the skin. When it occurs on the nipples, impetigo is very painful, but it can be quickly cured with an oral antibiotic or an antibiotic cream. Bactroban (mupirocin) is a prescription antibiotic cream commonly used to treat impetigo.

Breast Pain

Occasionally mothers complain of pain inside the breasts while nursing. You may feel pain in your breasts if you become engorged, which usually happens two to four days after delivery (see "Engorged Breasts," page 68). If your nipples are burning and pinker than normal, see "Irritated Nipples," page 77. If you feel a mild aching at the start of nursing, it may be related to the beginning of let-down.

Deep breast pains, sometimes described as "shooting," that occur soon after nursing may be related to the sudden refilling of the breast. These pains usually disappear after the first weeks of nursing. Shooting pain in the breast can also accompany plugged milk ducts (see page 187) and nipple irritation from yeast or dermatitis (see pages 182 to 185).

Leaking Milk

During the early weeks of nursing, milk may drip, leak, or spray from the breasts. This is a normal sign of let-down. While the baby nurses at one breast, milk often drips or sprays from the other. Let-down, and leaking, may occur frequently and unexpectedly between nursings as well. Milk may leak during sleep. It may be stimulated by the baby's sounds, by thoughts about nursing, or by any routines associated with feeding time. A shower may stimulate let-down. Dripping, leaking, and spraying usually lessen considerably after a few weeks of nursing.

Some mothers' breasts do not leak. Women who have nursed previously may notice that their breasts leak less with subsequent children. Both of these situations are usually normal.

Coping Measures for Leaking Milk

1. While nursing, open both bra flaps, and let the milk drip onto a small towel or diaper.

2. Change cloth or disposable nursing pads as soon as they become wet.

3. Try silicone LilyPadz (see Appendix A, page 361), which don't absorb milk but instead apply a gentle pressure on the nipple to prevent leakage.

4. Avoid routine use of plastic breast shells if you do not need them to improve the shape of your nipples. They may keep your clothes dry, but they can cause excessive leaking and keep your nipples moist. Milk collected in the shells between nursings is unsafe for feeding. Only if the shells are washed just prior to nursing and put in place during nursing can the milk be stored for later feedings.

5. Don't try to control leaking by habitually pumping your breasts. Pumping actually stimulates greater milk production and could make your breasts fuller and more prone to leaking.

6. If your breasts leak during the night, place extra cloth or disposable pads in your bra or use silicone pads, which adhere to the skin and don't require a bra to hold them in place (see Appendix A, page 361). Or simply spread a bath towel over the bed sheet to keep it and your mattress dry.

Let-down Difficulty

During the early weeks of breastfeeding, the let-down response is developing. Sometimes mothers are told that they must be happy, relaxed, and carefree for the let-down of milk to occur. If this were the case, few women would ever succeed at nursing. Although many mothers worry that their milk won't be available as needed, let-down failure is extremely rare among women who nurse regularly and often.

For the establishment and maximal functioning of the let-down reflex, nurse the baby every two to three hours around the clock during the first week. Make sure that she is positioned correctly and is compressing the sinuses beneath the areola, and that her feeding time is not limited. Ideally, the baby should be allowed—encouraged, if necessary—to drain one or both breasts well at each feeding.

It is important to make yourself as comfortable as possible for feedings. The milk may not release completely if you are experiencing much pain—whether from sore nipples or from the trauma of delivery. Taking a mild pain reliever such as acetaminophen (Tylenol) or ibuprofen (Motrin, Advil) a half hour or so prior to nursing may help.

The signs of milk release during the first week will vary for each woman. They may include

- mild uterine cramping during nursing;
- increased vaginal flow during nursing;
- dripping, leaking, or spraying of milk, especially during nursing;
- occasional sensations in the breast during nursing; and
- softening of the breasts after nursing.

The most reliable indicator of milk let-down is the baby's swallowing. As the milk releases, the baby will swallow after every one or two sucks. Most women, particularly first-time mothers, do not feel the let-down reflex during the first few weeks after birth.

Usually when a mother believes she is experiencing a let-down difficulty, the problem is actually with the baby's latch-on or sucking or with a low milk supply. See "Difficult Latch-on: Refusal to Nurse," page 95; "Sucking Problems," page 102; and "Underfeeding and Weight Loss," page 107.

Milk Appearance

Whereas colostrum is usually clear, yellow, or orange, mature breast milk is white, sometimes with a bluish tint. If it resembles skim milk from the dairy, this does not mean your milk is "weak"; breast milk normally looks thin. Occasionally a mother discovers that her milk is green, blue, or pink. Such coloring is due to her intake of vegetables, fruits, food dyes, or dietary supplements and is not harmful to the baby.

Blood in the milk can usually be traced to a bleeding nipple. Occasionally, bleeding from the breast occurs during pregnancy or when breastfeeding begins. Frequently, a benign papilloma is the cause, and the bleeding generally stops within several days. Blood in the milk will not hurt the baby, though substantial amounts may make him vomit. If you are advised against nursing, pump for a few days. The problem will clear up on its own in a day or so.

Difficult Latch-on:
Flat, Dimpled, or Inverted Nipples

Both mother and baby get frustrated when latching on to the breasts is difficult because of flat, dimpled, or inverted nipples. Typically, the problem is intensified if the breasts become engorged or overly full. When they do, even nipples that protruded before may suddenly flatten or dimple. Frequently, one nipple proves to be more troublesome than the other. Persistence and patience help most mothers through this problem.

Mothers with problem nipples are often more prone to soreness. This is because they tend to focus simply on getting the baby latched on rather than on getting the baby latched on well, with the nipple deep in the baby's mouth. A poor latch can lead to nipple soreness and even injury.

To help the baby latch on to an inverted nipple, place your thumb above the areola and your fingers below, and push your breast against your chest wall.

Don't squeeze your thumb and forefinger together, or the nipple may invert further.

Treatment Measures for Flat, Dimpled, or Inverted Nipples

1. Put the baby to the breast within the first two hours after birth. The timing of the first nursing may be critical when the nipples are flat, dimpled, or inverted. Many babies are able to latch on easily to problem nipples during this initial period, and they continue to do well.

2. To help the baby latch on to a flat nipple, make it stand out by pinching, stroking, or rolling it between your thumb and forefinger. Pinching a dimpled or inverted nipple could invert it further. To help the baby latch on to an inverted or dimpled nipple, place your thumb 1½ to 2 inches behind the nipple, with your fingers beneath, and pull back toward your chest. The crossover or football hold will allow you the most visibility and control. Consider trying "biological nurturing" (see page 50) to help the baby achieve a successful latch.

3. Express a few drops of colostrum or milk onto your nipple or onto the baby's lips if he is reluctant to latch on. Glucose water (available in hospital nurseries) dripped over the nipple may also entice the baby, although it sometimes makes the nipple too slippery. At home, in a pinch, you can mix a teaspoon of refined sugar in a cup of warm boiled water, then drip the solution over your nipple. But never use regular honey or corn syrup on your nipple, as they have been associated with infant botulism.

4. Stop nursing if the baby is frantic. Expressing a few drops of colostrum or milk onto the baby's lips or dripping glucose water on his lips can help calm him and regain his interest in latching on.

5. If a nurse or another helper is working with you, try using the side-lying position—or, if you're large-breasted, the football hold —to allow your helper maximum visibility and control. If your nipples are dimpled or inverted, ask the helper to pull back on the breast behind the nipple rather than pinching it. Sometimes these sessions become intense and upsetting, so let your helper

know when you or your baby needs a break. If you are in the hospital, let a variety of nurses or lactation professionals work with you; you can usually find one or two who are exceptionally skilled and sensitive.

Begin pumping and feeding by 24 hours after birth if your baby still has not latched on. A clinical-grade rental pump is usually the best choice for collecting milk and improving the nipple shape. Before the milk comes in, you may be able to collect even more colostrum by manually expressing it. You can read about manual expression and pumping in Chapter 5, page 225. You can also learn the technique of hand expression from a lactation consultant or by viewing a helpful video made by Dr. Jane Morton of Stanford University at http://newborns.stanford.edu/Breastfeeding/HandExpression.html.

6. Continue putting the baby to breast.

7. Try to avoid giving the baby an artificial nipple of any kind for the first couple of days. Whether or not your baby has succeeded at latching on at first try, this may be very important. An artificial nipple can make his subsequent attempts at the breast more difficult. Options for feeding a newborn manually expressed or pumped colostrum include a dropper, a spoon, a syringe, and a soft cup.

8. Many mothers consider using a nipple shield when they have trouble getting their babies to latch on to the breast. A nipple shield is a thin, clear, soft silicone cover worn over the nipple. Holes at the tip allow milk to flow to the baby. When you use a shield, your baby may latch on and suck, but the sinuses behind the areola will not be adequately compressed unless the shield is the right size for both your nipple and the baby's mouth and the baby is well latched on to the breast and not just the shaft of the shield. Without expert help, a shield can thus inhibit the flow of milk and adequate emptying of the breast, which could lead to a poor milk supply and insufficient milk intake for the baby.

A nipple shield

If you want to try using a nipple shield to make your nipples stand out, wait until a couple of days after the birth, to give the baby a chance to learn to latch on without the shield and for your milk to come in. When using a shield, take it off after the baby has sucked for 1 to 2 minutes, and try to get him to latch on without it. Pumping just before nursing may work just as well as a nipple shield in making the nipples stand out. Use a nipple shield throughout feedings only if your milk is in and either (1) a lactation professional determines the correct shield size and makes sure that the baby is taking enough milk while you're wearing the shield, or (2) you use a clinical-grade rental pump after each nursing to guarantee that your breasts are being well emptied and also have the baby weighed every few days to make sure he is gaining at least an ounce a day.

9. If you and your baby are discharged from the hospital before nursing has occurred, locate a clinical-grade rental pump (see Appendix A, page 361) and use it at least eight times a day. (See Chapter 5, page 227, for guidelines on pumping, and refer to Appendix B, page 370, for the approximate amount of milk your baby needs at each feeding.) Keep trying to nurse; at least three or four short practice sessions per day, on a soft breast when the baby is not frantic, should eventually pay off.

10. If you become engorged when your milk comes in, soften the areola by pressing on it, as described on page 68. You can also try wearing breast shells in your bra for at least a half hour before nursing; this is often essential for dimpled or inverted nipples.

Many hospital maternity units have breast shells. If yours doesn't, send your partner or a friend to a maternity shop or lactation clinic to purchase a pair. Lastly, you can briefly pump your breasts just before nursing to pull the nipples out enough for the baby to latch on.

If your baby continues to be unable to latch, there may come a time when it is best to begin feeding your milk by bottle. This may be when milk production begins and if it becomes too time-consuming to feed using other methods. In this situation, you may need a great deal of support and encouragement. Finding this support will make all the difference. Seeing a lactation professional may be very helpful. Remember that most insurance companies are required to cover lactation visits under the Affordable Care Act.

It is very common for a baby to suddenly latch on one day, rewarding his mother's persistence.

Fatigue and Depression

During this first week, make your life as simple as possible. Your partner or helper is essential to your recovery and adjustment. He or she can be most helpful in assuring your rest by taking over family and household duties and limiting phone calls and visitors.

Rest is necessary to your ability to cope during the postpartum period. Make a commitment to take at least one nap a day, to make up for sleep lost in labor and afterward. You may find that you are able to sleep better during naps and at night if you tuck the baby in with you. Babies often sleep better this way, too.

Turn off your cell phone, or mute it. An answering machine can be very helpful in preventing disruptions while you nap, if you adjust the number of rings. It's also handy when you are busy with nursing and baby care.

Eat a good breakfast; perhaps your partner can prepare it for you. If you lack an appetite at mealtimes, frequent snacking throughout the day on high-protein foods will assist your recovery and help maintain your energy level.

If you have had tearing or an episiotomy, or you have hemorrhoids, take several baths each day. Warm water is soothing and relaxing, and it will speed the healing of your perineum.

Don't expect to adjust to new parenthood on your own. Reach out for help or reassurance whenever you need it. Friends or relatives might welcome the opportunity to come and help out for a while, and you should feel free to call the hospital staff, a public health nurse, your childbirth instructor, or a breastfeeding counselor whenever you need assistance, reassurance, or support.

If you feel tired and overwhelmed, try not to keep it to yourself. Let your partner know; a good cry on someone's shoulder may leave you feeling much better. Avoid making your partner the target of your fears and anger. Instead of criticizing, let him know exactly what you need. One mother put it very well: "I just need him to give me hugs and let me know I'm doing okay." Your partner, after all, may be feeling as much stress as you are.

If you are alone with your baby during this first week, make a special effort to limit your activities. Perhaps you can have a friend come by to fix you lunch. Let the dishes soak all day, and tidy up the house for only 10 minutes at a time, if you must. Perhaps you can afford to pay for light housekeeping once or twice a week for a short period.

Feeling depressed over a birth experience is not uncommon. You may be able to resolve some of your feelings by talking to your childbirth instructor or birth attendant. In a week or two, you might try to locate a postpartum or cesarean support group.

Concerns about the Baby

Sleepy baby

Many babies are sleepy during the first several days after birth. They may be so sleepy that they refuse to wake for nursing or fall asleep after just a few minutes of sucking. Sleepiness during the first few days may be related in part to recovery following labor and delivery. Pain medications and general anesthetics given to the mother during the birth process also lessen the baby's wakefulness and interest in nursing. When newborns are wrapped snugly, too, they usually sleep for long periods of time (that's why nurses bundle them tightly). Babies may act too sleepy to nurse when they feel full from a water or formula supplement or an air bubble. The newborn with jaundice may also be somewhat sleepy.

Although it may seem unkind, after the first 24 hours the sleepy baby should be wakened and fed at least every two and a half hours (measured from the start of one nursing to the start of the next) during the day and evening, and every three to four hours in the night. The sleepy baby needs a "mother-led" rather than a "baby-led" schedule until she begins waking on her own. This is necessary not only for her nutritional well-being but also to ensure milk production and supply. Frequent feedings will also help minimize jaundice.

Treatment Measures for the Sleepy Baby

1. While in the hospital, take advantage of the baby's normal sleeping and waking cycles by keeping her with you as much as possible.

2. Avoid supplements, pacifiers, and nipple shields. All of these may decrease the baby's vigor at the breast.

3. Before attempting to nurse, wake the baby. Unwrap and undress her down to the diaper. Dim any bright lights, and sit the baby up on your lap by holding her under her chin. While talking to the baby, gently rub or pat her back (you may get a burp). Or place her against your bare chest and wait for her to begin rooting.

4. If the baby falls back asleep soon after latching on, massage or compress your breast to encourage more milk flow (see page 53). Babies are more vigorous at the breast when they are receiving milk.

5. Try the side-lying position; babies tend to nurse for longer periods in this position (get assistance, if needed, to help the baby latch on). The football hold can also be helpful in keeping a baby awake, though it is not as effective as side-lying.

6. Burp the baby after nursing at one breast to encourage her to take the other. Sitting the baby up in your lap and bending her slightly forward usually works best. If you don't get a burp after a couple

of minutes, there is probably none to be had. Change her diaper if needed.

7. If all else fails, try again in an hour.

8. Alert your physician if your baby is very lethargic and cannot be roused by the preceding techniques after five to six hours.

Bowel Movements

Your baby's first few stools are called meconium. Meconium is black, greenish-black, or dark brown, and it's tarry or sticky. By the second or third day, after several good colostrum feedings, the baby will have passed most of the meconium. He may have a few greenish-brown or brownish-yellow transitional stools.

Once milk production is established and the baby is nursing well, stools take on their characteristic yellow or mustard color. This usually occurs by the fifth day, unless the baby is jaundiced and receiving phototherapy, which makes the stools dark, or is not getting enough milk. Yellow stools by the fifth day are usually a sign that the baby is getting sufficient milk.

During the early days most babies have at least two bowel movements daily. The stools of a breastfed baby are generally the consistency of yogurt. They are soft or even runny, and they may appear curdled or seedy. This is not diarrhea. These stools have a sweet or cheesy odor.

Your baby may pass his stools easily, or he may fuss, grunt, and turn red in the face while having a bowel movement. This is not constipation. Constipation is not possible as long as your baby is totally breastfed.

If your baby doesn't have bowel movements every day, or if by the fifth day his stools are still dark, he may not be getting enough milk. See "Underfeeding and Weight Loss," page 107, for more information on determining if your baby is getting enough.

Jaundice

A yellowing of the skin and eyes, jaundice is caused by bilirubin, a yellow pigment that is present to some degree in all blood. The skin becomes yellowish when the amount of bilirubin is higher than normal.

Bilirubin comes from the red blood cells. These cells live only a short time; as they are destroyed, bilirubin is made. Bilirubin is then processed through the liver and finally eliminated in the stool. During pregnancy, the mother's liver processes bilirubin for the baby. After birth, the baby's liver has to begin doing the job. This usually takes a few days. Until the baby's liver is able to process bilirubin, it may increase in the baby's blood. This normal rise is referred to as physiologic jaundice. This is the most common form of jaundice, and about 40 percent of all babies develop it. It is usually noticed on the second or third day of life, and it generally disappears by one week of age.

Mild to moderate jaundice of this type will not hurt a baby, although many parents worry about it. However, the baby who nurses poorly or not at all during the first few days may become jaundiced from the lack of colostrum, which is important for the elimination of meconium. When meconium is retained in the bowel longer than usual, bilirubin cannot be eliminated as needed. The best way to treat this jaundice is to make sure the baby gets plenty of colostrum and breast milk (see "Underfeeding and Weight Loss," page 107).

Some babies develop jaundice for other reasons. One type of jaundice, ABO incompatibility, occurs when the mother's blood type is O and the baby's blood type is A, B, or AB. During pregnancy, maternal antibodies cross the placenta, break down red blood cells, and cause more bilirubin to be produced in the baby after birth. On the first or second day after delivery, the bilirubin level may rise rapidly. Other, less common blood incompatibilities also produce elevated bilirubin levels. Babies of Asian descent typically experience higher bilirubin levels.

Babies with any bruises resulting from the birth process commonly develop jaundice. Also more prone to jaundice are babies who are sick right after birth or born prematurely, at low birth weights, or to diabetic mothers. Twins, too, are especially susceptible. Some drugs that are used during labor, including Pitocin (see page 21), can also cause jaundice.

Another type of jaundice, common only to breastfed newborns, is known as breast-milk jaundice. It occurs in approximately one-third of all nursing babies, generally on the fifth day after birth. Breast-milk jaundice usually lasts four to six weeks but can continue for as long as eight to ten weeks. When a baby's skin stays yellow beyond the first week, breast-milk jaundice is diagnosed by laboratory tests to rule out other forms of jaundice. Breastfeeding need not be interrupted to make this diagnosis. The exact cause of this jaundice is still unknown, but it has never been known to cause any problem for a baby.

If your baby looks jaundiced, the doctor may order tests to measure the level of bilirubin in the blood and determine whether treatment is necessary. If the baby was born at term and is otherwise healthy, many doctors will not order treatment unless the bilirubin level is over 20 milligrams per deciliter. Frequent breastfeeding may be all that is necessary.

Some jaundiced babies are treated with phototherapy. The "bililights," along with frequent nursing, help to destroy excess bilirubin. The baby usually lies under these lights from two to four days, her eyes covered with a protective mask.

Often the bilirubin level will stay constant for 24 hours but drop by 48 hours. The treatment is discontinued as soon as the bilirubin level has dropped to a normal level. Usually a baby is hospitalized for phototherapy, but in some communities home phototherapy services are available.

Rarely, usually in cases of blood incompatibility, the bilirubin climbs rapidly to high levels. On these occasions an exchange transfusion may be done to reduce the bilirubin. Over an hour or two, small amounts of the baby's blood are taken out and replaced with donated blood.

Some doctors ask the mother to stop breastfeeding temporarily whenever a baby becomes jaundiced. This is generally unwise, since breastfeeding is usually one of the most effective ways of eliminating jaundice. Calling a halt to nursing is also unfortunate for the mother, who may wonder if her milk is really best for her baby.

Mothers are also commonly told that their nursing babies need water supplements to help get rid of jaundice. But water supplements do not lower the level of bilirubin in the blood. Some studies suggest, in fact, that water supplements are associated with higher bilirubin levels. In addition, babies who are routinely given water tend to be nursed less frequently, and they have a higher rate of early weaning.

Since 1994, the American Academy of Pediatrics has recommended a different approach: Healthy, full-term babies over 72 hours old with bilirubin levels below 20 milligrams per deciliter (or 340 micromoles per liter) should be nursed frequently, at least eight times every 24 hours, and should receive no water supplements.

Treatment Measures for Jaundice

1. Let the baby's physician know you prefer to continue nursing throughout the period of jaundice.

2. Nurse frequently, ideally every two to two and a half hours, and encourage the baby to suck for at least 15 to 20 minutes at each breast. If your baby needs phototherapy, taking her from under the bili-light for these feedings will not delay the effectiveness of treatment. Intermittent phototherapy is thought to be as effective as continuous exposure.

Nurse often during phototherapy; taking the baby from under the bili-light for feedings will not slow her recovery from jaundice.

3. If your baby is sleepy, as jaundiced babies sometimes are, see "Sleepy Baby," page 88, for effective measures to wake her for feedings.

4. Avoid water supplements, as these do not reduce bilirubin levels and may discourage the baby from nursing frequently.

5. To be sure your baby is getting enough milk, keep track of her bowel movements. She should have at least two each day, and preferably three or more. She should have lost less than 10 percent of her birth weight, and she should gain an ounce a day after the fifth day. If she isn't gaining this much, refer to "Underfeeding and Weight Loss," page 107.

6. If you are still hospitalized or you are welcome to stay in a hospital room while your baby is being treated, ask the nurses if you can have the baby's crib and light set up next to your bed so you can care for the baby and nurse frequently.

7. If you cannot stay 24 hours a day with your baby, express your milk every three hours using a clinical-grade rental pump (see Chapter 5, page 227, for advice on pumping). Take your milk to the hospital for the feedings you will miss.

8. If your doctor is firm in his or her desire for you to temporarily stop nursing, again, express your milk every three hours to keep up your supply. Freeze your milk, and save it for later.

9. If you are struggling to get your baby to latch on, you may find that she becomes upset even when you bring her near your breast. In this situation, you may begin to think that your baby does not want to nurse. Nothing could be further from the truth. If your baby cries at the breast and seems unwilling to try to latch on, know that she is simply frustrated. She is crying because she wants to latch on and suck but isn't getting the signal she needs. She cannot feel your nipple far enough back in her mouth.

Difficult Latch-on: Refusal to Nurse

Latch-on problems can originate either with the baby or with the mother. Some babies fail to latch on well because they are sleepy (see "Sleepy Baby," page 88). Many babies struggle to latch on when the breast becomes overly full or engorged (see "Engorged Breasts," page 68), when the mother and baby are not positioned well for latch-on, or when the mother has flat, dimpled, or inverted nipples (see "Difficult Latch-on: Flat, Dimpled, or Inverted Nipples," page 83). Problems other than these are as follows.

The baby who has nursed earlier. During the first week, a baby who has already nursed may suddenly refuse one or both sides. He may simply act uninterested although he is awake, or he may become upset when put to one or both breasts. This may be because he has been given a bottle or pacifier during the first week and has developed a preference for an artificial nipple. Such a baby will likely start nursing again after a few hours uncoaxed or after one or more of the following measures are taken.

Treatment Measures for the Baby Who Stops Nursing

1. If you are overly full or engorged, soften the areola by pressing it (see page 68) or by manually expressing or pumping a little milk (see Chapter 5, page 225) just before putting the baby to breast.

2. If the baby is frantic, calm him. A few drops of colostrum or glucose water dripped on his lips or over the nipple may alert and encourage him. Glucose water is available only in hospital nurseries, but at home, in a pinch, you can mix a teaspoon of refined sugar in a cup of warm boiled water to entice the baby. Occasionally a very upset baby may need to be tightly swaddled in a thin blanket.

3. Pay attention to proper positioning (see "Positioning at the Breast," page 44). When the baby turns his face from side to side with his mouth wide open, pull him in closer so his tongue can

feel the nipple. Consider trying "biological nurturing" (see page 50) to see if the baby can achieve a successful latch more easily in this position.

4. Try letting the baby suck on your finger for a few seconds just before putting him to breast.

5. If the baby seems to spit out the nipple with his tongue, try holding some covered ice against the nipple for a few minutes to firm it. This can be particularly effective for the baby who has become used to an artificial nipple.

6. Persist. The baby who is hiccuping, having a bowel movement, or staring at his mother or something else interesting will usually be reluctant to latch on. Try again in an hour or so.

7. Coax the baby who is suddenly refusing one breast by using the football hold on that side.

8. If you can't get the baby latched on, express your milk until you can, using a clinical-grade rental pump. This may be crucial to bringing in your milk supply and to maintaining high production. Refer to Chapter 5, page 227, for information on pumping milk, and Appendix B, page 370, for the approximate amounts of milk a baby needs at each feeding.

9. Get a lot of support and encouragement. If possible, see a lactation professional.

The baby who refuses one side. Some babies latch easily to one side but refuse the other. This may happen when one nipple is more difficult for her because of the nipple size or shape (see "Difficult Latch-on: Flat, Dimpled, or Inverted Nipples," page 83). Some babies may feel uncomfortable lying on one side. This can happen when a baby has a fairly common condition known as torticollis. Torticollis can be present at birth or take up to three months to develop, and most doctors believe it could be related to abnormal positioning of the fetus inside the uterus.

This condition puts pressure on a baby's sternocleidomastoid muscle, the large muscle that runs on both sides of the neck from the back of the ears to the collarbone. Extra pressure on one side of this muscle can cause it to tighten, making it difficult for a baby to turn his neck. Babies with torticollis will act like most other babies except when it comes to activities that involve turning. A baby with torticollis keeps his head in one direction when lying down and tilts the head in just one direction, and has difficulty nursing on one side. If you think your baby might have torticollis, ask your doctor to examine your baby, which involves seeing how far your baby can turn his head. If a diagnosis is made, the doctor will probably teach you neck stretching exercises to practice with your baby at home. These exercises help loosen the tight muscle and strengthen the weaker one on the opposite side. This will help to straighten out your baby's neck. In certain cases, the doctor may suggest taking your baby to a physical therapist for more intensive treatment. In the meantime, you may need to position your baby differently—for instance, using the football hold—for him to be able to latch on to the breast.

The baby who has not yet nursed. If a day or more has passed since the baby's birth and she still has not managed to latch on and suck, she may have one of the specific problems described as follows.

Recessed jaw. Some babies are born with a very recessed lower jaw. This can best be seen by looking at the baby's face in profile. A recessed jaw is problematic because a baby can latch on only if her chin reaches the breast before her upper lip; otherwise she can't take enough breast tissue into her mouth.

When you try to get a baby like this to latch on, make sure your breast isn't overly full. Extend the baby's head slightly backward as you bring her onto the breast so that her chin touches the breast first. Consider trying "biological nurturing" (see page 50) to see if the baby can latch on to the breast in this position. A baby with a recessed jaw will probably begin latching on and sucking between four and six weeks of age. In the meantime, you may need to pump your milk and feed it to your baby by bottle.

Tongue-tied. Some infants who can't latch on to the breast—mostly males—are tongue-tied. This means that the frenulum, or string-like tissue that attaches to the underside of the tongue, is so short or connected so close to the tip of the tongue that the baby may not be able to extend his tongue past his bottom lip. More important, he may not be able to raise his tongue high enough to express the milk from the breast. Although he may be able to suck on a finger or rubber nipple that extends well into his mouth, he may be unable to grasp the underside of his mother's nipple. Not only does he fail to get milk, but nursing may be very painful for his mother even when the baby is correctly positioned. Sometimes a clicking sound can be heard as the baby sucks. Occasionally a tongue-tied baby can manage to latch on to one breast but not the other.

The solution is simple: the frenulum should be clipped to release the tongue. Some physicians are reluctant or unwilling to perform this procedure, called a frenotomy, because studies conducted many years ago showed that tongue-tied infants rarely developed speech difficulties later in life; the studies concluded that tongue clipping was therefore unnecessary. Unfortunately, though, some tongue-tied babies are unable to breastfeed. If you cannot persuade your doctor to clip the frenulum, find another who will. A surgeon or dentist may do this in his office, and the procedure takes just a minute. You can see Dr. Jane Morton's photographs of a baby both before and after a frenotomy by following the link at http://newborns.stanford.edu/Frenotomy.html. Dr. Bobby Ghaheri's website also contains a wealth of information and resources for nursing the tongue-tied baby: www.drghaheri.squarespace.com.

The tongue-tied baby may not be able to extend his tongue far enough or high enough to latch on to his mother's nipple.

Upper lip tie

Upper lip tie. Some newborns are born with their upper lip "tied" to their upper gum. Usually this poses no problems with nursings. If severe, it can cause the baby's upper lip to turn inward instead of outward. This may be irritating to the nipple if severe enough. Few pediatricians recognize this problem, but some pediatric dentists believe that an upper lip tie can lead to a gap between the teeth later on or can cause a problem with dental decay. If it seems to be causing nursing pain, an evaluation with a pediatric dentist may be in order. Again, Dr. Ghaheri's website may be helpful.

Protruding tongue. A few babies have tongues that protrude. The tongue may look longer than normal; it may be visible between the lips much of the time. Some mothers have described the protruding tongue as forming a hump in the mouth that the nipple is not able to get past.

You may be able to teach the baby to nurse by encouraging her to open wide with her tongue down and pulling back behind the areola just before latch-on. The football hold is recommended for the best visibility and control.

If you manage to get the baby onto the breast, be sure she is sucking adequately. This means she does not come off the breast easily; she is taking long, drawing sucks; and she is audibly swallowing.

Tongue sucking. Other infants who have difficulty latching on to the breast are those who suck their own tongues. These babies usually slide off the nipple after one or two sucks, and their cheeks dimple with each suck. They may also make clicking noises. When the baby opens her mouth to root or to cry, you may notice that her tongue is far back in her mouth or is curled toward the roof of her mouth.

Attempt to get the baby to latch on only when she opens wide with her tongue down. Stimulating the lower lip or slightly depressing the chin may help the tongue to drop. Pull the baby in close. The crossover or football hold is best when you are alone, and side-lying will give more control and visibility when someone is assisting you.

When refusal persists. If you have followed the preceding suggestions and your baby still has not latched on, try the following measures.

Treatment Measures for Refusal to Nurse

1. Work with the baby in short, frequent sessions. If someone is assisting you, the side-lying position may give the greatest control and visibility. These sessions may become intense and upsetting for both you and the baby, so let your helper know if you need a break. If you are in the hospital, ask for help from various nurses or lactation professionals. You may find one or two who are exceptionally skilled and sensitive.

2. Encourage your baby by expressing a few drops of milk onto your nipple or onto his lips. Or try glucose water (available in the hospital) or, at home, a teaspoon of sugar—never corn syrup or honey—in a cup of warm boiled water (see page 84).

3. Try "biological nurturing" (see page 50) to see if the baby will latch on in this position.

4. If, 24 hours after birth, your baby still has not latched on, begin manually expressing or pumping (see Chapter 5, page 225) and feeding the baby your expressed colostrum. But don't feed it by bottle; an artificial nipple of any kind could make his attempts at the breast more difficult. Alternatives to a bottle are a dropper,

a spoon, a syringe, and a soft cup. Express your colostrum and feed it to the baby at least eight times in each 24 hours. Refer to Appendix B, page 370, for the approximate amount the baby needs at each feeding.

5. Continue pumping and feeding at least eight times in each 24 hours.

6. If your baby "shuts down" or gets upset at the breast, let him suck on a finger, nail side down. After a minute or two, quickly offer the breast, compressing it tightly so that it extends as far as possible into the baby's mouth.

7. Pump just before nursing to make your nipples stand out more. Some babies do better on a soft or half-empty breast.

8. If you use a nipple shield to help the baby latch on (see page 85), take it off after the baby has sucked for 1 to 2 minutes, and try to get him to latch on without it. Use a nipple shield throughout feedings only if your milk is in and either (1) a lactation professional has determined the correct shield size and made sure that the baby is taking enough milk while you're wearing the shield, or (2) you use a clinical-grade rental pump after each nursing to guarantee that your breasts are being well emptied, and you have the baby weighed every few days to make sure he is gaining at least an ounce a day.

9. If your baby seems to latch on but sucks only once or twice, he is probably not well attached. Take him off the breast and try again.

10. Continue short practice nursing sessions several times a day. Try to be patient but persistent; don't give up on your baby.

11. If your baby continues to refuse to nurse, there may come a time when it is best to begin feeding your pumped milk by bottle. This may be when milk production begins, if it becomes too time-consuming to feed using other methods.

12. Get a lot of support and encouragement. Ideally, see a lactation professional. Your insurance should cover this.

Many babies with latch-on problems overcome them during the first ten days, but a significant number first latch on at about one month of age. With this in mind, know that the most important thing to do until the baby finally latches is to keep your milk production as high as possible. See Chapter 5 for advice on how to do this.

Sucking Problems

Some babies seem to latch on to the breast well but suck poorly. With some, the suction is so poor that they easily slide off the breast or can be taken off effortlessly. A baby's cheeks may dimple with each suck, and frequent clicking noises may be audible. Such a baby isn't really sucking on the nipple but on her tongue, which may perhaps be a habit developed in the uterus. Other babies with poor suction may have one of the physical problems described under "The Baby Who Has Not Yet Nursed," page 97. Babies with poor suction receive only the milk that drips into their mouths.

Although most babies with sucking problems have them from birth, others may develop them if they lose much weight, usually close to a pound, by the end of the first week. If this happens, and the baby cannot correct her suck after several good attempts at latching on, express your milk and feed it to her for 24 to 72 hours, supplementing breast milk with formula as necessary. After the baby is rehydrated and has regained a few ounces, she may correct her suck on her own.

A baby may have difficulty sucking at one or both breasts because he is tongue-tied. In this situation, the tongue is tethered by the short piece of tissue beneath. No matter how hard the baby tries, he isn't able to reach his tongue forward and then up far enough to strip the milk from the breast. Not only may he fail to get milk, but nursing a tongue-tied baby may be very painful for the mother, even when the baby is correctly positioned. Sometimes a clicking sound can be heard as the baby sucks. To correct the problem, have your baby's doctor or dentist clip the baby's frenulum (see page 98).

Another group of babies who have difficulty sucking and getting enough milk are those with very high palates. When the roof of the mouth is very high, the baby has trouble compressing the breast against the palate to express the milk into her mouth. Many babies with high, arched palates do little swallowing at the breast and fail to gain weight well. Few health professionals, including pediatricians, yet recognize high palates as a potential problem for nursing babies. If it is difficult to see the very top of a baby's palate without placing your head close to the baby's chest, or if the shape of the roof looks much deeper than the curve of a teaspoon, the palate may be too high. If you can get the baby to suck on your little finger (nail side down), and you feel a frequent loss of suction between your finger and his tongue, or your finger isn't in firm contact with the roof of his mouth, the palate may be too high. Another sign of a high palate may be clicking sounds while the baby is sucking.

In the case of a high palate, the mother should use an electric pump right after each nursing to bolster her milk supply. After a few days the baby will usually start to swallow more at the breast and gain weight better, but as soon as the pumping stops, the baby may begin to take less milk and will again fail to gain sufficient weight. Usually supplemental pumping is necessary for several weeks, until the baby has grown enough to suck more efficiently. Using the football hold, or positioning the baby straddling your thigh, may help the baby suck better. Time is often the remedy for babies with sucking problems.

Dimpling of the baby's cheeks during nursing may signify an inadequate suck.

Lastly, babies whose mothers have large nipples—as large as or larger than a quarter—may be unable to suck effectively. Instead of latching on to the areola, behind the nipple, the baby compresses only the nipple itself, and so gets very little milk. In this case the mother needs to express her milk, using a clinical-grade rental pump, to build and maintain high production until the baby has grown enough to latch on to and compress the breast, not just the nipple. The mother will also need to obtain a large flange for effective pumping (see page 239).

Treatment Measures for the Baby with Poor Sucking

1. Remove the baby from the breast as soon as the faulty suck is evident.

2. Check the position of the tongue when the baby's mouth is wide open. If the tongue is curled against the roof of the mouth, try to lower it with your finger by stimulating the lower lip.

3. Using the crossover or football hold, compress the breast behind the nipple, and pull the baby in as close as possible for latch-on.

4. Try "biological nurturing" (see page 50) to see if the baby can achieve better suction in this position.

5. Work with the baby in short, frequent sessions. If someone is assisting you, the side-lying position may give the greatest control and visibility. These sessions may become intense and upsetting for both you and the baby, so let your helper know if you need a break.

6. If, 24 hours after birth, your baby still is not sucking well, begin manually expressing or pumping (see Chapter 5, page 225) and feeding the baby your expressed colostrum. But don't feed it by bottle; an artificial nipple of any kind could make his attempts at the breast more difficult. Alternatives to a bottle are a dropper, a spoon, a syringe, and a soft cup. Express your colostrum and feed it to the baby at least eight times in each 24 hours. Refer to Appendix B, page 370, for the approximate amount the baby needs at each feeding.

7. Try manually expressing or pumping just before nursing. Some babies do better on a soft or half-empty breast.

8. If you use a nipple shield to help the baby latch on (see page 85), take it off after the baby has sucked for 1 to 2 minutes, and try to get him to latch on without it. Use a nipple shield throughout feedings only if your milk is in and either (1) a lactation professional has determined the correct shield size and made sure that the baby is taking enough milk while you're wearing the shield, or (2) you use a clinical-grade rental pump after each nursing to guarantee that your breasts are being well emptied, and you have the baby weighed every few days to make sure he is gaining at least an ounce a day.

9. Continue short practice nursing sessions several times a day. Try to be patient but persistent; don't give up on your baby.

10. If your baby continues to have sucking problems, there may come a time when it is best to begin feeding your pumped milk by bottle. This may be when milk production begins, if it becomes too time-consuming to feed using other methods.

11. If you are discharged from the hospital and the baby still isn't nursing well, use a clinical-grade rental pump (see page 232) for collecting your milk. Continue pumping your milk and feeding it to the baby at least eight times in each 24 hours.

12. Get a lot of support and encouragement. Make an appointment to see a lactation professional. Your insurance carrier should cover visits with a lactation consultant for you and your baby.

Like babies with latch-on problems, those with sucking problems often overcome them during the first ten days, but many improve only at about four to six weeks of age. With this in mind, know that the most important thing to do until the baby finally overcomes the problem is to keep your milk production as high as possible. See Chapter 5 for advice on how to do this.

Fussiness and Excessive Night Waking

It can come as a surprise when your baby suddenly becomes fussy after spending most of his first few days sleeping. It is difficult to listen to your baby's cry; it may feel like an alarm going off in your body. Sometimes parents are told it is healthy for babies to cry or that babies will become spoiled if tended to every time they fuss. But comforting your infant and responding to her needs is very important to her well-being and her development of trust. Babies are really unspoilable.

Newborns cry for a variety of reasons. Often they are fussy during the first night home from the hospital. They may be hungry as often as every hour, especially when your milk is just starting to come in, or when feedings have been limited because of their sleepiness or for other reasons. Some babies seem to need more sucking time than others. Some seem to pass a lot of gas, which causes them discomfort. Many newborns become upset when they are not kept snugly wrapped. Perhaps they miss the close, secure feeling of the womb.

Then there are the babies who sleep most of the day and wake frequently during the night. These babies are said to have their days and nights mixed up.

Coping Measures for Fussiness

1. Nurse your baby on demand, approximately every two to three hours for at least 10 to 20 minutes at each breast.

2. Massage or compress your breasts while you nurse to increase the flow of milk (see page 53).

3. Burp the baby after he finishes at each breast.

4. Wrap the baby snugly in a light blanket after each feeding.

5. Avoid water or formula supplements.

6. If the baby seems unsatisfied after a feeding, nurse him some more, or rock him or walk with him next to your body and then nurse him again in an hour or two.

7. If the baby frequently seems discontent after nursings, refer to "Underfeeding and Weight Loss," page 107.

Newborns normally wake about every three hours during the night. If your baby wakes more often than this, nurse her more often during the daytime and evening, every two to two and a half hours. If the baby has been sleeping through feeding times, wake her. See "Sleepy Baby," page 88.

Your baby may be crying at night not because she is hungry but because she wants to be close to you. Try tucking her in with you for at least a few nights. You may both sleep better.

Underfeeding and Weight Loss

During the first week, you may wonder if your baby is getting enough to eat. You may worry about whether your milk is adequate—especially if the baby seems to be nursing all the time or is fussy after feedings. Some mothers wonder if their milk has dried up when they observe the normal softening of the breast that occurs as the initial engorgement recedes.

Seeing if the baby will take a bottle of water or formula after nursing is not a reliable method of determining if he is getting enough breast milk. Most babies will take a couple of ounces of water or formula if it is offered, even when they have had enough milk from the breast.

A baby can lose too much weight, though, when the milk doesn't come in by the third or fourth day, when nursing is infrequent, or when he has had trouble latching on and nursing well during the period of initial engorgement. Excessive weight loss can also occur when a mother uses a nipple shield over her nipple for nursing, when a newborn has a faulty suck, and, certainly, when a baby is sick. Babies who have high palates or who are tongue-tied may fail to express milk well while nursing and thus get too little milk (see "Sucking Problems," page 102). Other women who may be unable to produce enough milk are those with insufficient glandular (milk-producing) tissue, or hypoplastic breasts (see page 116), and some with polycystic ovary syndrome, or PCOS (see page 119). Sometimes laxatives the mother has taken can cause a baby to have excessive bowel movements and to lose weight or gain too slowly.

Signs of adequate milk intake are listed on page 218. If you and your baby don't show all these signs, have him weighed. If you find that your baby has lost 10 percent or more of his birth weight within the first five days after birth, or if he isn't gaining an ounce per day after the fifth day, take the following measures.

Treatment Measures for Underfeeding

1. See a lactation professional. Again, your insurance provider should cover these services.

2. To estimate the amount of milk you are producing and to increase your milk supply, obtain a clinical-grade rental breast pump (see Chapter 5, page 232). Any other pump might be inadequate for estimating milk production and rebuilding a low milk supply.

3. To estimate your milk production, pump immediately after nursing the baby. If you have a double collection kit, which is ideal, pump for a total of 10 to 20 minutes, or longer if the milk continues to flow. If you are pumping one breast at a time, pump each twice, for a total pumping time of 20 to 30 minutes, or longer if the milk is still flowing. Feed your baby this milk and any necessary formula. See Appendix B, page 370, to determine how much milk your baby needs per day.

   Exactly two hours after completing this pumping, pump again instead of nursing. You may very well get less milk at this second pumping than at the first. Multiply the number of ounces collected at the second pumping by 12. This will give you an estimate of how much milk you are producing over a 24-hour period; if you collect 1½ ounces, for example, you are producing about 18 ounces per day. Offer the pumped milk to the baby. If you determine that you have enough milk for your baby and yet she has not been gaining well, it may be that she is not taking all of the milk available at some or many of her feedings. This can happen with newborns who were born prematurely, who tend to drift off to sleep while nursing, or who have sucking difficulties.

4. Review the video recommended in Chapter 2 (see page 48) to be sure your baby is latching on well. Consider using "biological nurturing" (see page 50) to see if she can achieve a deeper latch this way.

5. Nurse at least eight times in every 24 hours, even if this means waking the baby for feedings (see "Sleepy Baby," page 88). Nurse for 10 to 15 minutes at each breast, or for as long as the baby is swallowing. If the baby swallows for only a few minutes, compress your breast (see page 53) to increase the flow. You can also switch the baby from breast to breast each time the swallowing stops.

6. If you're not producing as much milk as your baby needs, stimulate greater milk production by pumping your breasts right after each nursing. Pumping both breasts at the same time not only takes less time but is more effective in stimulating increased milk production. Use a double collection kit, if you have one, for 5 to 10 minutes, or pump each breast separately for 5 minutes, and then return to each breast a second time for a few more minutes. You can also spend a few minutes hand-expressing milk from both breasts after pumping to help insure more complete emptying (see Chapter 5, page 225).

7. After pumping, feed the baby whatever breast milk you've collected, along with formula as necessary. If the baby needs supplemental formula (see step 3), divide the amount of supplement needed daily by the number of feedings the baby is getting each day (usually eight). A baby who needs 3½ ounces of formula, for example, should get a bit less than ½ ounce after each of her eight daily nursings. The goal is to offer about the same amount of breast milk and formula at each feeding so that the baby wants to nurse at regular intervals.

8. Some mothers consider using donated breast milk from friends, relatives, or even strangers. For more information on the possible risks of using donated milk, see pages 167 and 366.

9. Consider using herbs to stimulate greater milk production (see page 72).

10. Ignore any suggestions to drink a beer or two to help increase milk production. Drinking beer can in fact lessen milk production.

11. If your milk production remains low even with the use of herbs, consider using a pharmaceutical drug, like domperidone, to stimulate more production (see page 112 and Appendix A, page 363).

12. As long as you must provide supplemental feedings, find a method that suits you. Many lactation professionals, fearing that bottle-feeding might interfere with the baby's ability at the breast, suggest using a nursing supplementer (see Appendix A, page 362), a cup, a soft tube with a syringe or finger, or an eyedropper. If one of these methods is recommended to you and it works well, good. But if you find it too frustrating or time-consuming, use a bottle. After the first few days of breastfeeding, supplementing by bottle rarely causes "nipple confusion."

13. Weigh your baby every few days to make sure that she is gaining well.

14. After each weighing, re-estimate your baby's milk needs. Then, two hours after your most recent pumping, express your milk instead of nursing and re-estimate your milk production (see step 3). If your production has increased enough to match the baby's needs, you can decrease or even eliminate any formula supplementation.

15. Consider renting a highly accurate electronic baby scale (see Appendix A, page 365). Use the scale before and after feedings to determine how much milk the baby takes from the breast. One gram of weight increase is equal to one milliliter of milk intake.

16. Once your baby is gaining well, her nursing seems more vigorous, and you are supplementing nursings only with your breast milk, you might try eliminating some of the supplement. For a few days, offer the baby only half of the milk that you are expressing, and freeze the rest. If the baby gains well over these few days, continue pumping, but don't offer her any of the expressed milk. If the baby continues to gain an ounce a day without any supplement, gradually stop pumping. Continue to have your baby weighed weekly.

If treatment fails. Although the technique just outlined will normally reverse a case of underfeeding within a few days, sometimes, when breast engorgement has been severe and little milk has been removed during this critical period, the decline in milk production can be difficult to reverse. In unusual instances, a mother fails to produce enough milk even after weeks of both stepped-up nursing and pumping. This can occur if the placenta was not completely delivered at the time of the birth (see page 70). It sometimes happens to women who have had breast surgery, particularly if the surgical incision was made around the areola (see "Nursing after Breast Surgery," page 119). Other women who may be unable to produce enough milk are those with insufficient glandular (milk-producing) tissue, or hypoplastic breasts (see page 116), and some with polycystic ovary syndrome, or PCOS (see page 119).

In any of these situations, lack of support from family, friends, and health professionals can make matters worse. But even with all of the best information and support, things sometimes don't turn out as we hope. If after giving breastfeeding your best effort you end up having to feed formula, you have not failed as a mother. Be proud of your efforts to nurse, and concentrate on providing your baby with all of the cuddling and loving that you can. Detailed information about formula and bottle-feeding can be found in *The Nursing Mother's Guide to Weaning* (see "Suggested Supplemental Reading," page 414).

Some mothers with insufficient milk production have found that continuing to nurse with a nursing supplementer has been a rewarding experience. Others have found nursing supplementers to be cumbersome and frustrating. Another option, particularly if the baby has become frustrated at the breast, is to bottle-feed and then nurse. "Comfort nursing"—nursing just after bottle-feedings, in between bottle-feedings, or during the night—may be a pleasant experience for both mother and baby.

Drugs that Stimulate Milk Production

Two pharmaceutical drugs used to help build the milk supply are metoclopramide (Reglan) and domperidone.

Metoclopramide is prescribed in the United States primarily for gastric reflux. But several studies have shown it to be effective and safe for increasing a mother's milk supply, although the U.S. Food and Drug Administration (FDA) has not approved the drug for this use. Metoclopramide has not been shown to cause any problems for a nursing baby; in fact, it is occasionally prescribed for infants. It may, however, make the mother sleepy. More worrisome side effects, such as agitation and uncontrolled muscle movements, are uncommon; if they occur, the drug should be discontinued. The typical dosage is 10 milligrams every six to eight hours for 14 days. If taken for longer than a few weeks, metoclopramide can lead to depression and other problems that may not resolve simply by discontinuing the medication. It should therefore never be taken for more than two to four weeks.

Although domperidone is marketed only for gastrointestinal disorders, studies show that it safely increases milk production, and the American Academy of Pediatrics has approved this drug, as well as metoclopramide, as safe to take while nursing. Domperidone apparently works by stimulating production of prolactin, the hormone that stimulates the breast to produce milk.

Because domperidone does not enter the brain tissue in significant amounts, it has far less frequent and serious side effects in the nursing mother than does metoclopramide. The side effects that can occur—headache, abdominal cramps, and dry mouth—are extremely uncommon when the drug is taken orally in normal doses for stimulating milk production, no higher than 40 milligrams four times per day. (The FDA issued a warning about domperidone after reports of sickness when the drug was administered in high intravenous doses as treatment for gastrointestinal disturbances. According to Thomas Hale, a professor of pediatrics and pharmacology at Texas Tech University School of Medicine, this use of the drug caused blood levels 80 to 150 times higher than that of women who take domperidone orally in normal doses.)

Although domperidone is not manufactured in the United States, it can be made here in compounding pharmacies, which operate in most areas. But the drug is much less expensive, and available without a prescription, when ordered through InHouse Pharmacy in Vanuatu (see Appendix A, page 364).

SPECIAL MOTHERS, SPECIAL BABIES

N URSING CAN BE A SPECIAL CHALLENGE in certain circumstances—situations that may result from a longstanding
condition or that may take you completely by surprise. Either
way, you may be tempted to give up the idea of breastfeeding
altogether. The specific guidelines in this chapter should help you make a
realistic appraisal of your situation and find, I hope, the happiest solution
for you and your baby.

SPECIAL MOTHERS

Medical Conditions and Breastfeeding

Although most medical conditions a mother might have pose no harm to
her nursing infant, a few are reasons to delay or even forgo breastfeeding.

A mother with active **tuberculosis** should not breastfeed—or have
any physical contact with her baby—until treatment has been administered for one to three weeks, after which she can no longer transmit
the infection. During this period, she can express her milk to maintain
her supply, but she should discard the milk she expresses (see Chapter 5). Afterward she can safely be reunited with her infant, and she
can breastfeed.

A woman with **hepatitis** can generally breastfeed safely. If she has
viral hepatitis, also known as infectious hepatitis or hepatitis A, her baby
should be immunized with gamma globulin. If she has an active case of
hepatitis B or persistent hepatitis B surface antigen (HBsAg), her baby
should receive hepatitis B–specific immunoglobulin (HBIG) immediately after delivery. She can begin breastfeeding as soon as the shot is
given, but her baby should also receive the first in a series of hepatitis

B vaccines within 24 hours of birth. For women with hepatitis C, the Centers for Disease Control and Prevention, the American Academy of Pediatrics, and the National Institutes of Health all support breast-feeding. Although it is theoretically possible to transmit hepatitis C to a baby through breastfeeding, several research studies have shown that breastfeeding does not increase the risk of transmission. A nursing mother may be more likely to infect her baby, though, if her nipples bleed. In this situation a mother can pump her milk (see Chapter 5) and discard it until the nipples are healed, and then breastfeeding can be resumed.

Mothers with HIV **(human immunodeficiency virus)** are discouraged from breastfeeding until more is known about transmission of the virus.

A woman infected with **cytomegalovirus (CMV)** can safely breast-feed her baby if he was born at full term. If the baby was born prematurely, he may be CMV-negative; that is, he may not have received antibodies against the disease during pregnancy and so may be vulnerable to the infection. The virus can be destroyed, however, by freezing the breast milk at −4 degrees F. for at least three days.

A mother with **herpes simplex,** in the form of either cold sores on or near the mouth or genital lesions, can nurse her baby. It is important, however, that anyone with a herpes sore take certain precautions in handling a baby to avoid transmitting the infection (see "The Mother with Herpes," page 131).

Breastfeeding is also safe when a woman is infected with **toxoplasmosis.**

A mother infected with **Lyme disease** should be immediately treated, and so should her baby. The mother can breastfeed if she has begun antibiotic treatment and her baby is healthy.

Because **human T-cell leukemia virus type 1 (HTLV-1)** can be transmitted through breast milk, a woman infected with this virus should forgo breastfeeding. (HTLV-1 is rare in North America, but it is increasingly common in other parts of the world. It is associated with the development of leukemia and lymphoma.)

A woman who develops **chicken pox (varicella)** within six daysbefore deliveryshould be isolated from her baby, although someone else can feed the baby the mother's expressed milk. The mother and baby canWbe reunited after the mother becomes noninfectious, typically after seven days.

Insufficient Glandular Tissue (Breast Hypoplasia)

Although the overwhelming majority of women can produce a full supply of milk for their infants, even after a setback due to infrequent nursing or inadequate sucking (see page 102), a few mothers are unable to produce enough milk. One condition that causes this is **insufficient glandular tissue,** or breast **hypoplasia.** Perhaps because of a congenital abnormality, hypoplastic breasts contain insufficient milk-making tissue and so are typically unable to produce enough milk.

Usually the mother finds that her breasts did not enlarge during pregnancy and did not undergo any changes (such as becoming heavier or fuller or leaking milk) during the first week after delivery. Most often she has tubular breasts, with 1½ inches or more between them—in fact, it seems to be that the greater the space, the more severe the condition. The majority of mothers with hypoplasia have one breast that is significantly smaller than the other, and most also have stretch marks on their breasts despite their lack of growth.

Many times, a mother does not realize she has insufficient glandular tissue and assumes that nursing is going well until her newborn experiences a weight loss of more than 10 percent, or he fails to gain an ounce a day after the fifth day and fails to regain his birth weight by 10 to 14 days of age. Unfortunately, many health-care providers do not recognize this condition either.

In 2000, my colleagues and I published the results of a research study in a lactation journal for health professionals (see www.sonic. net/_mollyf/igt/). We worked with 34 women whom we suspected of having breast hypoplasia. For six weeks we had each mother pump after every nursing and take three fenugreek capsules three times a day to try to stimulate more milk production. Many of the mothers who had mild cases of hypoplasia achieved normal milk production by six weeks post partum, but none of the mothers with the most severe form of hypoplasia achieved adequate production.

As time went on, we added other therapies to help these mothers produce more milk. Specifically, we had them take domperidone and Motherlove Herbal Company's More Milk Special Blend (a combination of fenugreek, blessed thistle, nettle leaf, fennel seed, and goat's rue), both of which boosted the women's overall milk production. Domperidone is not manufactured in the United States, but it can be made in a compounding pharmacy or mail-ordered (without a prescription and less expensively) from InHouse Pharmacy in Vanuatu (see Appendix A, page 364). More Milk Special Blend is available from local distributors or directly from the manufacturer (see Appendix A, page 363).

Through our research, we also discovered that some mothers who had had breast augmentation surgery to enhance the size and shape of their breasts in fact had breast hypoplasia. Breast augmentation surgery

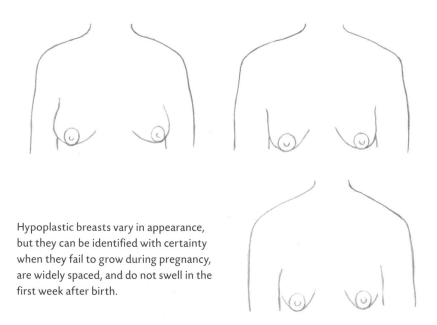

Hypoplastic breasts vary in appearance, but they can be identified with certainty when they fail to grow during pregnancy, are widely spaced, and do not swell in the first week after birth.

does not improve the milk-making tissue of the breast, so whenever a mother tells us that she has breast implants and that her infant is failing to gain weight well, we ask about the appearance of her breasts prior to having the surgery.

With the help of a lactation professional, if possible, monitor your milk production and your baby's weight (see page 107). If you can't build an adequate milk supply, you can still continue breastfeeding, but you'll need to provide supplemental formula while you nurse. Some mothers supplement their babies after nursing, by bottle (see "Underfeeding and Weight Loss," page 107), while others choose to use a nursing supplementer system (see Appendix A, page 362). A supplementer, with its thin, soft tubing attached to a bottle-like container of formula or expressed milk, allows the baby to be fed supplemental milk while nursing at the breast. This may be the best way to supplement if the baby fusses at the breast or simply drifts off to sleep.

We saw some women with breast hypoplasia again, years later, with a new baby. Surprisingly, we found that these mothers produced more milk with their subsequent babies than with their firstborn.

As the baby nurses, she can get immediate satisfaction through a supplementation device.

SPECIAL MOTHERS, SPECIAL BABIES

Polycystic Ovary Syndrome

Another condition that can sometimes cause a low milk supply is **polycystic ovary syndrome (PCOS).** Occurring in up to 8 percent of women, PCOS is a complex syndrome of ovarian and other metabolic and hormonal abnormalities that develop during adolescence. Women with PCOS can have an array of problems, including ovarian cysts, menstrual irregularities, infertility, obesity and large waist size, excessive hair growth in a male distribution pattern, acne, insulin resistance and adult-onset diabetes, and depression. Not all mothers with PCOS have low milk production; some actually have overabundant milk. But it's a good idea for all mothers with PCOS to ensure good milk production by working with a lactation professional and pumping after feedings. Some women with PCOS have succeeded in increasing their production by taking the medication metformin, which reduces insulin and testosterone levels, and some have reported improvement using herbs like fenugreek and goat's rue, both of which are components of More Milk Special Blend capsules and extract (see page 72).

Nursing after Breast Surgery

When performed prior to a woman's giving birth, minor breast surgery such as a biopsy or removal of a lump seldom affects the woman's ability to nurse unless the incision was made on the nipple or areola. A woman who has undergone a mastectomy can nurse on the remaining breast, and by nursing frequently she may be able to provide most or all of the milk that her baby needs. A breast that has been subject to radiation therapy produces little or no milk, but, again, the other breast should produce milk normally.

When a surgical implantation has been performed to alter the size and shape of the breasts, milk production is usually not affected unless the milk ducts have been severed (this may be the case if the incision was made along the edge of the areola). In the case of a breast reduction, milk production depends on the extensiveness of the surgery. When the nipples have been relocated on the breasts, some or all of the ducts have usually been severed, and so the milk supply is often threatened.

When a mother's milk ducts may have been severed, her baby should be observed closely for signs of low milk intake. I recommend a weight check by three to four days of age and every couple of days thereafter. A weight loss of 10 percent or more, or failure to gain an ounce a day after five days of age, indicates that a baby needs supplemental feedings.

If you have had breast surgery involving an incision around the areola, you may benefit from securing a breast pump and using it starting on the third day after birth. Pump for 5 minutes or so on each breast right after each daytime and evening nursing; if possible, pump both breasts at once. This can help bring in a more plentiful milk supply. For further guidance, see Chapter 5, page 227, as well as "Underfeeding and Weight Loss," page 107.

I have worked with many women who have brought in a full supply of milk after breast reduction surgery. For many of these women, using a breast pump after each nursing helped a great deal in building an initially low supply. Herbal preparations such as fenugreek and blessed thistle capsules and More Milk Special Blend tincture have also helped boost production (see page 72). Some of the mothers have found that using a nursing supplementation device (see Appendix A, page 362) helped to increase production as well. In all cases, however, two to eight weeks' effort was required before milk production entirely met the baby's milk needs.

When the milk supply is clearly insufficient and shows no signs of increasing, a mother can still continue breastfeeding indefinitely, if she wishes. A nursing supplementation device may help keep the baby from preferring the bottle.

Nursing after Gastric Bypass Surgery

Mothers who have undergone gastric bypass surgery to lose weight need nutritional guidance for both pregnancy and breastfeeding. This surgery reduces the body's intake of calories both by making the stomach smaller and by bypassing part of the small intestine, where nutrients are absorbed. Iron, folate, zinc, vitamin B_{12}, and calcium are the nutrients most often lost. Everyone who has undergone bypass surgery needs daily vitamin and mineral supplements, and pregnancy and breastfeeding increase nutritional demands even more. Particularly important are iron and vitamin B_{12}; a deficiency of either of these nutrients can lead to anemia in the mother during pregnancy and lactation, and even in the infant (signs of B_{12} deficiency in breastfed infants include diarrhea, vomiting, constipation, and poor weight gain). Ordinary prenatal vitamins may not be adequately absorbed after gastric bypass surgery, and the mother's impaired ability to absorb fat can make her milk too low in fat and calories. For these reasons, a doctor must carefully monitor both mother and baby from the start of pregnancy through weaning.

Mothers who have undergone a gastric lap-band procedure do not need to worry about lost nutrients, as this procedure does not affect the small intestine.

Nursing an Adopted Baby

More and more mothers who are planning to adopt babies are considering breastfeeding them. An infant's suck can stimulate milk production whether or not the mother has ever had or nursed a baby before, and even if she has reached menopause. Most adoptive mothers, however, need to supplement their breast milk, many for the entire time they are nursing. Probably the safest and most convenient way to supplement breastfeeding is with a nursing supplementation device specifically designed for this situation (see Appendix A, page 362).

Some women's enthusiastic claims of producing abundant milk for their adopted babies may set up other adoptive mothers for disappointment. It is impossible to predict whether an adoptive mother will be able to produce milk, or how much she will produce, even if she is currently nursing or has recently nursed another baby. Adoptive nursing will be most successful if you focus on the relationship between you and your baby, rather than on your milk production. Measure your success by whether the experience truly helps make the baby yours.

Before the baby arrives, it is wise to learn as much as possible about breastfeeding and adoptive nursing. Be sure that the pediatrician you're choosing for your baby will be supportive of your efforts. A lactation professional may be able to refer you to other adoptive mothers who have nursed their babies.

Nursing an adopted baby doesn't require any advance preparation; you can simply put the baby to the breast and see what happens. In this case, though, you may or may not eventually produce significant amounts of breast milk. But if you know at least several weeks in advance that your baby is coming, you may be able to increase your chance of producing ample milk by following one of the treatment plans developed by Jack Newman, a physician, and Lenore Goldfarb, a lactation professional. These protocols are described on pages 123 to 127.

When your baby arrives, he may be easily persuaded to begin nursing, or he may require a great deal of patience and persistence. In general, the younger the baby is, the easier the transition from the bottle to the breast will be. See page 95 for assistance in getting the baby to nurse.

Most adoptive mothers need to supplement their milk with formula. Some women try to increase their milk production by using formula in only minimal amounts or by overdiluting it. But these practices often result in stress and underfeeding for the baby.

If you've decided to use a supplementation device, you may be hoping for donations of breast milk to use in it, and perhaps you've already received offers of donated milk. But don't expect others to continue donating indefinitely. It can be a real effort for a nursing mother to collect extra milk. There is also the remote possibility that infectious diseases, including HIV and hepatitis, could be transmitted through donated milk.

Women who have breastfed adopted children often say that it has been one of the most memorable and rewarding experiences of their lives. You may especially enjoy nursing your adopted baby when she is older and you needn't concern yourself so much about milk production.

Moments spent soothing a tired, hurt, or frustrated baby or toddler at the breast are priceless for any nursing mother.

The Newman-Goldfarb Protocols

These regimens have helped over 4,000 adoptive mothers, relactating mothers, and "intended" mothers (those who have used surrogates to carry a baby to term) to bring in substantial milk supplies. Each protocol involves pumping, preferably with a clinical-grade rental pump and a double collection kit (see Chapter 5), and taking both an oral contraceptive, to hormonally mimic pregnancy, and a galactogogue, a medication that stimulates milk production. There are three protocols: a regular one, an accelerated one, and a third just for postmenopausal women. As a rule, the longer you follow your protocol, the more milk you will produce.

The protocols described here are designed to mimic what happens before and after pregnancy. During pregnancy a woman's body produces increasing amounts of progesterone, estrogen, and lactogen, via the placenta, and prolactin, via the pituitary gland. These hormones ready the breasts for breastfeeding. Once pregnancy is completed, progesterone and estrogen levels drop and prolactin levels increase, resulting in lactation.

Oral contraceptives can provide the estrogen and progesterone needed to simulate pregnancy (they do not supply prolactin or lactogen). To induce lactation, you will need to take monophasic oral contraceptives—that is, all active ones, with no sugar pills—every day, without breaks. Each pill should contain at least 0.035 milligram ethinyl estradiol (estrogen) and at least 1 milligram norethindrone or an equivalent progestin. Acceptable oral contraceptives include Ortho-Novum 1/35, Necon 1/35, Demulen 1/35, Norethin 1/35E, Norinyl 1+35, Zovia 1/35E, and Microgestin.

Women who have a history of thrombosis, cardiac condition, or severe hypertension shouldn't take oral contraceptives, and other women can't tolerate their side effects. Some women have tried estrogen patches, estrogen lotion, or progesterone cream instead. If you have mild hypertension, you may be able to reduce it enough by taking methyldopa (Aldomet) to make oral contraceptives safe for you. Methyldopa has the added benefit of increasing milk supply, and it is approved by the American Academy of Pediatrics for use in breast-feeding mothers.

Since oral contraceptives sometimes cause depression, women with a history of depression are generally advised not to take them. But several such women have followed the protocols while taking the antidepressant sertraline (Zoloft), which studies show to be safe during breastfeeding.

The galactogogue that should be taken along with the oral contraceptive is domperidone (see page 112 and Appendix A, page 363). For best absorption, take domperidone a half hour before meals. Adoptive nursing mothers may need to take domperidone for the entire time they are nursing.

Consult your doctor before beginning to follow one of the protocols. If your doctor is not familiar with the process of inducing lactation, find an experienced lactation professional who is. See Appendix A, page 358, for help in locating one or, if you will be present at the baby's birth, ask if one is available at the hospital or birthing center. If you use a lactation professional, be sure your physician knows that you plan to breastfeed and receives a copy of the protocol.

The regular protocol. This plan is suitable for a mother expecting a baby via surrogacy or for an adoptive mother with a long lead time. Women who follow this protocol are generally able to meet most, if not all, of their babies' needs for milk until the babies are weaned.

1. At least six months before the baby is due, take an active oral contraceptive (that is, one containing hormones and not the "filler" pills provided with each monthly pack) daily and 10 milligrams domperidone four times per day for one week.

2. After a week, increase the domperidone dosage to 20 milligrams four times per day, and continue taking the oral contraceptive. Your breasts will swell, although the oral contraceptives will actually suppress milk production, as happens during pregnancy. Don't pump or take any milk-augmenting herbs.

3. Six weeks before the baby is due, stop taking the oral contraceptive, but continue taking 20 milligrams domperidone four times a day. You should experience vaginal bleeding; if you don't, you may need an exam to find out if you're pregnant.

4. Begin pumping your breasts, every three hours if possible during the day, and at least once at night. Pump 5 to 7 minutes on the low or medium setting, and then massage, stroke, and rapidly shake both breasts.

   Stopping the oral contraceptive while continuing to take domperidone and beginning to pump your breasts should cause a rapid decrease in the level of progesterone in your blood and a rapid increase in the level of prolactin. By mimicking what happens after pregnancy and birth, this process should cause your milk to come in.

   Once you have started pumping, you can take some other measures to augment your milk supply. Three times a day, with meals, take three capsules each of blessed thistle (390 milligrams per capsule) and fenugreek (610 milligrams per capsule). For more information on these herbal preparations, see page 72. Try also to eat oatmeal at least three times a week, since women following the protocols have noticed significant increases in their milk supplies when they eat oatmeal regularly. You should also avoid caffeine and drink water whenever you are thirsty.

   Your milk may come in over just a few days, or it may take a week or two; everyone responds differently. The milk will first appear as clear drops, which will gradually become an opaque white. Then the milk will begin to spray while you pump, and finally to flow in a steady stream. Save the milk for your baby (see "Collecting and Storing Your Breast Milk," page 250).

5. When the baby arrives, nurse as soon as possible. Nurse the baby often, whenever he seems hungry or at least eight times in 24 hours. Supplement your milk as necessary with formula or donated milk, fed by bottle or through a nursing supplementation device (see "Underfeeding and Weight Loss," page 107). Until

you have an ample milk supply, it's a good idea to pump for 10 minutes after each feeding.

Continue taking domperidone—20 milligrams four times per day—and fenugreek and blessed thistle until your milk supply is well established. Once you have an ample milk supply, you may be able to decrease the domperidone and even eliminate it completely. To avoid dramatic drops in your milk supply, however, you should decrease the dose very slowly, by one pill per day.

The accelerated protocol. Jack Newman and Lenore Goldfarb recommend this plan for mothers expecting babies through surrogacy and adoptive mothers who have less than six months to prepare.

1. Take an active oral contraceptive (that is, one containing hormones and not the "fillers" provided with each monthly pack) daily for 30 to 60 days nonstop, along with 20 milligrams of domperidone four times a day. For this protocol, it is highly recommended to take Microgestin or Ortho-Novum 1/35. Expect that the rapid start of medications will cause fatigue.

2. If breast changes occur within 30 days, stop taking the oral contraceptive but continue taking domperidone. Otherwise, continue taking both medications until your breasts swell. Then begin pumping as in the regular protocol, with a fully automatic pump and a double-pump kit, and taking the herbs and oatmeal as described for the regular protocol. Store as much breast milk as you can (see "Collecting and Storing Your Breast Milk," page 250).

3. When you begin nursing, continue taking domperidone. Nurse the baby often, whenever he seems hungry or at least eight times in 24 hours. Until you have an ample milk supply, it's a good idea to pump for 10 minutes after each feeding. Supplement your milk as necessary with formula or donated milk, fed by bottle or through a nursing supplementation device (see "Underfeeding and Weight Loss," page 107).

The menopausal protocol. If you've reached menopause naturally or had your reproductive organs surgically removed, you may still be able to bring in a milk supply and breastfeed. All you need are breasts and a functioning pituitary gland. This protocol can be started just as soon as you know a baby is on the way to you. However, if you are over the age of 35, note that there are health risks associated with the use of estrogen-progesterone oral contraceptives that you need to discuss with your doctor. If you are unable to use Microgestin or Ortho Novum 1/35 as described below, replace it with either Provera (2.5 milligrams) or Prometrium (100 milligrams), and take that along with the domperidone.

1. If you're undergoing hormone-replacement therapy, stop. Instead, take either Microgestin or Ortho Novum 1/35 once a day. The Microgestin or Ortho Novum 1/35 contains enough estrogen and progesterone to keep your menopausal symptoms at bay while also readying your breasts for milk production. You also need to take domperidone—10 milligrams four times a day for the first week and then 20 milligrams four times a day thereafter.

2. Stay on the combination of Microgestin or Ortho Novum 1/35 and domperidone for at least 60 days, until your breasts swell by one cup size and begin to feel full, heavy, and tender. At this point, begin pumping your breasts, following the guidelines for the regular protocol above. Take the dietary measures described for the regular protocol, too.

3. If your menopausal symptoms resume, you can reduce them by consuming soy products, especially soy milk and soy butter, which contain phytoestrogens. Consume only as much soy as you need to stop your hot flashes; too much would decrease your milk supply.

Deciding Whether to Use a Protocol

The decision whether or not to follow a Newman-Goldfarb protocol may depend on how much time you have. The regular protocol might increase your milk supply more than other measures would, but only if you can follow the regimen for six months or more. This may be easy if you're using a surrogate mother, in which case you'll know about the pregnancy from the beginning. If you're adopting internationally, also, you may learn about your baby several months before you bring the baby home. But sometimes a baby's homecoming is postponed, for as long as two months or more. A baby four months old or older who has been regularly bottle-fed is likely to refuse the breast. Unless you're willing to go to great lengths to persuade him to nurse, you may not want to take on the protocol.

Many adoptive parents don't know until weeks or just days in advance that they can bring their baby home. Sadly, the earlier in the pregnancy that an adoptive family is told they have been matched with a baby, the more likely it is that the birth mother will change her plans. Many women start the protocol in anticipation of adopting and then end up with no baby to nurse, or they continue pumping month after month with no news of the baby. Even those who are able to pump an impressive amount of milk find they cannot bear to keep up the pumping indefinitely.

For every mother who follows the regular protocol, brings in a good milk supply, and then acquires a baby to nurse within a reasonable amount of time, several others run into problems. Side effects can be difficult. Some women following the protocols experience weight gain, depression and tearfulness, exhaustion, swollen legs, and extremely sore and swollen breasts. Some fail to get a full milk supply even after four months or longer on the protocol. After such an investment of time and energy, this is a great disappointment.

The accelerated protocol often works well for women who have two to six months to prepare, but some lactation consultants feel that mothers who have less than 60 days to prepare will get a milk supply established faster by pumping and taking domperidone without birth control pills, which suppress milk production as long as they are taken and for several weeks afterward. In fact, some adoptive mothers bring in a full milk supply without domperidone, using only breast stimulation and herbs that promote milk production. An herbal preparation that is especially effective for adopting mothers is the More Milk Special Blend tincture (see page 72).

A potential risk for women who use the protocols is coming to view a nursing supplementer as evidence of failure, rather than as the important tool it is for both nurturing a baby and stimulating milk production. When a mother with a low milk supply nurses as much as possible, using a supplementer as needed, her supply often increases. More important, she establishes a long-term nursing relationship with her baby, which is beneficial in so many ways.

Relactation

For a variety of reasons, a mother may want to begin nursing after initially starting her baby on the bottle, or to resume nursing after weaning her baby.

In general, the less time that has elapsed since weaning, the easier bringing back a full milk supply will be. A mother with a five-day-old baby who has never nursed, or with a six-week-old who has been weaned for just a few days, should be able to bring in a full milk supply within several days. After longer periods without nursing or expressing milk, the ability to re-establish full milk production will vary from woman to woman.

Always critical to milk production is frequent and regular stimulation and emptying of the breasts. This means that either a vigorously nursing baby or a clinical-grade rental breast pump should drain both breasts at least every two and a half hours during the day and evening and twice at night. Even when a baby is willing to nurse, using a rental pump with a double-pump kit for 5 to 10 minutes right after nursing can be very helpful in stimulating further milk production. See Chapter 5 for guidance on expressing your milk.

Herbal preparations such as fenugreek and blessed thistle capsules and More Milk Plus capsules or tincture can be very helpful in rebuilding a milk supply. See page 72 for more information.

If you find that herbs do little to increase your milk production, consider using domperidone to stimulate more milk production (see page 112 and Appendix A, page 363).

Regardless of the time that has elapsed between weaning and attempting relactation, a baby will need supplemental feedings until full milk production has been established. You can continue bottle-feeding, but offer the bottle only after nursing and give slightly less formula than before. Or you can use a nursing supplementation device (see Appendix A, page 362), which allows you to feed your baby supplemental milk or formula while he sucks at the breast. This option may be most helpful if your baby acts frustrated while nursing.

Knowing how much supplemental milk and formula to give a baby can be a bit of a guessing game. If you are renting a clinical-grade pump, you can use the method described in "Underfeeding and Weight Loss," page 107, to estimate your milk production and your baby's supplemental milk needs. Without this type of pump, you will need to rely solely on weight checks.

Whether or not you're using a rental pump, have your baby weighed every day or two during the first week or so after you start trying to relactate. Until your baby is three months old, he should gain an ounce a day. Gaining less than this amount indicates that he needs more supplemental breast milk or formula; gaining more may mean that the supplement should be cut back a little. Always weigh your baby naked, on the same scale, at about the same time of day, and just before a feeding.

Very accurate electronic baby scales for home use are available for rent. Such a scale can also be used before and after feedings to determine how much milk the baby takes from the breast. See Appendix A, page 365, for information on renting a scale.

The Mother with Diabetes

Many diabetic mothers enjoy the advantages of nursing. For them, breastfeeding often stimulates a remission-like response, resulting in a decreased need for insulin and an increased need for calories. Babies of diabetic mothers are less likely to develop the disease themselves later in life if they are breastfed rather than formula-fed.

If you are diabetic, your requirements for insulin and calories will need to be closely monitored—especially during the early hours after delivery, when your insulin needs will drop dramatically.

For the first day or two, your newborn's blood sugar must be closely watched as her body adjusts to receiving less glucose than it did during pregnancy. She may need frequent nursing, and possibly supplemental glucose by nipple or IV, until her glucose levels stabilize. Because the infant of the diabetic mother is commonly delivered a few weeks early, she may also have respiratory problems, and she is more prone to becoming jaundiced. If your baby is born three or more weeks early, refer to "The Near-Term Baby," page 136.

Throughout the months of breastfeeding, careful monitoring of your glucose level, insulin dose, and caloric requirements must continue. As the baby stimulates increased milk production, you and your doctor will need to adjust your insulin dosage and caloric intake to prevent insulin reactions.

You should take particular care to avoid sore nipples and breast infections. This means giving careful attention to correct positioning of the baby, watching for signs of thrush (yeast) in the baby's mouth and on the nipples (see page 182), and getting plenty of rest. Yeast infections are very common in the diabetic mother and her infant. Plugged ducts and other early signs of breast infection should be treated promptly (see page 187).

When weaning begins and milk production declines, you'll need to readjust your insulin dosage and diet again. This will be easier if you wean the baby slowly.

The Mother with Herpes

If you have an active genital herpes lesion or a positive culture near your due date, you will probably deliver by cesarean section. So long as the lesion is well covered and you wash your hands thoroughly before feedings, you can nurse the baby safely without gloves. There is no reason that you cannot share a room with the baby as long as you maintain these basic precautions. Should you have a herpes outbreak at home, the same principles apply.

Herpes type I lesions are generally those that develop above the waist, usually on the mouth. Frequently they appear as cold sores or fever blisters. If you develop such a lesion, it is important to wash your hands thoroughly before touching the baby and to avoid placing her in contact with the sore. Anyone else with a herpes lesion should do the same.

Occasionally a mother will develop a herpes lesion on her breast, nipple, or areola. In such a case, express your milk (see Chapter 5) until the lesion is gone.

The Mother with Epilepsy

Most medications to control the occurrence of epileptic seizures are considered safe for nursing; however, it is best to check out any drug with your doctor. Major anticonvulsant medications are listed in Appendix D, where their safety is discussed (see page 379).

Dorothy Brewster (1979), a nursing mother with epilepsy, offers these suggestions for others:

- Have cribs or playpens available in various areas of the house; place gates across stairways and doorways.
- Nurse in a large upholstered chair, or pad the arms of a rocking chair.
- Use guardrails and pillows around the bed for night nursing.
- When alone on outings with the baby, tag the stroller or carrier with the name of the baby and the name of a person to contact in the event that you have a seizure.

Nursing and Thyroid Conditions

Hypothyroidism

Symptoms of an underactive thyroid gland may include extreme fatigue, poor appetite, and sometimes a low milk supply. Thyroid replacement quickly reverses these symptoms. The mother who is taking medication for hypothyroidism can breastfeed, as these drugs do not affect the baby.

Hyperthyroidism

Occasionally a doctor will discover that a nursing mother has an enlarged thyroid gland. Signs of hyperthyroidism include weight loss, increased appetite, nervousness, rapid heart rate, and palpitations. Nursing must be discontinued for at least 48 hours when radioactive iodine is used for diagnostic testing; however, other tests are available that do not require this interruption. If radioactive iodine is used, express or pump your milk (see Chapter 5) and dispose of it.

If you are taking medication for an overactive thyroid gland, you can breastfeed as long as the specific medication is considered safe for the nursing baby. PTU (propylthiouracil) is the drug of choice, since it has the least effect on a baby's thyroid gland. The baby's thyroid level should be monitored by a pediatrician.

Emotional Barriers to Breastfeeding

It has been estimated that an astounding 25 to 40 percent of women of childbearing age were sexually abused during childhood. Many of these women have emotional difficulty with the experiences of childbirth and breastfeeding, which can revive old feelings of shame, guilt, or both. Such feelings keep some women from even trying to nurse; they feel certain even before the baby is born that they will not be able to handle breastfeeding. Others discover uncomfortable feelings only once they begin nursing their newborns. Sometimes memories of abuse surface for the first time with the initiation of breastfeeding. Thankfully, some women who were sexually abused find childbirth and breastfeeding an empowering and healing experience. This is most likely for women who have undergone therapy to resolve their feelings about themselves and their bodies.

How a mother who has been sexually abused responds to the idea of breastfeeding depends on whether her breasts played a part in the abuse and how far along she is in her recovery. If you were sexually abused and are now beginning to breastfeed, the feeling of suckling may disturb you. You may feel as though you do not want to share your body, and you may dread feedings. You may feel helpless or out of control if your baby's frequent requests to be fed remind you of your abuser's inescapable demands. You may be tempted to postpone feedings or limit the baby's time at the breast, even if you know that either of these tactics could lessen your milk production and endanger your baby. You must find ways to meet your baby's needs while protecting yourself from being reminded of your abuse.

Should you find yourself having very mixed feelings about breastfeeding, during pregnancy or just after the birth, you might consider giving nursing a short trial. Even a few days of nursing is a boon to a baby's health.

If the feeling of your baby's sucking disturbs you, you might try using a nipple shield (see page 85) to lessen the sensations. Selecting the right size is important to ensure comfort for you and sufficient milk for your baby, so have a lactation professional assist you.

If your baby does too much "comfort sucking" for your comfort, you can safely use a pacifier after your milk supply is well established and your baby is gaining weight well. Offer the pacifier after a good feeding, not when the baby seems hungry.

Night wakings may be particularly disturbing for women who were wakened during childhood with sexual demands. In this case, it may be preferable to put the baby to sleep in a cradle or crib rather than in your own bed, and to have your partner bring you the baby when he cries or even set an alarm and go to the baby before he is likely to begin crying.

While many mothers feel uncomfortable nursing in front of others, you may have a heightened sense of modesty if you were sexually abused. You may feel more comfortable if you wear a specially made nursing top to expose less skin, cover up with a shawl or a light blanket (or a "nursing cover" specially made for this purpose), or bottle-feed breast milk when other people are around.

If your feelings about past sexual abuse continue to make breastfeeding difficult, consulting a psychotherapist may help. Or you might try www.solaceformothers.org, an online support group monitored by a psychotherapist, that helps mothers who are dealing with trauma, including past sexual abuse.

New mothers who have experienced sexual abuse are more likely than other women to suffer postpartum anxiety or depression (see page 196). If this happens to you, your regular physician or a psychiatrist can prescribe medications that are safe to use while breastfeeding.

If your feelings about past sexual abuse continue to make breastfeeding difficult despite expert help, a good solution may be to pump your milk and feed it to the baby by bottle (see Chapter 5). Some women gladly do this for many months, even though it is more time-consuming than breastfeeding.

If you find even pumping stressful, feeding formula may be best for you and the baby. If people ask why you are not breastfeeding, you can use an excuse like "My baby hasn't been able to latch on."

No matter how you choose to feed your baby, a postpartum support group may be helpful to you. You may want to speak with the leader privately, however, to be sure you will not be ostracized for whatever choices you have made.

SPECIAL BABIES
Medical Reasons for Not Breastfeeding

Infants born with **galactosemia,** a rare inherited disorder, lack the enzyme necessary to break down the sugar found in all milk, including milk-based formulas, other dairy products, and breast milk. These babies must be fed a special lactose-free formula. Newborn screening tests done at discharge from the hospital or birth center detect most cases of galactosemia.

Infants with **phenylketonuria (PKU),** another rare metabolic disorder, require a diet with little phenylalanine, an amino acid. Because breast milk is low in phenylalanine, a baby with PKU may be breastfed part-time provided she is also fed phenylalanine-free formula. Her blood level of phenylalanine must be monitored to be sure that it remains between 5 and 10 milligrams per deciliter. A pediatric dietitian can help set up a regimen that includes limited breastfeeding.

The Near-Term Baby

Barring any health complications, babies who are born three to five weeks before the due date are usually treated like any other newborns by physicians and nurses, and parents are encouraged to do the same.

Like full-term infants, near-term infants tend to breathe more regularly, maintain a higher blood-sugar level, and cry much less if allowed to rest unswaddled against the mother's bare chest immediately after birth. If your baby is healthy at birth, you will probably be permitted to hold him skin-to-skin right after he is dried. Your baby may crawl to your breast and latch on to it unaided within the first hour or two of life. Bathing, weighing, and eye treatment can be postponed for an hour or so or until you and your baby are able to complete the first feeding.

It is important to understand, however, that a baby born a few weeks early doesn't behave exactly like a baby born at term. You may find that your baby tends to be extra sleepy and to nurse inconsistently. He may be vigorous at some feedings and inefficient at others. He may fall asleep at the breast before he has taken in sufficient milk. Unless you wake him every two and a half to three hours, he may sleep too long between feedings. He may fail to gain weight; he may even lose weight.

A few days of sluggish nursing and limited milk removal could have a devastating effect on your milk production. To ensure a plentiful supply for a near-term baby, I strongly recommend using a clinical-grade rental pump with a double collection kit. Starting on the third day after birth or earlier, pump each breast for 5 to 10 minutes right after each daytime and evening nursing (freeze the milk you collect for later use). This will help you build an abundant milk supply, which in turn will help the baby get sufficient milk even when he is sleepy at a feeding. See Chapter 5 for more information on pumping milk.

When your baby stops sucking during a feeding, compress your breast (see page 53) to increase the flow. This will also help the baby drink more milk.

Watch your baby closely for the signs of adequate milk intake—vigorous sucking and swallowing and frequent stools. Weigh the baby at four to five days of age, and at any time you are concerned about his milk intake, to be sure that he has not lost an excessive amount of weight. Refer to Appendix B, page 370.

If the baby is gaining about an ounce a day or has regained his birth weight at 10 to 12 days, without any supplemental feedings, you can gradually stop pumping over a few days. Weigh the baby once again before returning the pump to the rental station, to be sure he has continued to gain an ounce a day.

If the baby's weight loss nears 10 percent or if he is not gaining at least an ounce a day, offer him the milk you're pumping plus any necessary formula. To determine how much supplement the baby needs, see Appendix B, page 370.

A baby born three to five weeks early who is sick may be unable to nurse at first. If this is the case with your baby, you can express your milk for him until he is well enough to begin nursing. In this way he will still benefit from your milk, and you will have established your supply by the time he is ready to begin breastfeeding. For more information, see Chapter 5 and the section that follows.

The Very Premature or Sick Baby

When a baby is born sick or very immature—that is, more than five weeks early—the first days after the birth can be overwhelming. In such a case you may have doubts about many things, including your ability to nurse the baby. If your baby is too immature or weak to breastfeed, know that expressing your milk for your baby is very important to his well-being.

Your milk is easier for your baby to digest than formula, and it is particularly suited for a preemie's special growth needs. The fatty acids in human milk promote eye and brain development, which is measurably superior in preterm infants fed mother's milk than in those fed formula. Mother's milk may also reduce a premature baby's risk of developing cerebral palsy (Lucas, 1992).

Premature infants are at greater risk than full-term infants for developing infections, and preemies are less able to cope with infections when they arise. As you already know, breast milk helps protect a baby against infections. Most protective is the earliest milk, colostrum, which as a preterm mother you'll be making longer than a full-term mother. Doctors think of colostrum as a medicine for preterm babies. As a medicine, colostrum has multiple benefits: It contains a high concentration of antibodies; it creates an environment in the intestinal tract that impairs the growth of harmful bacteria; and it has components that directly attack dangerous germs.

The first drops of colostrum contain the highest concentrations of antibodies, the second drops the next highest, and so on. For this reason, you should number each batch you collect and feed the batches in the sequence in which you have collected them. A nurse or lactation professional can show you how and where to store your colostrum.

Kangaroo Care

Just as a kangaroo baby, born very undeveloped, is carried and fed in its mother's pouch, a premature human baby benefits from being held next to his parent's body. More and more intensive-care nurseries are allowing and even encouraging parents to practice "kangaroo care": The preemie, dressed only in a diaper and hat, is placed upright between the mother's or father's breasts, inside the parent's shirt or under a blanket. The baby's head is turned to one side, with his ear above the level of the parent's heart. Premature babies held this way for two hours or more once or twice a day have one-quarter the rate of apnea, or temporary cessation of breathing, of other premature infants. Even a premature baby on a ventilator can be safely moved to the mother without an increase in oxygen. Preemies held kangaroo-style experience no lowering of the heart rate, or bradycardia; in fact, their heart rates are much more stable while they are being held. Their temperatures are stabilized, too, by the warmth of the parent's body. The babies gain weight more rapidly than those kept full-time on a warming bed or in an incubator, perhaps because babies cared for kangaroo-style sleep more deeply, conserving their energy. Faster weight gain means shorter hospital stays; the length of hospitalization for a kangaroo-care baby is reduced by as much as 50 percent. Finally, the skin-to-skin contact not only contributes to parent-baby bonding but also tends to increase the mother's milk production.

Babies who are not yet ready for feedings but are receiving intravenous fluids instead may benefit from having just 0.1 milliliter of colostrum placed in each cheek every three to four hours. This tiny amount will not be swallowed but instead will be absorbed into the baby's lymphatic system to help protect her respiratory and intestinal tracts. If your baby is getting intravenous fluids in place of feedings, be sure to ask if she can have a small amount of colostrum swabbed inside her mouth.

Let the hospital staff know about any medications you take, including any over-the-counter medicines or herbal preparations. Although most medications are safe to take while nursing, a few could harm a sick or premature infant.

If you develop a breast infection (see page 190), you will need to discard any milk you collect, because preterm infants are more susceptible than other babies to bacteria in breast milk.

Refer to Chapter 5 for information on expressing milk in general and for a premature or sick baby in particular, on feeding hindmilk (see below), and on pumping for longer than a few weeks (see page 246).

Supplementing Breast Milk

Although breast milk alone is the perfect food for a full-term infant, a preemie, because of her small size and immaturity, may have somewhat different nutritional needs. Many premature infants need supplemental nutrients, especially calcium, phosphorus, and protein. The nurses may mix commercially prepared fortifiers with your milk to provide for these special needs. Usually, the fortifiers are discontinued about the time the baby should have been born. But a preemie needs supplemental iron and vitamins even after discharge from the hospital.

Many premature babies also need a more concentrated source of calories than breast milk. In this situation, a baby may be fed a special preemie formula along with breast milk. A possible option is to feed

Collecting Hindmilk for a Premature or Sick Baby

Very small premature babies and babies with heart or lung problems may be able to take only small amounts of milk at their feedings. To compensate for smaller feedings, these babies may require higher-calorie milk to grow well. When milk lets down, it starts out as low-calorie *foremilk* and gradually becomes more and more fatty. The milk expressed or fed last contains the most fat. This milk is referred to as *hindmilk*. Feeding hindmilk can be very helpful in achieving good weight gain in a preemie or a baby who has heart or lung problems.

To collect hindmilk separately from foremilk, pump for about 2 minutes after the milk lets down, and then stop pumping and switch collection bottles. Pump again until the breast is completely drained. Label the first bottles as foremilk, the second as hindmilk. Provide the hindmilk for the baby's immediate needs, and freeze the foremilk for the future (for use during separations or for supplementation).

hindmilk—the fattier milk produced after the first few minutes of pumping (see page 140). Feeding hindmilk exclusively will speed the weight gain of premature infants.

When Breastfeeding Begins

The preterm or sick newborn is ready to begin feedings at the breast when his overall condition is stable. It's impossible to know just when a baby will reach this point. If he has poor muscle tone, if he still requires a ventilator, or if he is not yet able to coordinate sucking, swallowing, and breathing, he may not be ready for breastfeeding.

When a baby is ready for oral feeding, breastfeeding is far better for him than bottle-feeding. Studies show that preemies at the breast have better respiratory rates, heart rates, and blood oxygen levels than preemies fed from a bottle. Many doctors tell mothers that breastfeeding is more stressful for preemies than bottle-feeding, but in fact the opposite is true. If there is doubt about the safety of your breastfeeding your preemie, the baby's heart rate and respiration can be observed on the electronic monitor during feedings.

When you begin nursing, try to keep your expectations modest. Preemies' abilities at the breast vary greatly, but most are unable to complete an entire feeding at first.

Have a nurse or lactation consultant help you during the first few sessions. Your goal is to position the baby well for nursing and to encourage her to latch on to the breast. These early practice sessions go best when the baby is awake and alert and the breast is not overly full. Keeping the baby snugly wrapped in a blanket could discourage her interest; it's better to hold her undressed against your skin, with a blanket draped over both of you. The nurse can check the baby's skin temperature after 5 to 10 minutes.

The crossover hold and the football hold (see pages 46 to 49) are the positions of choice for nursing a premature baby as both of these positions support the baby's head. Place your hand around the baby's head with your fingers behind and below her ears. Support her neck and shoulders with the palm of your hand and your wrist. With your thumb at the point where the baby's nose will touch the breast, compress the breast with your fingers. Lightly stroke the baby's upper lip with your nipple to signal her to open her mouth wide. As soon as she does, pull her head and shoulders toward you so that the nipple is on top of her tongue and far back in her mouth.

While you are nursing your baby, you should eventually be able to hear her swallowing. This means she is sucking effectively and getting your milk. If you do not hear swallowing, make sure the baby is actually latched on to the breast. Her suction should be so strong that it is hard to pull her off. You should not see dimples in her cheeks or hear clicking noises as she sucks. These signs would indicate she was sucking on her tongue and not on your breast. Gently squeeze the breast while the baby is latched to increase the amount of milk the baby receives.

Once latched on to the breast and sucking, a preemie may fall asleep after just a few minutes. Again, preemies' abilities at the breast vary greatly, so be patient. As long as you have positioned your baby correctly and are encouraging her to open her mouth, you have been successful.

Getting a preemie to latch on requires extra effort: Use the crossover or football hold.

If the baby sucks well at the first breast and seems ready for more, you can simply transfer her to the other side without turning her, or you can reposition her in the opposite arm using the football hold.

Until she is sucking vigorously at the breast, the baby may need a supplement after nursing. Most hospitals give nursing preemies supplements by bottle; others give them by passing a soft tube through the nose or mouth into the stomach, to avoid "nipple preference." Be sure to pump after feeding sessions and collect your milk so it can be fed to your baby as a supplement. Until your baby is nursing without any supplemental feedings, you will need to continue expressing milk after each nursing to maintain your milk supply.

Difficult latch-on. Many premature infants have difficulty latching on, due to their immaturity as well as having received rubber nipples as pacifiers or for feedings. Some babies have trouble learning to lower their tongue to latch on, whereas others seem unable to identify their mothers' nipples in their mouths.

Premature infants who are having trouble latching on or drawing milk from the breast may do better with a small-sized nipple shield (see page 85). Nipple shields seem to help immature babies recognize that there is something in their mouths, and this recognition stimulates them to begin sucking. You will want the help of a lactation professional in determining exactly which size shield works best for your nipples and the baby's mouth.

If your baby is unable to latch on to the breast even with a nipple shield, refer to "Difficult Latch-on: Refusal to Nurse," page 95. In my experience, a premature infant typically learns to nurse after a period of daily practice approaching the mother's due date.

The Transition To Full-Time Nursing

While you and the baby are establishing nursing, you may wonder how much milk the baby is taking. Although mothers and health professionals often try to gauge the baby's milk intake by how long he nurses, how much swallowing can be heard, or whether the baby will take supplemental milk, none of these methods are accurate. The best way to determine the baby's milk intake is to weigh him before and after nursing, in the same diaper and clothing, on an electronic gram scale. Each gram of weight gain equals 1 milliliter of milk intake.

How much breast milk a baby should take at each feeding can be calculated by multiplying the baby's weight in kilograms by 22.5 (a pounds-to-kilogram conversion chart is in Appendix B, page 370). This will give you in milliliters the amount of milk the baby needs at each of eight daily feedings. For example, if a baby weighs 2.2 kilograms, he will need 49.5, or approximately 50, milliliters of milk each time he nurses, for a total of eight times per day. If the baby takes 30 milliliters during the nursing session, he will need an additional 20 milliliters after nursing to gain an adequate amount of weight.

While you are in the hospital, have your baby weighed on the nursery's scale before and after nursings. If you do this at each nursing, you should begin to develop a sense of how much milk the baby is taking at any feeding. Once at home, you may need weight checks only every two days or so to help you judge how much supplement the baby needs. If you want to continue pre- and post-feeding weight checks at home, rent a highly accurate electronic scale (see Appendix A, page 365).

Nursing More Than One

Needless to say, caring for two or more babies takes a tremendous amount of time and energy. Breastfeeding multiples is not only more healthful and economical than giving them formula, but in many ways it is more convenient. Mothers of twins often say that nursing is easier and less time-consuming than preparing and feeding bottles, particularly when a woman has mastered the skill of nursing two babies at the same time.

Although many mothers worry about being able to produce enough milk for more than one baby, most women are capable of producing plenty of milk for two and even three babies.

As soon as you become aware of the twins during pregnancy, you should begin some special preparations. You will want to arrange for as much help as possible for the first several weeks after the birth. It's also a good idea to get to know other mothers who have successfully nursed their twins. Many communities have organizations for mothers of twins. You might also contact your local breastfeeding support group; such a group usually provides literature on caring for and nursing twins.

Approximately half of all twins are born prematurely. During pregnancy you can do much to lessen the risk of premature delivery and other complications by maintaining a diet high in calories—at least 2,900 a day—and protein—at least 110 grams a day. Talk with your health-care provider about monitoring yourself for signs of preterm labor. Identifying regular contractions, even if they are mild, is important to prevent premature birth.

Establishing an Abundant Milk Supply

Making enough milk for two or more babies depends on the frequent and complete drainage of the breasts. Multiples who are born early or of low birth weight may not consistently nurse effectively enough to stimulate abundant milk production. For this reason I recommend using a clinical-grade rental pump, with a double collection kit, whenever multiples are born three or more weeks before the due date or weigh less than 6 pounds each. See Chapter 5 for guidelines on expressing milk for near-term and very preterm infants. Even if your babies are healthy and latching on to the breast frequently, pump for 5 to 10 minutes after each nursing to ensure complete drainage of the breasts and to stimulate abundant milk production. Read "The Near-Term Baby," page 136, for more information on nursing premature babies and Chapter 5 for guidelines on expressing milk.

If the babies are in a special-care nursery and are unable to nurse, use the clinical-grade pump at least eight times every 24 hours. Read "The Very Premature or Sick Baby," page 138, and see Chapter 5 for information on expressing milk. You should aim to produce 20 to 24 ounces of milk per day for each of your babies.

You can nurse twins simultaneously using the cuddle hold, the football hold, or a combination of the two.

Breastfeeding Two or More

You should nurse each of your babies at least eight times in every 24 hours. This may mean waking smaller babies every three hours during the day and evening for feedings, and every four to five hours in the night, until they are gaining weight well without any supplementation.

Some mothers prefer nursing their babies together as much as possible, whereas others choose to nurse them separately. Nursing two at once certainly saves time, and it may be necessary when both of the babies are hungry. If you want to nurse the babies together, there are three basic positions you can try:

- both babies in the cuddle hold with their legs side by side or crossed over each other,

- one baby in the cuddle hold and the other in the football hold, or
- both babies in the football hold.

During the early weeks, you may need assistance getting the babies on the breast at the same time. You will also probably need a few pillows for positioning. (Special pillows are available for nursing twins. See Appendix A, page 364, for ordering information.) It may be easier to position the baby who nurses less vigorously first and then put the vigorous nurser to the breast. Nursing the twins simultaneously should get easier as they get older and need less head support and assistance latching on.

Nursing the babies separately, each baby on one breast only, may be easier to manage and will allow you more time with each individually. You may decide to feed each baby whenever she seems hungry, or you may prefer to encourage the babies to eat and sleep on approximately the same schedule. To maintain a similar routine for both babies, simply offer the breast to the second baby, waking her if necessary, after nursing the first. Although most twins eventually develop a preference for one breast over the other, it is wise to alternate the babies at each feeding during the early weeks so the breasts will be evenly stimulated; this is particularly important when one baby is more active than the other. Keeping a simple written record may be helpful at first.

Mothers of triplets generally nurse two babies simultaneously and then the third baby from both breasts, or else another caregiver gives the third baby a bottle. Again, alternate the babies from one feeding to the next.

During the early weeks, if the babies are gaining weight adequately, substituting bottle-feedings for nursings is best avoided. You want to be sure your breasts are stimulated by the babies' sucking so that milk production remains adequate. Forgoing the bottle also helps minimize the occurrence of plugged ducts and breast infections.

Caring for Yourself

For the mother who is nursing two or more babies, getting plenty of rest, food, and drink is essential. Most nursing mothers are naturally more hungry and thirsty than usual. If you take on too much and become fatigued, though, you may lose your appetite and too much weight. Nutritionists recommend that a mother nursing twins consume at least 3,000 calories daily. Your diet should include high-protein foods and a quart or more of milk a day, the equivalent in other dairy products, or a calcium supplement. Vitamin C and B-complex supplements or brewer's yeast may also be beneficial.

The Baby with Noisy Breathing (Laryngomalacia)

A baby born with this abnormality has "squeaky" breathing. The larynx, or voice box, is malformed, causing the tissues to flop over and partially block the airway opening. The cause of this condition is thought to be congenital, but relaxation of the upper airway or low muscle tone may also be factors. When the baby breathes in, the larynx is partially obstructed, and you hear a high-pitched, squeaky sound known as stridor. This is the most common cause of noisy breathing in infants.

Typically this noise begins during the first two months of life, often in the very first days. Sometimes the sound is confused with nasal congestion, but no nasal discharge is present, and the sound persists. For most infants, laryngomalacia is not serious. Despite having noisy breathing, they are able to eat and grow. The stridor is often more pronounced when the baby is lying on his back or crying, and sometimes during and after feedings. Some infants with laryngomalacia also have problems with reflux (causing spitting up and vomiting), because they have more stomach acid than other babies. The stridor commonly seems to get worse between four and eight months of age, and most babies outgrow it by 18 to 20 months, when the laryngeal structures develop more.

Babies with mild stridor may do better with short, frequent feedings in a more upright or forward-leaning position—that is, with the mother reclined and the baby lying on top.

A small percentage of babies with laryngomalacia do struggle with breathing, eating, and gaining weight. Symptoms that require prompt attention include not breathing for more than 10 seconds, turning blue around the lips, or the baby's chest pulling down, also known as retracting, without relief after being wakened or repositioned. Some babies may choke while feeding or inhale milk into their lungs. Infants with reflux may be given medications that may worsen the laryngomalacia symptoms. If the symptoms are severe, other tests are often done to evaluate the condition. A few infants may require tube feeding or even surgery.

A website devoted to helping parents whose infants have laryngomalacia can be found at www.copingwithlm.org.

The Baby with a Birth Defect

A baby with a birth defect may need breast milk, and the comfort and security of the breast, even more than other infants. Nursing such a baby is usually possible, but the mother must be supported in her efforts. Although some mothers of babies with birth defects have been discouraged from even attempting breastfeeding, many have gone on to nurse their babies successfully.

Depending on your baby's problem, you may be able to begin nursing right after birth, or you may need to express milk for a while (see Chapter 5). Whatever the circumstances, it may be helpful to seek guidance from a lactation professional.

Heart Defect

Infants with minor heart defects generally have little trouble breastfeeding. The exception is the baby with a severe defect, who may become easily fatigued or stressed during feedings; he will start breathing rapidly, his heart will beat faster, and his overall color may change. His growth may be greatly affected by his heart abnormality. He may also be more prone to infections and therefore in greater need of breast milk than other babies.

A baby who is getting a normal amount of breast milk but is gaining insufficient weight may grow better if he receives extra high-calorie hindmilk. Provided your milk supply is abundant, pump for 2 minutes or so to remove the lower-calorie foremilk, and then nurse the baby. This will provide him with a feeding that is higher in calories.

If your baby becomes stressed during feedings, nurse him more frequently for shorter periods of time. He may also be more comfortable if you hold him upright for nursing, as in the football hold.

Cleft Lip and Palate

The baby born with a cleft lip, palate, or both may have difficulty latching on and sucking effectively, so feeding her may present special challenges. Breastfeeding may be possible, depending on the location and extent of the cleft, but most of these babies, particularly those with cleft palates, are unable to get enough milk from nursing alone. Yet breast milk helps reduce the number and severity of ear and respiratory infections, which are more common in these babies than in others. Many mothers of babies with clefts, therefore, pump their milk and feed it to their babies using whatever method works best for the baby.

The baby born with a cleft lip alone may have little difficulty nursing. Until the lip is repaired, usually when the baby is several weeks old, she may need to be positioned with the cleft sealed, to permit suction. You may be able to create a complete seal just by pulling the baby close against your breast so that your breast occludes the cleft. If you find that your baby has more difficulty nursing on one side than the other, try using the football hold on that side.

Whether a baby with a cleft palate can nurse usually depends on the location and extent of the cleft. When it is in the soft palate only, the baby may or may not be able to nurse without much difficulty. It's best to position her so her head is raised; milk may come out of her nose if you feed her while she is lying flat. Ask the baby's doctor or a lactation professional about devices and techniques to help with feedings. An infant can be fitted with an obturator, a plastic dental appliance that covers the cleft and allows for adequate sucking. Some lactation professionals have reported success with the use of a nursing supplementation device (see Appendix A, page 362) and certain positioning techniques.

If the baby has a cleft palate and is unable to latch or effectively create suction, use a fully automatic electric breast pump every two to three hours around the clock, to stimulate and maintain an abundant milk supply. A clinical-grade rental pump with a double collection kit is most efficient and requires the least amount of pumping time. See Chapter 5 for more information on expressing milk.

Bottle-feeding a baby with a cleft lip or palate can also be challenging. The nursing staff should have special feeders of various types that you can try while you are in the hospital. The SpecialNeeds Feeder (formerly called the Haberman Feeder) has worked well for some of my clients. See Appendix A, page 365, for ordering information.

A cleft palate is generally not repaired until the baby is one to two years old. In the meantime, nursing can be difficult or even impossible. In this case, you will probably need to express milk for some time. Pumping and feeding your milk is far cheaper than feeding formula and may be very helpful in preventing ear infections.

Whether your baby has a cleft lip, a cleft palate, or both, closely monitor her weight to make sure that she is getting enough to eat. If you are exclusively bottle-feeding, see Appendix B, page 370, to determine how much milk she needs at each feeding. If your baby is able to latch on and suck but you're unsure whether she is getting enough milk, weigh her every couple of days, and adjust the amount of supplement as needed to maintain a weight gain of about an ounce a day. Renting an electronic scale for a few weeks may be helpful; you can use the scale before and after nursings to determine how much milk the baby is getting, or simply use it daily to check her weight. See Appendix A, page 365, to locate a scale.

Developmental and Neurological Problems

Babies with Down syndrome, hydrocephalus, spina bifida, cerebral palsy, and other neurological problems benefit greatly from breastfeeding. Because nursing provides frequent physical contact, it may be especially valuable to such a baby's development.

If the baby's sucking ability is affected, teaching him to nurse will require a great deal of patience. You may need guidance from a lactation professional experienced with such problems and also from a physical therapist. In this case, start out using the pump after each nursing to bring in and maintain an abundant milk supply. Once the baby is feeding well and gaining weight at the rate of an ounce per day, you can gradually stop pumping.

If your baby is unable to suck, you may need to feed him with a feeding tube. But some babies may be able to nurse with a nursing supplementation device (see Appendix A, page 362) or to drink your expressed milk from a special bottle like the SpecialNeeds Feeder from Medela (see Appendix A, page 365).

Down Syndrome

Many infants with Down syndrome are able to nurse. Not only does nursing further their development, it also provides them with much-needed protection from illness, as they are at greater risk than most babies for developing infections.

Some babies with Down syndrome have difficulty learning how to latch on and suck effectively. The baby may have weak muscle tone; he may act sleepy and uninterested in the breast. In this case, rouse him frequently for nursing (see "Sleepy Baby," page 88) and pump after nursings until he is gaining weight as expected.

Typically, the baby with Down syndrome grows slowly. If your baby's suck is weak and inefficient, you may need to pump out the milk he leaves in the breast. Regular pumping will allow you to maintain sufficient milk production and provide the baby extra milk, which you can feed as a supplement after each nursing.

Hydrocephalus And Spina Bifida

These birth defects are usually corrected surgically as soon as possible. Until the baby can begin to nurse, the mother must express milk (see Chapter 5). For many such babies, positioning at the breast requires special attention so that they are protected and comfortable.

Cerebral Palsy

Babies with cerebral palsy may also be able to nurse, depending on the severity of their condition. Breastfeeding problems that occur are usually related to either (1) poor muscle tone and a weak suck or (2) excessive muscle tone (rigidity and abnormal posture), tongue thrusting, clenching of the jaw, and difficulty swallowing. Both of these situations usually lead to slow weight gain. Some infants with cerebral palsy are able to breastfeed successfully with a nursing supplementation device (see Appendix A, page 362). A baby with cerebral palsy who struggles with bottle-feeding may do well with a SpecialNeeds Feeder (see Appendix A, page 365).

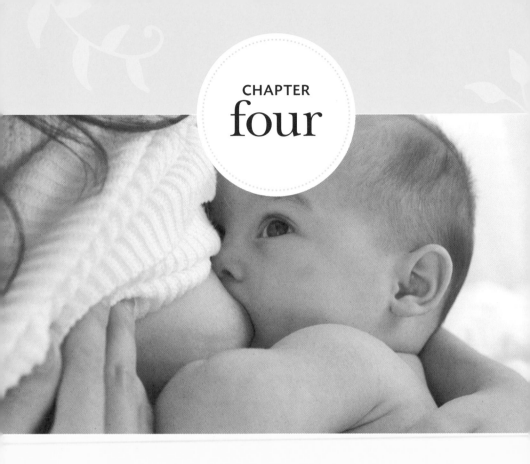

THE LEARNING PERIOD: THE FIRST TWO MONTHS

A FTER THE FIRST WEEK, you may already be feeling energetic and confident in your abilities as a new mother—or you may be exhausted, overwhelmed, and perhaps troubled by some aspect of breastfeeding. In any case, it is important to realize that the first two months after giving birth are a time for adjustment and learning. Mothers normally have questions and concerns about themselves, their babies, and nursing during this period.

NOW THAT YOU ARE POST PARTUM

Caring for Yourself

During the six weeks after birth, all of the many changes of pregnancy are reversed. Virtually every system in your body will go through some readjustment. As your uterus shrinks in size and the inner lining is shed, a new layer is formed. The vaginal flow, or lochia, decreases in amount and progresses to pink or brown and then to white. Many women continue bleeding throughout the first month. Intermittent spotting is common. Too much activity may cause the lochia to become heavier and turn red again—a signal that you should slow down.

If you have had a vaginal birth, your vagina, perineum, urethra, and rectum have undergone considerable stress. Frequent warm baths will speed healing and help relieve discomfort—unless you have hemorrhoids, in which case ice packs may be preferable. Menstrual pads soaked with witch hazel and then frozen are very soothing for hemorrhoids.

Kegel exercises will help this area return to normal by strengthening the entire pelvic floor. These exercises are simple and can be done anytime, anywhere. Several times a day, tightly squeeze the muscles around your anus, then around your vagina and urethra. Gradually work up to 100 "kegels" a day.

If you have had a cesarean birth, keep in mind you are recovering from major abdominal surgery. Most likely, you will need to take pain medication for the first week or so. Using a mild pain reliever such as acetaminophen (Tylenol) or ibuprofen (Motrin, Advil) every few hours may be enough to keep you feeling comfortable. If you are prescribed a narcotic pain reliever, use it only when over-the-counter medications are not enough. Taking a narcotic pain reliever often and for more than one week could make your baby sleepy and could possibly even cause you to have withdrawal symptoms—depression and anxiety, crying, difficulty sleeping, nausea, vomiting, diarrhea, excessive sweating, and dilated pupils—when you stop taking the medication.

You may be bothered by an uncomfortable sensation that your abdominal organs could fall out. A lightweight girdle or a wide band such as the Belly Bandit or the Cinch (available in maternity stores and online) might provide some welcome support.

Constipation is a common complaint in the weeks after giving birth. You can best prevent it by drinking plenty of fluids, eating foods with a lot of fiber, and getting regular exercise. Be aware that some laxatives could affect the baby through your milk, causing cramping, excessive stools, and even weight loss. For advice on safe laxatives, see Appendix D, page 385.

Night sweats are very common in the first few days after birth, and they sometimes continue for several weeks.

Starting at approximately six to twelve weeks after birth, some women experience generalized hair loss (*telogen effluvium*). Because of the hormonal changes following birth, hair follicles simultaneously move from the growing phase (which they were in during pregnancy) to the resting phase of their development. Postpartum hair loss is seldom severe, and women never go bald because of it. The period of hair loss lasts three to six months. It has no relationship to breastfeeding.

Most women experience emotional changes during the postpartum period, and some notice problems with mental function, too. Anxiety, moodiness, and irritability are common responses to the hormonal changes that occur after giving birth, as well as to the tremendous responsibility of caring for a new baby. Forgetfulness, inability to concentrate, and difficulty expressing thoughts are also common complaints. All of these problems normally pass with time, good food, plenty of rest, and social support.

Because of the rapid physical changes of the postpartum period and the tremendous amount of time and energy needed to care for and nurse a baby, rest should take high priority for all new mothers. Fatigue can slow recovery from birth and may lead to tension, inability to cope, poor appetite, and depression. Try to take at least one nap every day during these important first weeks. Do essential household chores and activities while the baby is awake so that you can nap together. Tucking the baby in with you at naptime and bedtime may help you both sleep better. Getting plenty of rest now will contribute greatly to your sense of well-being and your breastfeeding success.

After a couple of weeks, some light exercise can do much to renew your energy. A brisk 20-minute walk with the baby can be invigorating; the fresh air will do you both good. Many community centers offer exercise programs for new mothers. Often the babies are included in the exercises, and sometimes infant care is provided. Some people have claimed that exercise causes lactic acid to build up in breast milk, and that this makes babies refuse to nurse, but in fact moderate exercise has little or no effect on the composition or volume of breast milk. With whatever activity you choose, however, you will want to start out slowly.

You may feel isolated as a new mother, especially if you have left work or school—and most of your friends—to care for the baby. You need adult companionship. Check with your childbirth educator or public-health nurse about groups for new mothers. Attending La Leche League meetings, taking a mother-baby exercise class, or socializing with women from your childbirth class are excellent ways of getting out with the baby and getting to know other new mothers.

New mothers' groups provide opportunities for socializing as well as learning about infant development.

Your Nutritional Needs

Drinking Enough

Maintaining an adequate intake of fluids is usually not a problem for the nursing mother. Most women are naturally more thirsty while they are breastfeeding. Contrary to popular belief, forcing fluids beyond satisfying natural thirst does not increase milk production. But when a nursing mother does not drink six to eight glasses of fluids every day, dark, concentrated urine and constipation usually result. You may need to make a conscious effort to increase your fluid intake.

Eating Well

Provided you established good eating habits during pregnancy and gained an adequate amount of weight, you probably won't need to change your diet much at all. Nursing mothers are often told to add about 500 calories, including 65 grams of protein, to their pre-pregnancy diets. Recent

Don't expect to be able to get into your old jeans for several weeks, at least.

research, however, indicates that many mothers may not need this much food, so don't feel you must eat more than you want. You can get extra nutrients in between-meal snacks, perhaps during nursings: Half a sandwich and a glass of milk or a half cup of nuts will supply about 500 calories. Some mothers experience a temporary loss of appetite during the first couple of weeks after delivery. Eating smaller, more frequent meals or snacks may be more appealing than three big meals each day.

You may feel discouraged that your shape is not back to normal. The clothes in your closet may seem as if they belong to someone else. Although you lost some weight when you delivered, you are probably still pounds away from your usual weight. During the early months of breastfeeding, this extra fat is a useful energy store. If you let your appetite guide you as you continue nursing, you will probably lose the excess weight gradually and feel good while doing it. Dieting during the early weeks is not a good idea.

If you prefer to monitor your caloric intake closely, you can estimate your daily caloric needs by multiplying your current weight by 15. Add 500 to your total to meet the caloric needs of nursing (if you are nursing twins, add 1,000 calories).

Example:

$$
\begin{array}{r}
135 \ \ \text{pounds} \\
\times\ 15 \quad\quad\\
\underline{2{,}025} \ \ \text{calories} \\
\underline{+\ 500} \ \ \text{calories} \\
2{,}525 \ \ \text{calories}
\end{array}
$$

A moderately active woman can expect to lose a pound every two to three weeks on this caloric intake. If you are very active and have no problem controlling your weight, or if you burn calories slowly, you will need to adjust the figures somewhat: Multiply your weight by 17 (high activity) or 13 (low activity). The minimum safe food intake for a nursing mother of average size is about 1,800 calories per day.

Milk production is largely independent of nutritional intake during the first few months of breastfeeding. This is partly because the fat accumulated in pregnancy is available as a ready supply of calories. When a mother's diet is inadequate, however, milk production usually continues at her expense—leading to fatigue, listlessness, and rapid weight loss. Some women have trouble finding time to fix nutritious meals for themselves when they are at home alone with the baby. If you find yourself in this situation, start the day with a good breakfast, and then snack throughout the day on nutritious foods such as hard-boiled eggs, leftover chicken or beef, cheese, peanut butter, yogurt, seeds, and nuts. Don't forget the fiber: Whole-wheat bread, whole-grain crackers, and raw fruits and vegetables will provide it. Some mothers have developed their own favorite recipes for high-energy blender drinks using ingredients such as milk, yogurt, nuts, and bananas or other fruits.

Low-carbohydrate diets are not recommended while nursing. Whole grains and other high-carbohydrate foods supply nursing mothers with vitamins, minerals, and energy. Low-carbohydrate diets are dehydrating, and they often cause constipation, fatigue, and sleeping problems.

Avoid snacking on foods or drinks that are high in sugar. Refined sugar provides only "empty" calories—empty, that is, of vitamins and minerals. Soda, cookies, and candy will not provide sustaining energy and may diminish your desire for more nutritious foods.

Mothers who are vegetarians can certainly maintain a diet to support their nutritional needs. But since vitamin B_{12} is found only in foods that come from animals, deficiencies may occur with a vegan diet, which excludes eggs and milk products as well as meat. For vegans, supplementation with up to 4 milligrams of vitamin B_{12} per day is recommended.

Although most nutritionists recommend that a nursing mother drink three 8-ounce glasses of milk a day, there is no need to drink milk if you don't like it or can't tolerate it. A woman's bone density tends to decrease somewhat during lactation even when her calcium intake is relatively high. This causes no long-term harm. The bones grow denser again after weaning, and some studies suggest that women who breastfeed actually reduce their risk of developing osteoporosis later in life.

SERVING	MILLIGRAMS CALCIUM
yogurt (8 oz.)	288
cheese (1 oz. cheddar or Swiss)	222
cottage cheese (½ cup)	110
tofu (½ cup)	68
corn tortillas (2)	84

Still, nutritionists recommend that breastfeeding women consume 1,000 milligrams of calcium per day. If you don't drink milk, make sure you're getting enough calcium from other sources, such as those listed in the table above.

Although dark green vegetables in general are rich in calcium (100 milligrams per half cup), the calcium they provide is poorly absorbed by the body. Broccoli is the one exception to this rule. If you do not use dairy products at all, calcium supplements may be necessary. The least expensive supplement, with the highest concentration of calcium, is calcium carbonate. Avoid bone meal, dolomite, and oyster shell, as some types have been found to be contaminated with lead.

Dietary Supplements

If you are well nourished, vitamin supplements are unnecessary while you are nursing, although you may need iron supplements if you are anemic after birth. Also, some nursing mothers develop vitamin B deficiencies, experiencing depression, irritability, impaired concentration, loss of appetite, and tingling or burning feet. A daily B-complex supplement is often prescribed to reverse these symptoms.

Sometimes nursing mothers are advised to take brewer's yeast, a natural source of B vitamins, iron, and protein. Some mothers feel it improves their milk supply or increases their overall energy level. Health-food stores carry brewer's yeast in a powdered form that can be mixed with juice or milk.

If you decide to take vitamin supplements or brewer's yeast, remember that they are no substitute for a varied diet of nutritious foods, and in large quantities they can sometimes be dangerous. There have been reports of fussiness in babies whose mothers take brewer's yeast or large doses of vitamin C. Vitamin B_6 supplements in large doses have been reported to reduce milk production.

Foods and Other Substances You May Be Wondering About

There are no foods that should be routinely avoided by nursing mothers, but occasionally a baby will be bothered by something the mother has eaten. Some babies fuss for up to 24 hours after their mothers have eaten garlic, onions, cabbage, broccoli, Brussels sprouts, cauliflower, or chiles. Citrus fruits and their juices, chocolate, and spices such as chili powder, curry powder, and cinnamon can also bother young nursing babies. If your baby has unusual symptoms such as sudden or persistent refusal to nurse, vomiting, diarrhea or green stools, gassiness, redness around the anus, fussiness at the breast, or colic symptoms, see "Concerns about the Baby," page 201.

Caffeine in the mother's diet has been known to cause irritability and colic symptoms in some babies. Caffeine is present in coffee, tea, and many soft drinks. You may want to limit your intake of these beverages.

An occasional glass of wine or beer is not believed to harm a nursing infant. Because alcohol passes through the breast milk, however, moderation is essential.

Mothers who smoke have lower levels of vitamin C in their milk than nonsmokers. Also, secondhand smoke increases a baby's risk of contracting bronchitis, pneumonia, and ear infections and succumbing to sudden infant death syndrome (SIDS). If you smoke, try to limit the amount, and don't do it in your home or anywhere around the baby. Don't let others smoke around the baby, either.

NURSING YOUR BABY

Your Nursing Style

During the early weeks, each mother develops her own style of nursing. Many women feel comfortable putting their babies to breast whenever the baby signals the desire to nurse. Others expect their babies to fall into a predictable feeding schedule. They may be troubled when their babies nurse irregularly or want to nurse again soon after being fed. These mothers may worry that perhaps they have too little milk or that it is somehow inadequate. Sometimes they feel they must hold the baby off until a certain number of hours have passed since the last feeding. But the breasts do not need to rest for any period of time to build up a supply for the next feeding; they produce milk constantly. The expectation that a baby should nurse on some type of a schedule usually leads to frustration for both mother and baby—and sometimes to breastfeeding failure.

Because breast milk is digested quickly, the newborn infant nurses often—typically between eight and twelve times in a 24-hour period, or about every one to three hours. Not only must a baby nurse frequently to satisfy her hunger and thirst, she also seeks out the breast to satisfy her needs for sucking, security, and comforting. Human infants want to nurse so often that they have been described as continuous feeders.

It is a common misconception that the breast empties in a certain number of minutes, and that a baby should be taken from the breast after those minutes have elapsed. In fact, most mothers experience the release of milk several times during a feeding. The length of time required to complete a feeding varies from baby to baby. The all-business nurser, who swallows continuously with few pauses, may be done in 10 minutes, whereas the dawdler may take up to 40 minutes. The length of nursing time may vary in the same baby from feeding to feeding. Before long, most mothers can tell when their babies have had enough.

Some babies nurse from only one breast at a feeding some or most of the time. This is fine, so long as the baby seems satisfied and is gaining weight adequately. You may prefer to offer only one breast per feeding, in fact, if you have an abundant milk supply. Your baby is more likely to drain the breast completely this way, and complete drainage helps prevent plugged milk ducts and breast infections. Your baby will also be sure to get the rich hindmilk, which is produced in increasing amounts as a feeding progresses.

I strongly recommend that your baby be weighed at 10 to 14 days of age. Although many infants are not scheduled for a routine well-baby exam until three to four weeks of age, a weight check at two weeks can be very beneficial. If the baby is back to her birth weight or beyond, you can be reassured early on that your nursing relationship is progressing well. On the other hand, if the baby has not yet regained her birth weight, you can usually correct this quite easily. When a poor weight gain is not discovered until three or four weeks, it is more likely to upset everyone and may be harder to correct than it would have been at two weeks.

You may find that nursing is the most enjoyable part of your day—a time to sit back, relax, and simply enjoy being with your baby. But it may be difficult at times for you to break away from what you are doing or sit still long enough for the baby to have a leisurely nursing. It may help to make a special little nursing nook for yourself—or two or three nooks in different parts of the house. You might include a book, some magazines, or a notepad within reach. Having the phone nearby may also be handy. Some mothers routinely grab a snack or something to drink just before sitting down to nurse.

Many babies seem to get hungry whenever food is served. To avoid interruptions at dinnertime, you might offer the baby the breast just before preparing your meal. Some parents have found that taking the baby for a walk just before dinner lulls her to sleep so that they can eat without interruption.

Your Milk Supply

During these early weeks your milk production may seem somewhat erratic. At times your breasts may feel as if they are bursting with milk. At other times you may worry that there is not enough milk, especially if your breasts seem empty and your baby wants to nurse all the time. Many mothers notice this happening around two to three weeks post partum and then again at six weeks, when a baby normally experiences appetite spurts and nurses more often to stimulate increased milk production. You can expect fluctuations in your milk supply as production becomes regulated according to the baby's requests.

By six to eight weeks after birth, many mothers notice that their breasts seem smaller or feel less full. This does not usually mean that less milk is being produced, but only that the breasts are adjusting to the large amount of milk within and to the baby's feeding pattern.

Some mothers misinterpret their babies' increased requests and their own softer breasts, and begin offering supplemental bottles. Usually, this marks the beginning of the end of breastfeeding. The mother begins to assume that she cannot make enough milk for her baby, and she offers more and more formula instead of allowing the baby to increase the mother's own supply of milk. After receiving formula, the baby sleeps longer and nurses less often. He becomes increasingly frustrated at the breast as his mother's milk supply dwindles, and breastfeeding is soon over.

Some mothers try to satisfy their babies' hunger with solid foods. But introducing solids during these early weeks is inappropriate, because a young infant is both physiologically and developmentally unable to manage them. His digestive system and kidneys are not mature enough to handle cereals and other baby foods. Because his immune system is still immature, he may develop allergies to solid foods given during this period.

Fluctuations in the fullness of your breasts and in your milk supply will probably pass by the end of the second month after birth. In the meantime, you can be reassured that your milk supply is probably fine if you are nursing at least eight times in each 24-hour period and letting the baby suck for as long as he wants. If you are worried about your milk supply, though, have your baby weighed. A weight gain of at least an ounce a day will tell you that your baby is getting plenty to eat. If you have additional concerns about your milk supply, see "Underfeeding," page 218.

Donating to a Milk Bank

While some women are unable to produce sufficient milk, others produce more than their babies can use. Therein lies the beauty of a milk bank, which serves both those in need of milk and those who wish to donate it. If you are considering donating your milk, it is best to wait until your baby is nursing well and gaining weight as expected. Your doctor may even be required to confirm that your baby is thriving before you are permitted to donate. It is also wise to freeze an extra supply of milk for your own baby in the case of an unexpected need, and definitely if you will be returning to work or school. Or you may be a mother who decides to wean and later regrets doing so because your baby is not tolerating infant formula.

Milk banks save babies' lives. The 18 accredited nonprofit milk banks in the United States and Canada help protect the most medically vulnerable infants, who are usually in hospitals. Donors are not paid; rather, the cost of the milk (which is sometimes covered by insurance or by the state) goes to the screening of donors, bacteriologic testing of the milk, pasteurization of the milk, and monitoring a chain of control from the donor to the receiving infant. (There are also for-profit milk banks, like Prolacta, which solicits milk to make a human milk fortifier for premature babies.)

If you are blessed with an abundant milk supply, consider donating some of your milk to a nonprofit milk bank. Like blood banks, milk banks very often experience serious shortages of human milk. Nonprofit banks send milk most often to the sickest babies, whose need for your milk could make the difference between life and death, or serious disability. Visit the Human Milk Banking Association of North America at www.hmbana.org to locate a milk bank site near you, and see Appendix A, page 366. You can be a breast milk heroine!

Casual Milk Sharing

If you are a mother considering accepting milk from a casual milk-sharing organization (such as Eats on Feets or Human Milk 4 Human Babies), keep in mind that someone else's milk may contain toxins, including medications, illegal drugs, tobacco, or alcohol. Certain diseases can be transferred through breast milk as well. Are donor mothers always honest about their intake of tobacco, illegal drugs, and medications? Are all mothers aware of their health history or that of their partners? There is some evidence that this is not always the case. Many milk banks find that donated milk is contaminated with bacteria and must be discarded. Casual peer-to-peer sharing of breast milk could cause harm to a baby receiving milk that has not gone through the process of maternal screening, and culturing and pasteurization of the donated milk. Furthermore, casual milk sharing diverts much-needed milk away from the accredited milk banks, where it can be given to the most medically needy infants.

Scheduled Feedings

Some parenting books and classes have promoted a philosophy of scheduled breastfeeding. Called Parent Directed Feeding, the program teaches parents to feed babies on a rigid three- to four-hour schedule and to eliminate nighttime feedings at an early age. The purpose is to relieve parental anxiety and instill a sense of order and discipline in the infant. Although most parents like the idea of predictable, widely spaced nursings and full nights of sleep from the early weeks on, these practices are often associated with low milk production, poor weight gain in the baby, and early weaning. Some babies subjected to this method have become dangerously thin and dehydrated.

Babies do best if they are nursed when they seem hungry. Parent Directed Feeding fails to take into account two important facts about breast milk and breastfeeding. First, nature has designed breast milk to be taken frequently. Low in protein, it is easily and quickly digested. Second, a mother's milk supply depends on frequent, complete drainage of the breasts. If she nurses fewer than seven times in a 24-hour period, her milk production generally declines. Although some mothers can meet their babies' needs with fewer than seven daily feedings, most cannot.

The American Academy of Pediatrics, and every other organization that supports breastfeeding, recommends that babies be fed whenever they show signs of hunger.

Infant Dietary Supplements

Supplements sometimes given to nursing babies include vitamin D, iron, and fluoride.

Vitamin D

Known as the "sunshine vitamin," vitamin D is actually a hormone manufactured by the body when the skin is exposed to sunlight. Dietary sources also provide some vitamin D; fatty fish, especially salmon, herring, and tuna, provide high amounts of the vitamin if they are eaten two to three times a week. Some other foods, such as cow's milk, orange juice, and dry cereal, are "fortified" with small amounts of vitamin D.

Vitamin D is important in multiple ways. Because it promotes calcium absorption in the intestinal tract, it is essential for the health of bones. Infants and children who get too little vitamin D are at risk for developing rickets, a painful bone-softening disease that has recently been reported in some American babies. Vitamin D is also a vital part of the immune system and so may make babies less prone to infection. A deficiency of vitamin D is associated with the onset of type 1 diabetes, multiple sclerosis, rheumatoid arthritis, and cancer.

Sunlight, not food additives or supplements, is "the biologically normal and most common way for humans of all ages to develop adequate levels of the hormone 'vitamin D,'" according to Cynthia Good Mojab, a research associate at La Leche League International. The amount of sunlight exposure needed to prevent vitamin D deficiency depends on such factors as latitude, season, altitude, weather, time of day, air pollution, how much skin is exposed, whether sunscreen is applied (since sunscreen prevents vitamin D production), and skin pigmentation. In general, babies achieve adequate vitamin D levels when exposed to sunlight for 30 minutes per week while wearing only a diaper or for two hours per week while fully clothed without a hat. Infants living in northern latitudes may need more sun exposure than this; infants living closer to the equator may need less. Dark-skinned infants may need more sun exposure than light-skinned infants, although researchers have yet to ascertain this. In any case, the exposure must be direct; sunlight that has passed through window glass, Plexiglas, or almost any other plastic does not allow the body to produce vitamin D, because these materials absorb ultraviolet B radiation.

Pediatricians and dermatologists, however, warn parents to keep their babies out of the sun, particularly during the first six months of life. Because sun exposure in infancy has been associated with an increased risk of skin cancer later in life, the American Academy of Pediatrics (AAP) now recommends that all children, including babies who are exclusively breastfed, consume at least 400 IU (international units) of vitamin D per day beginning as soon as possible after birth and continuing through childhood. All infant formulas, like commercially produced cow's milk, are fortified with vitamin D, and babies fed at least 500 milliliters (17.6 ounces) of formula daily get as much vitamin D as the AAP recommends.

But breast milk contains little vitamin D unless the mother takes the vitamin orally in high doses. For exclusively breastfed babies, vitamin D is available in over-the-counter liquid supplements, to be given to the baby by dropper. D-Vi-Sol, made by Enfamil, contains 400 IU of vitamin D per dose; Tri-Vi-Sol, made by the same company, contains vitamins A and C as well as 400 IU of vitamin D. Because breastfed babies don't need supplemental A and C, D-Vi-Sol is generally the better choice between these two. Although the daily dose of each of these preparations is only 1 milliliter, it must be given slowly so that the baby does not gasp, gag, and cough.

Cod liver oil, a supplement much hated by children of generations past, also contains vitamin D as well as vitamin A. The oil is no longer recommended for babies, however, because it can contain mercury and can be toxic at high doses.

There is some controversy about giving oral vitamin D to babies. According to Cynthia Good Mojab, no one has investigated the potential risks, such as aspiration of the liquid, harmful changes in the baby's gut, or increased susceptibility to infection. Since vitamin D is often given in combination with other vitamins, future studies should include the risks of supplementing with those vitamins, too.

An alternative to liquid vitamin-D supplements are the more concentrated Baby Ddrops, which are made by Carlson Laboratories and available at health-food stores and through online pharmacies. One daily drop, providing 400 IU of vitamin D, is placed on the nipple for the baby to take while nursing. The drops are odorless, tasteless, and colorless.

The AAP recommends that a breastfed baby be given supplemental vitamin D until she is weaned to infant formula or, preferably, until she is at least a year old and is drinking at least 2 cups of whole milk per day.

If you want to avoid giving your baby vitamin D supplements, you have a couple of choices. While you're pregnant, you can get plenty of sunshine and dietary vitamin D. This will ensure that your baby is born with enough vitamin D stores to last two months even if she is never exposed to the sun. Then you can postpone giving supplements at least until your baby is two months old.

After your baby is born, you can also take supplemental vitamin D yourself, in the amount of 4,000 to 6,000 IU per day. This will increase the amount of D in your milk enough to protect your baby. The recommended form of supplemental vitamin D is cholecalciferol, or vitamin D_3.

Iron

The full-term newborn has sufficient stores of iron for at least the first six months after birth. The small amounts of iron in breast milk are very well utilized by the nursing infant, so iron supplementation is unnecessary. Furthermore, iron supplements can interfere with the anti-infective properties of breast milk.

The baby born prematurely, however, is likely to use up her iron stores earlier than the full-term infant. Supplemental iron is recommended for the premature infant beginning at two months of age or earlier.

Fluoride

This mineral, taken from infancy in water or in supplemental drops, has been shown to reduce childhood dental cavities by 50 to 65 percent. Because little fluoride reaches a baby through breast milk even if the mother drinks fluoridated water, fluoride supplements have sometimes been prescribed for exclusively breastfed babies. Too much fluoride, however, can cause spotting of the developing tooth enamel, and some infants are reported to become fussy and irritable and to have gastrointestinal upsets after being given fluoride. For these reasons, the American Academy of Pediatrics recommends delaying fluoride supplements until a baby is six months old and then using them only if the local drinking water is severely deficient in fluoride, with less than 0.3 parts fluoride per million.

The usual dose of supplemental fluoride is 0.25 milligram per day. Fluoride is available by prescription, either alone or in combination with vitamins A and C, which breastfed babies don't need.

LIFE WITH YOUR BABY

Sleeping with Your Baby

Although mothers and babies have slept together at least as long as mammals have roamed the earth, recent warnings about the dangers of bed sharing are worrying new parents. The American Academy of Pediatrics (AAP) has stated that bed sharing can be hazardous under certain conditions, and in 1999 the Consumer Product Safety Commission recommended against parents and babies sleeping together at all. But many physicians, scientists, parents, and sudden infant death syndrome (SIDS) researchers—including one of the Safety Commission members—disagree with this recommendation.

SIDS, or crib death—that is, sleep apnea resulting in a baby's death—has many risk factors. The most common is placing a baby to sleep on her stomach. The second most common is the mother's smoking, either before or after the baby's birth. Formula feeding and overheating are other risk factors, and another is putting the baby to sleep alone in a room. The largest SIDS study to date has shown that infants who sleep alone in a room are more than twice as likely to die from crib death as are infants who share a room with parents. In countries where bed sharing is common, where smoking is not, and where breastfeeding is the norm, SIDS is rare.

Anthropological and developmental studies suggest that mothers and infants are biologically and psychologically designed to sleep next to each other. Parents who sleep with their infants report that they enjoy this closeness and find it makes nighttime parenting easier. Being close to the baby in the night means being more aware of her cues and therefore more responsive to her needs. Even though bed-sharing mothers and babies wake more frequently, they go back to sleep sooner and so get more sleep overall than mothers and babies who sleep separately. Babies who sleep with their parents also cry significantly less than babies who sleep alone.

Because bed-sharing mothers nurse more frequently, they produce more milk than they would otherwise. This can be especially important to women who must spend time apart from their babies during the day. Women who work outside the home also often find that bed sharing helps them feel more connected to their infants.

The AAP recommends that babies sleep in the parents' room for the first six months. James McKenna, an anthropologist at the University of Notre Dame and an expert on infant sleep, also urges parents to sleep in the same room with the baby, if not the same bed, for at least the first six months of life. Dr. McKenna believes that a parent's close breathing may help regulate an infant's own breathing pattern, and that bed sharing may thus reduce instances of SIDS. His review of studies suggests that when a mother and her baby are close enough during nighttime sleep to sense each other in at least two of four ways—sight, scent, sound, and touch—the baby's risk of succumbing to SIDS is significantly decreased. As Dr. McKenna points out, the sharpest recent decline in rates of SIDS and other infant deaths has occurred among middle-class whites, the very group that has most increased its rate of parent-child bed sharing over the same period.

In his sleep laboratory at Notre Dame, Dr. McKenna has found that bed-sharing mothers and their infants are extremely sensitive to each other's movements and physical condition throughout the night, across all sleep stages. For instance, healthy, full-term babies whose air passages become blocked alert their bed-sharing mothers and, under normal circumstances, maneuver out of danger. Babies who sleep alone, Dr. McKenna has found, spend more time in deeper stages of sleep, which may be harmful for babies with inherent arousal deficiencies.

Other researchers have suggested that babies who sleep with their mothers develop into children who are independent, sociable, confident, and well able to handle stress. Children who have never slept in their parents' beds are, according to their parents, harder to control, less happy, more prone to tantrums, more fearful, and more dependent.

There are certainly hazards to avoid in bed sharing, but there are hazards in laying the baby to sleep anywhere. Wherever the baby sleeps, the dangers are mostly the same: pillows, toys, and quilts that could suffocate; cords and ties that could strangle; gaps in which a baby could become wedged; heights from which she could fall; and overheating. Bed sharing poses the additional risk of "overlying"—accidental smothering—but this is generally a concern only when other children are sleeping in the same bed or a parent is intoxicated or extremely exhausted. Generally, adults have a sense of their own boundaries even when asleep; this is why you don't fall out of bed.

If you smoked during pregnancy or if your baby isn't exclusively breast-fed, room sharing, rather than bed sharing, may be the safest sleeping situation for your baby, studies show. The reasons for this are unclear.

For most of the benefits of bed sharing with no risk of overlying, you might try placing your baby's bed very close to your own. You can even buy a baby bed that attaches to an adult bed so you can reach your baby without getting up even though she is sleeping on a separate surface (see Appendix A, page 366). Or you can put your baby in a small bed on top of your own (see the Snuggle Nest at www.babydelight.com).

Following are some guidelines for safe infant sleep, with the parents or in a separate bed:

- Use a firm mattress that fits the bed or crib frame well, without gaps in which a baby could become wedged.

- Stretch the sheet tightly around the mattress.

- Avoid nightclothes with strings or ties, both for the baby and, if you're sharing the bed, for yourself and your partner.

- Keep the baby's face uncovered.

- Leave off the comforters, feather beds, stuffed animals, lamb skins, and other soft things that could pose a risk of suffocation. The baby doesn't need a pillow.

- Put the baby on her back or side to sleep.

- Don't smoke, and don't let other people smoke in the house.

- Avoid overheating the room in which the baby sleeps, and avoid overdressing the baby. Keep the room cool if you share a bed so that the warmth of your body combined with the warmth of the covers does not overheat the baby, or have the baby sleep outside the covers.

- Avoid laying the baby to sleep near dangling cords or sashes.

- Don't leave a young baby, especially one born prematurely, to sleep in a car seat or infant seat. If the baby's upper body is inadequately supported, her airway may become blocked.

If your baby sleeps in a crib, follow these guidelines:

- Make sure the rails are no farther than 2⅜ inches apart.

- If you use crib bumpers, make sure that they have at least six ties. The ties should be no longer than 6 inches long.

- When the baby learns to sit, lower the mattress so that she can't fall out or climb over the side rail.

- Hang any crib mobile well out of the baby's reach, and remove it when the baby starts to sit or reaches five months of age, whichever comes first.

- When she learns to stand, set the mattress at its lowest level and remove any crib bumpers.
- When she reaches a height of 35 inches or the side rail is less than three-quarters of her height, move her to another bed.
- Remove any "crib gym" when a baby can get up on all fours.
- Dress the baby in a blanket sleeper instead of using a blanket. If you do use a blanket, make sure the baby's head remains uncovered.
- Consider using a baby monitor with the speaker turned toward the baby during naps. Background noise from the monitor may protect the baby as well as bed sharing.

If your baby sleeps with you, follow these guidelines:

- Don't place the bed against the wall or against other furniture, since the baby could become trapped in between.
- If your bed has head- or footboard railings, they should be spaced no wider than 2⅜ inches apart.
- Don't leave the baby to sleep alone in your bed.
- Fasten back your hair, if it is very long.
- After drinking or taking drugs that may cause you to sleep too soundly, and at any time that you are extremely exhausted, put the baby to sleep in a separate bed.
- Don't use bed rails in the baby's first year, since she could become wedged between the mattress and the rail.
- Don't let an older sibling share a bed with an infant younger than one year old.
- Don't share a waterbed with your baby, since the surface could hamper breathing if your baby were to turn face down.
- Consider bed sharing carefully if you or your partner is obese. Your weight might create a depression in the mattress that the baby could roll into. Sleeping on a very firm mattress might be safer in this case.
- Don't sleep with the baby on a sofa or overstuffed chair.

Different sleeping arrangements may work best for you at different times. You might place your baby in a bassinet at bedtime but move her into your bed later for night feedings. You might instead nurse the baby to sleep in your bed and then move her to her own bed afterward. Or you might put the baby to sleep in the nursery but then sometimes end up sleeping there all night yourself. You might follow a certain pattern for many months or change more often as your baby grows and your own needs change.

Illnesses: Yours and the Baby's

When you come down with a minor illness such as a cold or flu, you need not interrupt breastfeeding. Most likely your baby will have already been exposed to the virus that caused you to get sick. In fact, the antibodies you produce against the illness will reach the baby through the milk and may protect him from getting the same sickness. Even though you may not feel much like eating, try to drink extra fluids to keep from getting dehydrated. Should you need to take a medication, even an over-the-counter drug, be sure to check on its safety for the baby (see Appendix D, page 374). Some over-the-counter cold remedies contain pseudoephedrine, which can decrease milk production, sometimes permanently.

Temporary weaning is also unnecessary if you suspect you have a case of food poisoning, provided your only symptoms are vomiting, diarrhea, or both.

Your milk supply may seem low during or just after an illness, but a few days of frequent nursing will usually bring milk production back to normal.

Should you require hospitalization or surgery, you can continue breastfeeding. If you know ahead of time that you'll need a hospital stay, you can pump and save milk for any time that you may be unavailable to your baby. You may be able to arrange to have your baby stay with you, although the hospital will probably require that another adult be there to care for the baby. Ask if the hospital has a fully automatic breast pump for you to use when you cannot nurse; if not, arrange to bring one along, with a double-pump kit. The hospital may even have a lactation professional on staff who can assist with any breastfeeding problems that arise during your hospitalization.

You won't need to express and throw out milk contaminated by an anesthetic or pain medication. By the time you awaken from anesthesia, there will not be enough of the drug in your body to be a problem for your baby. Pain medications are also safe. If you take this book to the hospital with you, you can refer to Appendix D for information on other medications.

When you are not able to nurse your baby, express your milk every two to three hours during the day and evening and as often during the night as you usually feed the baby. Ask the nurses to wake you as often as you need to pump. They should be able to refrigerate your milk in clean containers that you can take home to your baby.

Should your baby become ill, nursing should certainly continue. Breast milk is the best source of fluids and nourishment for recovery and nursing the best source of comfort. But be aware that sickness often changes a baby's nursing pattern. He may nurse more than usual, or he may lose interest in nursing. Ear infections, sore throats, and fever blisters may make nursing painful for the baby. As long as he is nursing infrequently or is refusing to nurse, be sure to express your milk every couple of hours to keep up your supply.

Colds and stuffy noses can make nursing difficult for a baby. Holding your baby upright while feeding, using a humidifier in the room, or administering saline nose drops and cleaning out his nose may make nursing more comfortable for him. Try the NoseFrida, a safe, gentle nasal aspirator that captures the baby's nasal discharge and prevents it from contaminating the device, unlike a traditional bulb aspirator. The NoseFrida is available at many stores and online.

Fever is a sign of infection. During the first four months, a temperature above 99 degrees F. if taken in the armpit, or 101 degrees F. if taken rectally, should be reported to the baby's doctor. If, besides having an elevated temperature, the baby doesn't act like his usual self or he nurses poorly, he should be checked by the doctor. The severity of a fever does not always correspond with the seriousness of an illness; a high fever may appear with a minor infection, and a low fever may accompany a serious infection. Because a fever may lead to dehydration, frequent nursing is very important.

Diarrhea in the breastfed baby, although less common and usually less severe than in the formula-fed baby, is characterized by frequent (12 or more per day), extremely loose or watery bowel movements. Often the stools are foul smelling, and they may contain mucus or blood. Since babies lose a great deal of fluid with diarrhea, they can easily become dehydrated, so frequent nursing is important. With its high water content, breast milk helps replace the lost fluids. Diarrhea generally improves within three to five days. Fever, infrequent feedings, or signs of dehydration (dry mouth, few wet diapers, listlessness) are reasons to notify your doctor. In cases of severe diarrhea, doctors occasionally recommend supplements of an electrolyte solution, such as Pedialyte, in conjunction with nursing.

The First Two Months: What's Normal?

During the first two months you can expect your baby will nurse between 8 and 12 times a day, including at least once at night. If your baby sleeps four to six hours at a stretch at night or takes a three- to four-hour nap during the day, she will probably want to nurse often during the next few hours to make up for the meal she missed. The baby who is nursing fewer than eight times in a 24-hour period or who is sleeping longer than six hours at a stretch at night is typically the infant who fails to gain enough weight during the early weeks of nursing.

Generally, eight or more wet diapers a day are a sign that the baby is getting enough milk. By two weeks, most nursing infants have regained their birth weight. A gain of at least an ounce a day is normal.

The breastfed baby typically has very loose and seedy-looking stools. During the first month most infants have at least one bowel movement daily. After the first month it is not uncommon for a baby to go several days without a bowel movement. As long as the baby seems comfortable, there is probably no need for concern; your baby is unlikely to be constipated or underfed. The baby who is not getting enough to eat typically has small, and usually infrequent, brown or greenish stools and is gaining less than an ounce a day.

Many mothers continue to experience dripping or spraying milk during or between nursings. But some women stop leaking altogether after the first several weeks, and most gradually notice less leakage.

At some point during the first two months you will probably start to experience the sensations of milk let-down. You may notice this tingling, pins-and-needles feeling in your breasts just before or during a feeding or at any time your baby signals you with his cry.

Occasionally babies spit up after a feeding. Some babies spit up after every nursing. This is usually due to an immature digestive system; what comes up is normally just a few teaspoons. If your baby spits up more, the cause may be certain foods or beverages in your diet (see "Spitting Up and Vomiting," page 201, and "Fussiness, Colic, and Reflux," page 204). In any case, spitting up passes with time; until it does, keep a diaper or small towel handy.

A baby cries for any of a number of reasons. She may be hungry or tired, or she may just want to suck and be held. Sucking at the breast is soothing and comforting for her. Babies usually have a fussy period in the evening. Although many theories have been suggested to explain why this is, most babies are comforted by extra nursing. Try not to assume your milk is somehow lacking. Many mothers who interpret their babies' cries this way begin supplementing with formula and soon find the babies weaned. See "Fussiness, Colic, and Reflux," page 204, for more on why babies cry and how to cope with crying.

During the appetite spurts at about two to three weeks and six weeks of age, your baby may act more fussy than usual and want to nurse more often. After a few days of frequent nursing, your milk supply will increase to meet her needs and she will return to her usual nursing pattern.

Some babies cry hard, as if in pain, for prolonged periods every day. They are said to have *colic*, which is just a name for extreme irritability that continues day after day—for any of a number of reasons. Some cry at the breast or refuse nursing entirely. If your baby has colic symptoms, see "Fussiness, Colic, and Reflux," page 204.

You may have heard that tending to your baby each time she cries will spoil her or will reinforce her behavior and cause her to cry more often. Nothing could be further from the truth. Babies do not cry to exercise their lungs, but because they are in need of something. If your baby's needs are met in infancy, she will develop a sense of security, and she will grow to trust in you and others as well.

During these early weeks, while you are learning about your baby, caring for her needs, and learning to breastfeed, you are apt to experience some feelings of concern, confusion, and perhaps even inadequacy regarding your mothering abilities. Motherhood and breastfeeding may not be exactly what you expected. Your baby's crying and the unpredictability of her sleeping and wakeful periods may be upsetting. The baby's nursing schedule (or lack thereof) and her many needs may make it impossible to feel organized or productive. Perhaps you are disappointed by the lack of help from your health-care providers. Early motherhood may also bring feelings of loneliness and isolation.

It is normal to have mixed feelings about nursing. Try to keep in mind that new motherhood brings a period of uncertainty and adjustment, and that nursing, like mothering, gets easier with time.

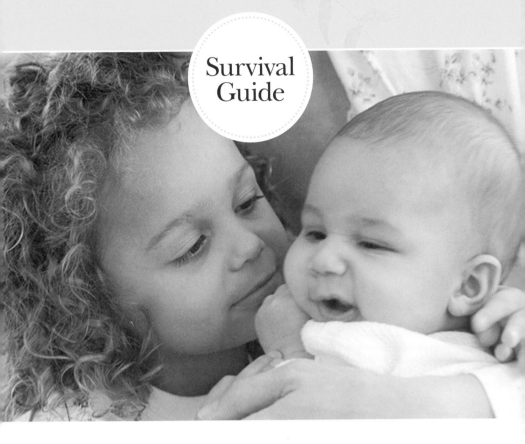

THE FIRST TWO MONTHS

Concerns about Yourself

- Sore Nipples
- Breast Pain
- Plugged Ducts
- Breast Infection (Mastitis)
- Breast Abscess
- Breast Lumps
- Leaking Milk
- Overabundant Milk
- Lopsided Breasts
- Nausea or Headache

- Depression and Anxiety
- Dysphoric Milk Ejection Reflex (Bad Feelings while Nursing)

Concerns about the Baby

- Spitting Up and Vomiting
- Pulling Away from the Breast
- Refusal to Nurse
- Fussiness, Colic, and Reflux
- Underfeeding

Concerns about Yourself

Sore Nipples

It can certainly be discouraging when sore nipples persist beyond the first week. If this happens to you, review the information on sore nipples (see page 73) in "Survival Guide: The First Week." It may be helpful to have your partner or a friend observe your latch-on technique and compare it with the descriptions of latch-on in "Positioning at the Breast," page 44. Babies who are tongue-tied may also cause painful nipples (see page 98). But don't discount the possibility that your nipples are irritated due to thrush or another dermatologic condition.

Thrush nipples. If your nipples suddenly become sore after a period of comfortable nursing, thrush is the most likely cause. This problem occurs when a yeast (monilia) infection in the baby's mouth spreads to the mother's nipples. The nipples become shiny, reddened, swollen, tender, and sometimes cracked. Occasionally, peeling or a red, dotty rash can be seen on the nipples. Some mothers complain of itching; others complain of burning. Thrush sometimes begins after the mother has taken a course of antibiotics or when she has had a vaginal yeast infection (symptomatic or not).

If you suspect a case of thrush, carefully inspect the baby's mouth. You may see white patches on the inside of the cheeks, inside the lips, and possibly on the tongue. Sometimes a baby will have no symptoms in the mouth but will have a diaper rash caused by yeast. A yeast rash often resembles a mild burn; it may be scaly and peeling. It is usually well defined, very red, and a bit raised, but sometimes it looks like just a patch of red dots. It usually appears in the genital area but may also be noticeable in the folds of the baby's diaper area. A yeast rash will not respond to typical remedies like frequent cleaning and the usual diaper rash creams. For treatment, see page 207.

Treatment Measures for Thrush Nipples

1. The treatment baby doctors usually recommend for thrush is
    1 milliliter nystatin suspension (Mycostatin) by dropper into the

baby's mouth after every other nursing, or four times daily, for 14 days. Wait a few minutes after nursing before giving this prescription medication so it won't be washed out of the baby's mouth by the milk. Half the dose should be dropped into each side of the mouth. Even if the symptoms are gone after a few days, continue the treatment for the full 14 days.

2. To prevent reinfection, the nipples must be treated at the same time as the baby's mouth. The best remedy is nystatin cream or ointment, which, like nystatin suspension, is available by prescription only. (The oral medication can be applied to the nipples instead, but it is usually ineffective.) Your baby's doctor may prescribe nystatin cream for your nipples (and for your baby's diaper rash, if present); if not, call your own doctor for a prescription, or use an over-the-counter antifungal cream such as Lotrimin AF, Micatin, or Monistat 7. Apply the medication after each nursing. Some lactation professionals recommend rinsing the nipples, for the first few days of treatment, with water or a mild solution of vinegar (1 tablespoon vinegar to 1 cup water) before applying the medication.

3. Because nystatin inhibits yeast growth for only about two hours after you swab the baby's mouth, it is often ineffective when used as prescribed. If your baby's mouth isn't clear of thrush after five to six days of treatment, ask your doctor about more frequent dosing, or try using gentian violet, as described in step 4, instead.

4. A 1 percent solution of gentian violet can be purchased without a prescription at most but not all drugstores, so call around before making the trip, or have the pharmacy order it for you. If you can find only 2 percent gentian violet, you can have the pharmacist dilute the solution, or you can do it yourself by placing a few drops in the cap and adding an equal amount of water. Thoroughly swab the affected areas in the baby's mouth using a cotton-tipped applicator, once or twice a day for three days. The solution will stain the baby's mouth purple; take care in applying it so that nothing else turns purple. Some lactation professionals recommend painting the mother's nipples with gentian violet, too, but I don't recommend this treatment if the nipples are tender.

5. Canadian pediatrician and breastfeeding specialist Dr. Jack Newman recommends using grapefruit seed extract (available at most
health-food stores) as a nipple solution. Mix five to ten drops of
the liquid into 1 ounce of water and rub some of this solution on
the nipples and areolas after nursings. The concentration of the
grapefruit seed extract can be increased gradually to up to 25
drops in 1 ounce of water. You can use this solution in addition to
any topical antifungal cream by alternating it with the cream. If
you find that your nipples begin flaking, stop using this solution.

6. If the weather allows, briefly expose your nipples to the sun two
or three times daily to hasten healing.

7. Sanitize your breastfeeding supplies to prevent reinfection. If
you're using nursing pads, change them at each feeding. If you
are using a pump, wash all the parts thoroughly after each use.
Bottle nipples, plastic breast shells, and pump parts that come in
contact with the breast or the milk should be boiled in water for
5 minutes daily. If your baby uses a pacifier, make sure you boil it
daily as well.

8. If thrush and accompanying sore nipples aren't cured by the
usual treatment measures, some mothers try fluconazole
(Diflucan), an oral antifungal agent. The usual dosage is 400
milligrams on the first day followed by 100 milligrams for the
next 13 days. This medication is very expensive, though, and I
find that most mothers can overcome yeast infections by using
antifungal cream on the nipples and treating the baby's mouth.
If you try a course of fluconazole and still suffer with nipple
soreness, yeast is probably not the problem.

9. If after the treatment just described your baby shows no signs of
thrush but your nipples are still irritated, see a dermatologist. In
the absence of visible thrush, pink, burning nipples may indicate
nipple dermatitis.

Nipple dermatitis. If you experience pink, tender nipples beyond the
first week of nursing and your baby shows no signs of thrush, you may

have another dermatologic condition. A dermatologist can probably both uncover the cause of the soreness and offer effective treatment. Before seeing a dermatologist, though, you might ask your regular physician to prescribe Dr. Jack Newman's all-purpose nipple ointment, or APNO. A topical medication that must be specially made up in a pharmacy, APNO includes 2 percent mupirocin ointment (15 grams), an antibacterial; 0.1 percent betamethasone ointment (15 grams), an anti-inflammatory; and 2 percent miconazole or clotrimazole powder, an antifungal. An optional fourth ingredient, ibuprofen, is helpful for pain relief. The ointment is applied sparingly after nursings or pumpings until the nipples are free of pain for a few days, and then gradually used less often.

If your nipples are still tender after treatment with APNO or an antibacterial ointment, I highly recommend seeing a dermatologist.

Painful, blanched nipples. Some women notice that their nipples become painful and pale at the end of nursing sessions. Often this pain and blanching results from poor positioning of the baby at the breast. The compression of the nipples probably causes a vasospasm—a spasm in the blood vessels—which prevents blood from getting to the nipples. You may be able to solve this problem by correcting your latch-on technique (review "Positioning at the Breast," page 44) and by applying warm compresses to the nipples right after nursing.

Sometimes vasospasm in the nipples results from Raynaud's disease or Raynaud's phenomenon (these two are different; the less common Raynaud's disease occurs on its own, whereas Raynaud's phenomenon is associated with illness such as rheumatoid arthritis or repetitive trauma or injury and affects some 22 percent of 21- to 51-year-old women). In both conditions, blood-vessel spasms brought on by a drop in temperature prevent blood from getting to a particular area of the body. Most commonly, Raynaud's occurs in the fingers, typically when a person goes outdoors from a warm building on a cool day. In this case, the fingers turn white and the tips hurt.

When Raynaud's affects the nipples, it causes nipple blanching just after a feeding, probably because the ambient air is cooler than the inside of the baby's mouth. When the baby comes off the breast, the nipple is its usual color, but it very quickly turns white. This blanching is accompanied by burning pain. Then the nipple turns blue; this is caused by deoxygenation of the blood. As the blood starts flowing back to the nipple, the nipple returns to its normal color, and the mother may experience a throbbing pain. The three-phase color change—from white to blue to red—suggests a diagnosis of Raynaud's phenomenon rather than poor positioning. The nipple colors and the types of pain may alternate for several minutes or as long as an hour or more.

If you have Raynaud's phenomenon, avoiding cold is important. Your entire body needs to be kept warm. Breastfeed in a warm place, wear warm clothing, and avoid exposure to cold at all times. If you experience a painful vasospasm, applying warm, moist cloths to your nipples may help. Avoid smoking and caffeine.

Dietary supplements may help alleviate vasospasms caused by Raynaud's phenomenon. Some women have used a combination of calcium (2,000 milligrams per day) and magnesium (1,000 milligrams per day). So far, however, no studies have tested the effectiveness of this remedy. Jack Newman, a pediatrician, reports that vitamin B_6 often helps with Raynaud's phenomenon and is safe to use. He suggests a dosage of 150 to 200 milligrams once a day for four days. If the symptoms don't lessen in this much time, vitamin B_6 probably won't help at all, Newman says. But if the pain resolves, he suggests taking a reduced dose of 25 milligrams once a day until you are pain-free for a few weeks. If the pain returns with the smaller dose, you can return to the higher dose (Newman and Pitman, 2006).

Various drugs have been investigated for the treatment of Raynaud's phenomenon. The most effective among them is nifedipine, which is primarily used to treat hypertension. Nifedipine is probably safe to use, since very little of the drug (less than 5 percent of the total dose) appears in the breast milk, and side effects in the mother are uncommon (the most frequent side effect is a headache). The usual dosage of nifedipine is one 30-milligram slow-release tablet per day for two weeks. If the nipple pain returns, as it does in about 10 percent of mothers, a second course can be taken. Women rarely require more than three courses.

Breast Pain

For a variety of reasons, your breasts may begin to hurt during nursing or become perpetually tender or sore. If this happens, it is important to identify the cause so that you can take any necessary action.

Uncomfortable engorgement can occur any time the breasts become overly full—when the baby misses a feeding, for example, or when he begins to sleep longer at night (see "Engorged Breasts," page 68).

Most mothers begin noticing normal let-down sensations during these early weeks. Let-down may be experienced as a mild ache at the start of nursing or a tingling, pins-and-needles sensation.

A deep pain, often described as "shooting," that occurs just after nursing is thought to be related to the sudden refilling of the breast. These pains disappear after the first few weeks of nursing. Blocked nipple pores can also cause stabbing pains (see below).

Pain during nursing, often described as burning or stinging, is usually associated with thrush. The nipples may be pinker than usual. Sometimes a rash may be visible. See "Thrush Nipples," page 182, for additional information on causes and treatment.

If you can feel a tender area or painful lump in your breast, see the following section.

Plugged Ducts

You may experience a plugged milk duct as a small, tender spot or as a large area of the breast that feels overly full and does not soften with nursing. If you look in a mirror, the skin over the area may appear reddened.

Occasionally a plug in one of the nipple openings blocks the milk flow and causes a backup of milk in the breast. If the nipple looks normal in color but you can see a white pimple (a "bleb") on the end of the nipple, particularly right after the baby comes off the breast, the problem may be a plugged nipple pore. Plugged nipple pores are often associated with stabbing breast pain, especially right after nursing.

Plugged ducts are most common during the early weeks of nursing, but they can occur at any time during breastfeeding. They occur for various reasons. In the early weeks and months, they frequently seem to be caused by incomplete drainage of the breast. Mothers with high milk production, including those nursing twins, tend to be more prone to plugged ducts. Interrupting the baby's nursing to switch to the other breast before the baby signals that he is finished may lead to a plugged duct. A plugged duct may follow a missed feeding or a long stretch at night without nursing. Overly tight bras, especially underwire types, may obstruct milk flow and lead to plugged ducts. Baby carriers with tight straps can also cause this to happen.

For unknown reasons, plugged ducts seem to be more common during the winter months. Some breastfeeding specialists feel that mothers who drink an insufficient amount of fluids, who become slightly dehydrated due to a cold or flu, or who are overly fatigued may also be more susceptible to developing plugged milk ducts.

Any breast lump that does not get significantly smaller within a week should be examined by a doctor.

Treatment Measures for Plugged Ducts

1. Remove your bra if there is any question that it may be too tight or may be pressing into part of your breast.

2. Before nursing, apply moist heat to the breast for 15 to 20 minutes.

3. Nurse frequently, at least every two hours. Begin each nursing on the affected breast.

4. While nursing, gently massage the breast just behind the sore area.

5. If you are following the preceding recommendations but notice no change in your breast after a feeding or two, try positioning the baby with his chin close to the plugged duct, if possible, to promote better drainage. If this doesn't work, get into the shower. With your breast well soaped, apply steady but gentle pressure behind the plugged area, pressing toward the nipple.

6. Increase your fluid intake so that you urinate more frequently.

7. If the blockage seems to be in the nipple, look for dried milk secretions or a clogged nipple pore, which may resemble a whitehead. If necessary, you can gently remove a visible plug from a nipple opening with a sterilized needle. (Wash your hands well. To sterilize a needle, place the needle in a cup of rubbing alcohol or hydrogen peroxide, and leave it there for 30 seconds. Wash your hands again, and then pick up the needle by the blunt end.) Using the needle to open the "bleb" may cause a little bleeding, but you probably won't feel any pain.

8. If nursing is too painful or if you suspect the baby isn't draining the affected breast well, begin pumping your breasts after or instead of nursing. Renting a clinical-grade pump for a couple of days may be best. If you are pumping instead of nursing, pump very often. Some mothers have found that using Pumpin' Pal Super Shields while pumping can clear up a plugged milk duct (see Chapter 5, page 276). Occasionally a mother who pumps with a plugged duct will get pink milk from a bit of blood coming from the plug opening up. There is no need to be alarmed, but avoid feeding that milk to your baby, as blood is a gastric irritant and can cause her to vomit.

9. Be alert for signs of a developing breast infection—fever, chills, and achiness—so you can treat it promptly. (See the section that follows.)

10. Should you get a second case of a plugged milk duct, see "Recurrent Plugged Ducts and Breast Infections" in "Survival Guide: Months Two through Six," page 314.

If a plug does not resolve after a few feedings with the above measures, some lactation professionals suggest using an old-fashioned treatment for swelling: Apply castor oil to a warm, moist washcloth, lay it over the sore area, and place a heating pad over the washcloth. Keep the compress and heating pad in place for about 20 minutes before nursing or pumping. This can be repeated before each feeding.

Breast Infection (Mastitis)

Up to 30 percent of all nursing women develop mastitis, or infection of the breast. It occurs most often in the first three months after birth and, interestingly, it is more common during the winter months.

A breast infection is caused by bacteria, often the same ones normally present on the nipples and in the baby's mouth. A breast infection often follows an untreated cracked nipple or a plugged milk duct. It is more likely to occur when the baby (or a pump) is ineffective at draining the breasts. Other possible causes include poor-fitting bras, skipped feedings, infrequent changing of wet breast pads, anemia, stress, and fatigue.

Since mastitis causes flu-like symptoms, women sometimes mistake it for the flu. Headache, general achiness, and a reddened area of the breast are the early symptoms; they are usually followed by fever (typically over 101 degrees F.), chills, and weakness. Usually only one breast is affected; it becomes quite tender in the infected area.

Women who promptly apply moist heat to the breast and work on getting it as empty as possible may recover quickly without antibiotics, usually in two days. In one study of women with mastitis, half used no antibiotics, and none of them suffered complications (Riordan and Nichols, 1990). I have come to believe, however, that prompt treatment with antibiotics is indicated whenever a nursing mother has flu-like symptoms and a reddened breast, especially if she has a fever. Some women have permanently lost their milk production from the affected breast following a breast infection, although this has usually occurred when treatment has been delayed. Late treatment can also result in an abscess, which may require surgical drainage. This risk may be greater if you are anemic.

Effective treatment with an antibiotic requires the right choice of antibiotic. The bacterium involved in mastitis is usually *Staphylococcus aureus,* or "staph," which is resistant to amoxicillin, penicillins G and V, and many other antibiotics.

Usually, the most effective antibiotics against this organism are cloxacillin and dicloxacillin, and cephalosporins, such as cephalexin (Keflex). Another frequently prescribed penicillin is Augmentin, a more potent form of amoxicillin. Erythromycin, clarithromycin, azithromycin, and clindamycin are used in women who are allergic to penicillin. All of these antibiotics are safe to take while breastfeeding unless the baby is allergic to them (the allergy usually causes a rash).

Recently, some staph infections have become resistant to all penicillins, so if you are not markedly better in three or four days, contact your health-care provider. You may need a different antibiotic, such as clindamycin, co-trimoxazole (Septra), or doxycycline. Mothers who fail to respond to antibiotics may have contracted MRSA, or methicillin-resistant *Staphylococcus aureus*. This bacteria has been cultured in the milk of some mothers who do not seem to be responding to the antibiotics normally used to treat mastitis. If you are still sick after a few days, speak with your doctor about this possibility.

In general, antibiotic treatment for mastitis should continue for 10 to 14 days. It is important to take the antibiotic until it is used up, even if you feel better, because you could develop a resistant infection if you stop too soon.

With prompt and proper treatment the symptoms usually subside within 48 hours. Nurse frequently during this period; discontinuing nursing would slow healing and might lead to the development of a breast abscess. Unless you are expressing milk for a premature or sick baby who is hospitalized, you don't need to worry that the baby will get ill, since the infection involves only the breast tissue, not the milk. Try to identify the probable cause of the infection so you can prevent a recurrence in the future.

Mastitis in both breasts, though rare, can be a sign of B-streptococcal infection, which is transmitted by the infant to the breasts. When both breasts are affected, the baby's doctor should be promptly notified so that the baby can be tested and treated, if necessary.

Treatment Measures for Mastitis

1. Go to bed, if you haven't already.

2. Remove your bra if you are more comfortable without it or if there is any question that it may be pressing into part of your breast.

3. Nurse frequently, at least every two hours, and begin each nursing on the affected breast. Giving up nursing could slow healing and lead to a breast abscess.

4. If nursing is too painful or if you suspect the baby isn't draining the affected breast well, begin pumping your breasts after or instead of nursing. Renting a clinical-grade pump for a couple of days may be best (see Chapter 5 for advice on expressing milk). If you are pumping instead of nursing, pump very often.

5. Call your doctor, who will probably prescribe antibiotics. Antibiotics should be taken for the entire time they are prescribed, even though the symptoms may disappear.

6. Increase your fluid intake enough that you notice an increase in urination.

7. Apply moist heat to the breast for 15 to 20 minutes before nursing or pumping and intermittently between feedings.

8. Monitor your temperature. A mild pain reliever such as acetaminophen (Tylenol) or ibuprofen (Motrin, Advil) may help reduce your fever and discomfort.

9. Consider taking vitamin C. Some women report that a dosage of 1,000 milligrams four times a day speeds healing and recovery.

10. After you have completed a course of antibiotics, watch for symptoms of yeast growth in the baby's mouth and diaper rash caused by yeast (see "Thrush Nipples," page 182).

11. See "Recurrent Plugged Ducts and Breast Infections" (page 314) if you have a recurrence.

Breast Abscess

On very rare occasions, a breast infection develops into an abscess. A breast abscess is an accumulation of pus walled off within the breast. It may occur when a mother stops nursing during a breast infection, when treatment for mastitis is delayed, or when a mother has trouble fighting a breast infection because she is anemic.

A breast abscess should be suspected whenever mastitis symptoms last for more than a couple of days and a lump persists. The lump may be hard or soft but does not change with nursing. An abscess must usually be drained by a physician, either in an office or a hospital. After it is drained, recovery is rapid.

Some doctors are willing to avoid surgical drainage by performing a series of needle aspirations, by which a needle is inserted into the abscess and the pus is withdrawn into a syringe. This is much less invasive than opening the abscess to drain over a period of a couple of weeks.

The development and treatment of an abscess can be traumatic. You may be advised to stop nursing entirely, or you may doubt yourself whether you should continue. Although you need not abandon nursing completely, you may be advised against nursing from the affected breast for the first few days after it is drained. In the meantime, you can rent a clinical-grade electric pump to maintain your milk flow until the baby resumes nursing on both sides. The incision may leak milk for a short while, but it will heal and close over. I developed an abscess six weeks after giving birth and went on to nurse successfully without any further difficulties.

Breast Lumps

Lumps in the breast are very common during the early weeks and are usually related to lactation.

The breast may feel generally lumpy when it is overly full or engorged. A tender lump that arises suddenly is usually a sign of a plugged milk duct or, when it is accompanied by fever and flu-like symptoms, a breast infection. A lump that appears just before nursing and seems to get smaller or disappear afterward is probably a small cyst that fills with milk.

Whenever a lump shows no change in size for longer than a week, it should be examined by a doctor. It is probably a harmless cyst or benign tumor; cancer is rarely the cause. But some breastfeeding women with persistent lumps have been found to have breast cancer, so see your doctor for a thorough breast exam as soon as possible. If further diagnosis is recommended, you don't need to wean your baby, although a doctor unfamiliar with the lactating breast may recommend doing so.

Some mothers may need a mammogram, ultrasound, MRI, or breast biopsy to rule out breast cancer. Mammograms and ultrasounds can be performed while you are nursing, but they are best done on an empty breast, so drain the breast as completely as possible just prior to these procedures. When a mother needs a breast MRI, the contrast agent used is generally considered safe to allow her to resume nursing after the procedure (see Appendix D, page 394). Needle biopsies, both fine-needle and core biopsies, can also be done while a mother is nursing, but mothers are often told to wean because a biopsy can cause a milk fistula. In reality, fistulas are very rare. Any necessary incisions should be done so as to avoid the nipple and areola, especially the lower outer border, to keep from injuring the fourth intercostal nerve. A radial (horizontal) incision is also recommended. The use of local anesthesia is safe for immediate nursing or pumping, and bottle or cup feeding the baby afterward is safe. In fact, the breast should be kept well drained after the procedure by nursing or pumping. Pumping may be preferable if there is much blood coming through the milk—blood can be irritating to the baby's stomach, so he might vomit up the milk.

Consider getting a second opinion whenever drastic measures are recommended.

Leaking Milk

See "Survival Guide: The First Week," page 80, for basic information on leaking, dripping, and spraying milk.

After a few weeks of nursing you may notice that leaking diminishes or stops entirely. This should not be a cause for concern so long as the baby is nursing frequently and gaining weight.

If continuing leakage becomes bothersome, you might want to try stopping it by pressing your wrist or the heel of your hand against your nipples whenever they start to drip. You might also try LilyPadz, sticky silicone pads that can be worn with or without a bra (see Appendix A, page 361).

If leaking at night continues to be troublesome, you might try nursing the baby just before you go to sleep.

Overabundant Milk

Some mothers seem to produce too much milk. Besides feeling weary of the jokes about being able to nurse twins, you may feel uncomfortably engorged much of the time. Leaking and spraying may be bothersome. Your baby may gasp and choke as the milk lets down.

Most women find this less of a problem after the first two months of breastfeeding. In the meantime, nursing your baby on just one side at each feeding should make your breasts feel more comfortable. When your baby is draining your breasts more completely, they will feel less engorged, even though each is nursed on less often. Decreasing your fluid intake is not recommended. Nor is wearing plastic breast shells or pumping after or between feedings, either of which would probably increase, not decrease, milk production.

If your baby has difficulty nursing because the milk lets down forcefully, see "Pulling Away from the Breast," page 202. Refer to "Overabundant Milk," page 316, if you continue to produce milk in overabundance after two months.

Lopsided Breasts

When one breast receives more stimulation than the other, milk production in that breast increases, commonly resulting in a lopsided appearance.

Providing more stimulation to the smaller breast will usually even out the size difference between the two. Start each feeding on the smaller side for a day or so. If your baby nurses there for only a few minutes, encourage her to take the smaller breast again after she has nursed at the fuller one. As soon as your breasts become closer in size, you can begin alternating the breast at which the baby begins each feeding.

Nausea or Headache

Rarely, a new mother experiences nausea when nursing her newborn. This is thought to be a gastric hormonal response to suckling. Eating something before nursing may help. Fortunately, nausea generally decreases in severity and frequency as nursing is established, and the problem usually disappears completely by six to eight weeks after birth.

Headaches in new mothers have various causes. A woman who has had spinal or epidural anesthesia may suffer from a severe headache whenever she raises her head. This occurs when spinal fluid, which cushions the brain, has escaped from the spinal canal, causing the brain to sag down into the opening at the base of the skull. Remaining in bed, increasing fluid intake, and drinking beverages containing caffeine may help. When spinal headaches continue for more than a day or two, some doctors offer a "blood patch," by which they inject the mother's own blood into the spinal canal. This often produces immediate relief.

Several case reports in medical literature have concerned "lactational headaches." These occur during feedings as the milk lets down and may be related to the hormone oxytocin. Some writers have said that pain relievers such as acetaminophen (Tylenol) and ibuprofen (Motrin, Advil) are helpful and that these headaches gradually become less severe and stop by two months after birth. But other writers have described cases in which relief came only with weaning.

Another type of headache associated with lactation occurs when one or both breasts are overfull. This type of headache may be a sign of an impending breast infection. Relief comes from draining the breasts well and heading off mastitis.

Other causes of headaches include a drop in hormones in the first week post partum; low blood sugar; eye, dental, or sinus problems; allergies; or migraine.

Regardless of the suspected cause of your headaches, you may want to consult with your doctor or a neurologist if they are frequent or severe. Keeping a headache log can be helpful in determining a diagnosis.

Depression and Anxiety

Many new mothers experience moodiness, mild anxiety, or an occasional "blue" day during the first two weeks after delivery. These feelings are due to the sudden hormonal changes that follow birth, fatigue from labor and lost sleep, and the stress that becoming a mother entails. But when emotional symptoms are severe, when they continue beyond the first two weeks after birth, or when they start later and last for more than two weeks, they may indicate postpartum depression or anxiety. Many new mothers who complain that they are depressed or anxious are told that their feelings are normal and to be expected. This is not true. Postpartum emotional disorders are often misunderstood or unrecognized by family, friends, and health professionals.

As many as one out of every nine or ten new mothers experiences postpartum depression, postpartum anxiety, or both. Much rarer is postpartum psychosis, characterized by delusions, hallucinations, or extreme mental confusion. Postpartum emotional disorders are more common in women who have had a stressful pregnancy or difficult birth, previous psychological problems, or relationship difficulties. Occasionally, a thyroid disorder may mimic postpartum depression.

Symptoms of postpartum depression or anxiety usually include several of the following:

- Change in eating habits (poor appetite or overeating)
- Change in sleep pattern (difficulty falling or staying asleep, oversleeping)
- Tenseness, nervousness
- Panic attacks with physical symptoms such as shakiness, palpitations, shortness of breath, or lightheadedness
- Fatigue or lack of energy
- Poor concentration, forgetfulness, or confusion
- Crying every day
- Feelings of hopelessness
- Withdrawal, lack of interest in usual activities
- Excessive worry or guilt feelings
- Recurrent disturbing thoughts or compulsive behaviors that cause distress or take up a great deal of time
- Failure to keep appointments

Symptoms that call for immediate assistance from a mental-health professional include these:

- Thoughts of suicide
- Fears of harming the baby
- Sounds and voices heard when no one is around
- Thoughts that seem not your own or out of your control
- Sleeplessness lasting 48 hours or longer
- Inability to eat
- Inability to care for the baby

There are many helpful books available on the topic for mothers suffering from postpartum depression or anxiety. I especially like *This Isn't What I Expected: Overcoming Postpartum Depression*, by Karen Kleiman and Valerie Raskin (see "Suggested Supplemental Reading," page 414). Many women with mild cases have helped themselves without professional assistance. Try the coping measures that follow.

Coping Measures for Depression and Anxiety

1. Tell your partner, a supportive friend, or a relative how you are feeling. Although some people may not understand, you may find valuable support close by.

2. Talk to your doctor or midwife about how you are feeling. Ask about blood tests to make sure something else, such as a thyroid disorder, isn't the problem.

3. Call Postpartum Support International (800-944-4PPD) to find out whether there is a postpartum support group in your area. Or visit www.postpartum.net and click on "Get Help."

4. Make getting extra rest a priority; being tired makes depression and anxiety worse. Nap when your baby naps. Maximize your baby's sleep stretches at night by feeding him every two to two and a half hours during the day and evening.

5. Enlist the help of others to relieve you of some mothering and household duties. Eliminate or lessen your daily chores until you are feeling better. If you want to do some chores, set minimal goals for yourself.

6. Maintain a well-balanced diet. If you have little appetite, fix small, nutritious snacks for yourself throughout the day. Avoid all caffeine and sugary foods and beverages; these are associated with worsening symptoms. Increase your intake of foods made up of complex carbohydrates, such as whole-grain breads and cereals, potatoes, rice, and pasta. Eat more fruits and vegetables. Using powdered milk or yogurt, wheat germ, and fruit or juice concentrate, you can make nutritious blender drinks. If you find it difficult to prepare food for yourself throughout the day, your pharmacist can recommend a high-calorie nutritional supplement such as Ensure or Sustacal.

7. Consider increasing your intake of the long-chain omega-3 fatty acids DHA (docosahexaenoic acid) and EPA (eicosapentaenoic acid), which have been shown to help prevent and remedy postpartum depression and other mental problems in new mothers. The main dietary source of DHA and EPA is fish, but you would have to eat a great deal of fish every week to achieve the necessary levels. Kathleen Kendall-Tackett, a psychologist, suggests taking omega-3 supplements, which can be found at almost any drugstore or health-food store. To prevent depression, she recommends 200 to 400 milligrams of DHA daily. To treat depression, she recommends 1,000 to 2,000 milligrams of EPA daily. These levels are recognized as safe by the U.S. Food and Drug Administration.

8. Try to take time with your appearance every day. When you get up, make a point of getting dressed, fixing your hair, and putting on a little makeup, if you like it. Pamper yourself with a facial, a new hairstyle, or something new to wear. Looking good may help you feel better about yourself.

9. Get some exercise every day. Many people find that exercise has an antidepressant effect. Join an exercise or dance class; many offer free childcare. Take a brisk walk every day with or without the baby.

10. Nurture yourself as much as possible. Take long bubble baths, get a massage, ask your partner to hold you, spend the afternoon watching a video or reading a light novel.

11. Make an effort to spend time with other adults. Invite friends over, join a postpartum group, or make friends with other mothers from your childbirth class. Your childbirth instructor may have additional suggestions. If you have just moved to the area, ask at your pediatrician's or family practitioner's office about social resources for new parents.

If your distress is severe or unrelieved by these measures, consider seeking professional help. Low-cost mental-health care is available in most communities. If cost isn't an issue, ask your doctor, midwife, or childbirth educator to refer you to a therapist, ideally one who has a special interest in postpartum mental illness.

Depending on your symptoms, a therapist may recommend medication. Some antidepressants are safe to use during nursing; others may not be. Safe antidepressants include sertraline, which is sold under the trade name Zoloft; nortriptyline (Pamelor); and paroxetine (Paxil). All of these are also available generically. When nursing mothers take one of these drugs, it is usually undetectable in their babies' blood.

You may be tempted to try St. John's wort, a popular herbal remedy for depression. This herb, however, has not yet been proven safe to use during breastfeeding.

Unfortunately, many doctors who recommend that women wean their babies before taking antidepressants do so because they don't know about recent studies on the safety of particular drugs during breastfeeding. In Appendix D, you'll find what information is available about the safety of various antidepressants. You may need to share this information with your doctor before coming to an agreement about what is best for you and your baby.

Dysphoric Milk Ejection Reflex (Bad Feelings While Nursing)

Some nursing mothers experience negative emotions beginning just before their milk lets down and continuing from several seconds to as long as a minute or two. This newly recognized syndrome, called dysphoric milk ejection reflex (D-MER), is apparently caused by a sudden drop in dopamine, a hormone and neurotransmitter.

Mothers with D-MER variously describe a sinking feeling in the stomach; a low mood; a brief feeling of hopelessness, depression, apprehension, or dread; "an urge to get away"; or simply "a yucky feeling." A few mothers experience feelings of impatience, frustration, agitation, or anger. The feelings quickly disappear after the milk releases but may recur as the milk lets down throughout the feeding.

D-MER is not postpartum depression or a psychological response to breastfeeding; it is a physiologic response. Happily, many things can help with this problem. Some women just distract themselves while nursing. Others get relief by keeping well hydrated, exercising, sleeping more, or taking small amounts of beverages with caffeine. Nutritional supplements such as omega-3 fatty acids and evening primrose oil may also relieve symptoms. The prescription antidepressant bupropion (the active ingredient in Wellbutrin) may be helpful as well. The website at www.d-mer.org is full of helpful information on managing D-MER.

Concerns about the Baby

Spitting Up and Vomiting

Spitting up small amounts of breast milk is common; some babies do this after almost every nursing. Recently, it has become common for doctors to diagnose these babies with gastroesophageal reflux, or GER (see "Fussiness, Colic, and Reflux," page 204).

Occasionally a baby may vomit what seems like an entire feeding. Although there may be no apparent cause, this can sometimes be traced to something the mother recently ate. Vomiting can also be a sign of infection. You will want to notify your doctor if the baby has a fever or if the vomiting continues.

When a baby continues vomiting forcefully after most feedings, you should suspect that either he is sensitive to something in your diet or he has pyloric stenosis, a muscular obstruction of the bottom part of the stomach that typically develops at about two to four weeks of age. It is thought to occur in 4 of every 1,000 babies. Although this condition is most common in first-born males, it can occur in females, and one study found it is more common in babies with an allergy to cow's milk. Typically the vomiting becomes progressively worse; the baby eventually stops gaining weight, or loses weight, and may become dehydrated. In the breastfed infant the condition may go undiagnosed longer than in the bottle-fed infant, since breast milk is digested much more easily than formula. The baby's weight may not be affected until the obstruction becomes nearly complete. Frequently, waves can be seen moving across the baby's lower abdomen from the left side to the right just after a feeding and prior to vomiting. X-rays confirm the diagnosis.

The obstruction is corrected with a relatively simple surgical procedure. Breastfeeding can resume within a few hours after the obstruction is removed. At this time breast milk is especially good for the baby because of its digestibility. Some mothers notice a temporary reduction in the milk supply after the baby's surgery. Rest, frequent nursing, and switching the baby from side to side during the feeding usually reverse this situation.

Pulling Away From the Breast

Babies pull off the breast while nursing for a variety of reasons. Often it is because they have had enough to eat or they need to be burped. If your baby has a cold, she may pull away because she is having trouble breathing through her nose. Try to position her so her head is more elevated during nursing. A warm-mist humidifier can be helpful in thinning nasal secretions, as can saline nose drops. You can also use the NoseFrida (see page 177) to remove excess nasal discharge from the baby's nostrils.

Some babies pull away from the breast gasping and choking as the milk suddenly lets down. This is usually a temporary problem; the baby gradually learns to keep up with the rapid flow of milk. In the meantime, positioning the baby differently may help. Try sitting the baby up, using the football hold, or lying on your back with the baby's head over you. You can also try laying the flat of your hand against the breast and pressing inward until the flow of milk seems to subside. Some mothers manually express or pump milk until the initial spray has subsided, but this could work against you by increasing the overall production of milk, which would strengthen the let-down response.

If your baby pulls away from the breast and cries or refuses to nurse, see "Refusal to Nurse," which follows.

Refusal to Nurse

If your baby pulls away from the breast crying or refuses to nurse, don't assume he is ready to wean. There are a number of possible reasons for such behavior, but when it persists, it can frequently be traced to certain foods in the mother's diet to which the baby is sensitive. Typically this behavior starts when the baby is about two weeks old. He may also act fussy and have very frequent, sometimes greenish stools. Other symptoms may include gassiness, redness around the rectum, a mild rash anywhere on the body, or a stuffy nose. Fussiness while nursing and refusal to nurse may occur sporadically or may increase as the day goes on. Although the baby refuses the breast, he may eagerly take breast milk from a bottle. The reasons for this are unclear.

Babies with gastroesophageal reflux also sometimes refuse to nurse. When accompanied by frequent spitting up and fussiness, refusal to nurse is most likely caused by a painful irritation of the esophagus.

A baby who has developed a yeast infection, or thrush, may also become fussy at the breast and refuse to nurse. Besides having a characteristic white coating on the insides of his lips, cheeks, or both, the baby with thrush may be gassy. There may also be a bright red, dotted or peeling rash around the baby's genitals or on your nipples. Your nipples may burn or itch.

Babies with ear infections also sometimes fuss at the breast and refuse to nurse. Although ear infections are less common in breast-fed than in formula-fed babies, especially in the first two months after birth, even in this period an ear infection may accompany or follow a runny nose.

Occasionally a baby will refuse to nurse because his mother is wearing perfume or a scented deodorant.

When a baby has been fed supplemental formula and the milk supply has lessened, he may lose interest in the breast, preferring the immediate flow from the bottle. He may fuss and cry when his mother tries to breast-feed him.

Treatment Measures When the Baby Refuses to Nurse

1. As long as your baby refuses to nurse, express your milk every two to three hours so your supply will not be affected. Use a clinical-grade rental pump or a near-clinical-grade personal pump (see Chapter 5). Feed the baby by bottle.

2. See the next section, "Fussiness, Colic, and Reflux."

3. Check your baby's mouth and your nipples for signs of thrush. See "Thrush Nipples," page 182.

4. If you can find no reason for your baby's irritability and refusal to nurse, have a doctor examine the baby.

Fussiness, Colic, and Reflux

You may be surprised to learn how much crying a baby can do and how uncomfortable it can make you feel. The sound of a baby's cry is intended to be distressing so adults will be alerted to his needs and answer them.

Many mothers tend to blame themselves for their babies' crying, wondering if their inexperience, nervous feelings, or milk supply is somehow responsible. Keep in mind that most babies fuss and seek out the comfort of the breast when they are tired, bored, lonely, or uncomfortable as well as when they are hungry, and that all babies have fussy periods during appetite spurts.

If you are worried that the baby is not getting enough milk, have him weighed. A weight gain of an ounce a day or more means your baby is getting enough milk (see "Underfeeding," page 218).

Some babies are extremely irritable during the early weeks, with periods of intense crying. If your baby's crying makes you feel that something is wrong, trust your instincts. By all means have your baby examined by your doctor.

Outlined below are common reasons that babies cry and suggestions for relieving their distress.

Missing the womb. Harvey Karp, a California pediatrician, theorizes that much of the fussing babies do in the early weeks results from missing the uterine environment. In *The Happiest Baby on the Block: The New Way to Calm Crying and Help Your Baby Sleep Longer*, Dr. Karp suggests that parents calm their babies through the five *S*s:

Swaddling. Many societies have used this technique to imitate the secure feeling of the womb during late pregnancy. A baby is wrapped tightly in a thin blanket with his arms at his sides. Securing the arms and hands keeps the baby from flailing them and makes him more receptive to the other four calming techniques.

To swaddle your baby, lay the blanket out flat, turn in a corner, and place the baby's neck on the folded edge. With the baby's right arm straightened at his side, pull the right corner of the blanket tightly over his body, and tuck it under his lower back on the left side. With his left arm straight at his side, pull the bottom corner of the blanket up over the right arm and shoulder and tuck the blanket under his right side; don't worry about scrunching the baby's legs. Now wrap the left side of the blanket snugly across his body.

Side or stomach position. Although it is now known that laying a baby to sleep on his stomach raises his risk of succumbing to sudden infant death syndrome (SIDS), laying a baby on his back tends to make him startle—to extend his arms and cry out as if he feels he is falling backward. To prevent startling—or the Moro reflex, as it is sometimes called—swaddle the baby and lay him down to sleep on his side, or let him rest on his stomach over your lap or shoulder.

Shushing. Loud white noise calms a baby because it sounds like the flow of blood from the placenta. The louder a baby cries, the louder the shushing he needs. Hair dryers and vacuum cleaners work as well as vocal shushing sounds.

Swinging. Swinging is also reminiscent of uterine life. The swinging should be in rapid, small movements back and forth with the baby face down across your lap. You can swing your baby by wearing him as you walk, by rocking him, or by using a baby swing after the baby is one month of age (see "Coping Measures for Fussiness, Colic, and Reflux," page 217).

Sucking. You can calm a baby who is upset but not hungry by either nursing or offering a pacifier. If your baby seems to need a great deal of comfort sucking, a pacifier may be appropriate. You can introduce one when your baby is between two and six weeks old. Before two weeks a pacifier could interfere with the establishment of breastfeeding, and after six weeks your baby might be much less willing to accept it.

Appetite spurts. You will probably notice that your baby is more fussy at around two to three weeks and again at around six weeks, when most babies experience appetite spurts. During an appetite spurt a baby nurses more frequently for a few days, and this stimulates an increase in milk production. Fussiness in the late afternoon or evening is typical.

The baby's temperament. Every baby is born with her own distinct personality. Some babies tend to be quiet, whereas others are more active. Some babies are highly sensitive to their surroundings and overreact to any sudden stimulation. They are tense, jumpy, and often fussy. They may go almost instantly from sleepy or calm to full-blown crying. Once crying, they may be difficult to soothe. Although some of these babies need to be carried around or entertained continually, others may actually resist being held or cuddled.

Learning how to mother a highly sensitive baby takes time and patience. You will soon develop a sense of what your baby enjoys and what she does not, how much stimulation she can tolerate and how to help her settle down. If your baby does not enjoy touching, try not to take it personally. With time and a gradual increase in physical closeness, she will eventually be able to tolerate and enjoy being held. Most babies outgrow their early fussy months and grow to be happy children.

Diaper rash. A baby may fuss a lot if she has a diaper rash. At each diaper change for an entire day, gently wash the baby's bottom and apply a zinc oxide ointment (such as Desitin). Expose the baby's bottom to the air as much as possible, and leave off disposable diapers or plastic pants. The rash should improve dramatically, unless it is caused by yeast (see the following section).

If the baby's stools are green, he may be reacting to certain foods in his mother's diet. See "Colic and Reflux," below.

Yeast infection. Although common in infants, yeast infections are frequently overlooked as the cause of excessive fussiness. A baby with a yeast infection usually shows signs in his mouth—on his inner lips or cheeks, and sometimes also on the tongue. This is known as thrush. The baby is typically very gassy, as the yeast is frequently present in the intestinal tract as well. The yeast may also cause a dotty, red rash or a peeling rash that resembles a mild burn, typically in the genital area. The mother's nipples are often reddened; they may show a rash, and they may itch or burn. One nipple may be more affected than the other.

Nystatin suspension (Mycostatin) is usually the drug of choice when a baby has a yeast infection. Because the nystatin is swallowed, the yeast in the bowel is usually eliminated. Sometimes, however, a diaper rash appears only *after* treatment with the oral medication, and in other cases a rash gets worse during the first few days of treatment. Nystatin ointment can be used to treat both the mother's nipples and the baby's diaper rash.

The other common oral medication, gentian violet, kills only yeast in the mouth and therefore is not recommended for the baby who is fussy and gassy, unless nystatin seems ineffective after several days of treatment.

See "Thrush Nipples," page 182, for a complete discussion of treatment measures for yeast infections.

Colic and reflux. Colic is a catchall term for unidentified infant discomfort characterized by periods of intense crying and apparent abdominal pain. Although the causes of colic have been much debated over the years, doctors have often dismissed it as something parents must simply endure until the baby is three to four months old, when the symptoms are expected to lessen or disappear. In the meantime, the baby is unhappy, and her mother may wonder if breastfeeding is to blame.

Recently, many babies who might in the past have been labeled colicky have been diagnosed instead with gastroesophageal reflux, which is also called GER or simply reflux. Reflux is the backward movement of food and acid from the stomach into the esophagus and sometimes into the mouth and out onto your shirt. Nearly all babies have episodes of reflux; most parents consider it normal for their babies to "burp up" after feedings. Some babies who regurgitate frequently show no apparent discomfort. Others, however, seem to suffer painful heartburn, even if they don't spit up their milk.

The main reason babies spit up is that the lower esophageal sphincter isn't fully developed in infants. Also, babies take in a lot of milk relative to the size of their stomachs, and many also swallow a lot of air when they nurse or suck on a pacifier. When the baby burps, milk may come up with the air.

Breastfed babies generally have fewer and less severe episodes of reflux than bottle-fed babies. Sucking at the breast triggers peristaltic waves along the gastrointestinal tract; these muscular contractions help move the milk down into the stomach and on to the small intestine. Also, human milk digests more completely and almost twice as fast as formula. The less time the milk spends in the stomach, the less opportunity there is for it to acidify before backing up into the esophagus. In addition, breastfed babies are generally fed in a more upright position than bottle-fed babies. Gravity may help to keep the milk and gastric acid in the stomach, where they belong.

Still, breastfed babies can suffer painful reflux. Symptoms of this problem can include sudden or inconsolable crying, arching of the back during feedings, refusing the breast or bottle, frequent burping or hiccuping, bad breath, gagging or choking, frequent throat inflammation, poor sleep patterns, slow weight gain, frequent ear infections, and, less commonly, respiratory problems—wheezing, labored breathing, asthma, bronchitis, pneumonia, and apnea.

Some babies with reflux want to nurse all the time and therefore may grow very fast, although it may seem as if they spit up all the milk they take in. On the way down breast milk is very soothing, as is sucking itself. But if a baby overfills her stomach, her reflux symptoms can worsen. For such a baby, it may be helpful to nurse on one breast at a time; the slower flow of milk may soothe the baby's heartburn without overfilling her stomach. Some mothers have reported that pacifiers help such babies.

Other babies with reflux seem to find nursing painful. They not only cry after and in between feedings, but they fuss at the breast and sometimes refuse nursings altogether. Oddly enough, they may take the same milk from a bottle that they wouldn't take from the breast.

Many parents try to minimize reflux by keeping their babies upright or semi-upright for 30 to 45 minutes after feedings. Recent research has found, however, that putting a baby in an infant seat (elevated to 60 degrees) actually increases reflux. Reflux is reduced, the studies have found, when the baby is laid on her left side or on her stomach. But putting babies to sleep on their stomachs has been associated with a higher rate of sudden infant death syndrome (SIDS). Perhaps the best idea is to carry the baby on her left side in a sling, both to minimize reflux and to soothe the baby with the motion of your body. You might also try laying the baby stomach-down on your forearm; parents say that the pressure on the belly seems to be soothing.

Jostling or other rough or fast movement of a baby after feeding may add to the problem of reflux. Burp the baby before switching breasts, but don't jiggle her. Just hold her over your shoulder or sit her upright, and pat her back gently. Let her suck at the breast until she falls asleep.

Some babies seem to suffer more with lower belly discomfort than with regurgitation and heartburn. Besides crying, these babies' symptoms may include gassiness; stools that are very frequent or green, mucous, or even bloody; and redness around the rectum. A baby may have a stuffy nose or a rash on her face or upper body. She may want to nurse all the time.

Although streaks of blood in a baby's stool or diaper rarely indicate an emergency, for a parent they are alarming, and when they appear, it's a good idea to call the baby's doctor. In most cases, however, blood in the stool results from either an anal fissure or a food intolerance. An anal fissure—that is, a small tear in the anus—usually results from constipation and straining during a bowel movement. Since exclusively breastfed babies cannot be constipated, anal fissures are unusual for them. A sensitivity or allergy to something in your diet is the more likely cause. Some doctors may say that a baby with bloody stools should be temporarily weaned from the breast and fed hypoallergenic formula instead of breast milk, but this is usually unnecessary. In most cases, the bleeding stops after the mother removes the offending food from her diet and the baby's gut has time to heal.

Something in your diet. Whether or not your baby has bloody stools, if she exhibits colic or severe reflux symptoms every day or nearly every day, you should try writing down everything you have eaten and drunk during the past three days. Include any nutritional supplements or medications. Make notes, too, of any particularly fussy periods the baby has had during the past three days. If you are producing a lot of milk, also have your baby weighed to see how fast she is gaining. A baby who is gaining much more than an ounce a day may be having symptoms of what I call hyperlactation syndrome, which is described on page 214.

Most foods that bother breastfeeding babies, as either intestinal irritants or allergens, fall into one of several major food categories. When a baby has been fussy at particular times, a suspect food can often be identified by looking back one to two meal periods or about two to six hours back. If eating chocolate, say, seems to cause your baby's symptoms, you can try giving up chocolate and see if she does better. But because more than one food may be making your baby fussy, you might be wise to avoid all of the commonly offending foods for a while, and then reintroduce them to your diet one by one. This way, you'll know exactly what bothers your baby.

Completely eliminating all of the following foods for three days may bring speedy relief to your fussy baby. Be sure to check the ingredients in any commercially processed food before eating or drinking it.

- *Chocolate and spices.* The major offender in chocolate is theobromide; even in small amounts, this ingredient is a potent irritant in the digestive tract of many infants. In the example given on page 212, the chocolate frozen yogurt was probably responsible for this baby's (and mother's) difficult night. Many spices and other strong flavorings, including cinnamon, chiles, garlic, and curry, can also bother young infants.

- *Citrus.* A frequently overlooked cause of digestive disturbances is citrus fruits and their juices. Oranges, lemons, limes, tangerines, and grapefruits can all bother a baby's intestines. Other strongly acidic fruits, such as pineapples, kiwis, and strawberries, affect many babies similarly. In the chart, the mother had grapefruit juice at breakfast and pineapple juice in the afternoon. Her baby may have been bothered by these.

- *Gas-producing vegetables.* Certain vegetables can also cause temporary digestive problems for young babies. These include onions, broccoli, cauliflower, Brussels sprouts, cabbage, bell peppers, and cucumbers. Prepared mustard can cause a similar reaction. Onions, an ingredient in so many dishes, can cause gastric upset for a baby even when they are cooked, ingested in small amounts, or eaten as onion powder. The stir-fry dish in the chart contained one of these offending foods.

- *Cow's milk.* Some infants are allergic to cow's milk and cow's milk products, including cheese, yogurt, sour cream, cottage cheese, and ice cream. Researchers have estimated that nearly half of all cases of severe reflux and colic are associated with an allergy to cow's milk. If a baby is truly allergic to cow's milk products, cutting back on milk will probably not eliminate the baby's symptoms. You must eliminate from your diet all dairy products, including those in commercially processed foods like creamed soups, certain types of salad dressings, and puddings; cow's milk may be identified as "casein" or "whey" on the label. You should not feed the baby any infant formula made from cow's milk. The baby in the chart may or may not be reacting to dairy products.

THURSDAY	
8:30 a.m. Grapefruit juice Prenatal vitamin Granola with milk Toast with butter	10:30 a.m.–12:00 noon Fussy, spitting up
12:15 p.m. Roast beef and cheese sandwich, with mayonnaise and lettuce Potato chips Milk	2:00 p.m.–5:00 p.m. Crying
3:00 p.m. Pineapple juice	
6:45 p.m. Chicken–green pepper stir-fry Spinach and mushroom salad, Italian dressing Rice Milk	
8:15 p.m. Chocolate frozen yogurt	11:30 p.m.–2:00 a.m. Very fussy, vomited

Sample chart of a mother's diet and her baby's reactions

If possible, do without certain medications and dietary supplements while you're avoiding these four food categories. Laxatives taken by a nursing mother can disturb her baby's intestinal tract. Aspirin and the chemical phenylpropanolamine, a decongestant, can make a baby fussy; both of these drugs are in many headache and cold remedies. Certain dietary supplements taken by the mother or given directly to the baby, such as vitamin C, brewer's yeast, and fluoride, have been known to cause colic symptoms. Fluoride is very helpful in preventing cavities, but it is best delayed until the baby is six months old and need be given only if your water supply contains less than 0.3 parts per million.

During the three days of eliminating all the commonly offending foods from your diet, write down what you eat and drink along with observations of your baby. If the baby has particularly difficult times, look back one to two meal periods, or about two to six hours before the symptoms began, and try to identify any suspect foods. You may find that you ate something forbidden without realizing it, or perhaps another food seems to be at fault. Other foods that can cause reactions include tomatoes, eggs, peanuts and peanut butter, corn and corn syrup, wheat (in breads, crackers, cookies, cakes, and noodles), soy (the basis of some infant formulas and an ingredient in many processed foods), apples, and bananas. If you decide to eliminate any one of these foods, you should continue to avoid the original four food categories, too. More than one food group may be affecting your baby.

If your baby is much better after the three days and having very few fussy periods or other symptoms, try adding milk products back into your diet. Have a lot of milk products early in the day and then watch the baby for 24 hours. If the baby reacts, avoid milk products completely for the next couple of days.

After this period, you might experiment with small amounts of milk, cheese, yogurt, or ice cream to see which of these, if any, your baby can tolerate, and in what quantity. Although some babies cannot tolerate any milk products, others do fine when their mothers have hard cheese, and some can tolerate small amounts of any milk products as long as their mothers take them only once every few days. (If you must cut dairy products from your diet completely, be sure you are taking sufficient calcium in another form; see page 161).

After you have established which dairy products are safe, and in what quantity, add another food category to your diet every few days. Eat a lot of the food in question. If the fussiness recurs, eliminate the offending food category from your diet again. Continue adding food categories until you have tested all the foods that you had eliminated. Again, more than one food may be a problem for a very sensitive baby.

Hyperlactation syndrome. Researchers have also identified a kind of colic that is characterized by gassiness, frequent stools, spitting up, and general discomfort and fussiness (Woolridge and Fisher, 1988). Although these babies may seem to be sensitive to something in their mother's diet, they show little or no improvement with the elimination of suspect foods and beverages. Typically these babies nurse frequently from both breasts and are gaining more than an ounce per day. Their mothers often have overabundant milk supplies.

Some lactation professionals refer to these symptoms as overactive let-down syndrome. I don't think that let-down is really the problem. More likely, the underlying cause of the colic is the baby's dispropor-tionate intake of low-fat foremilk, the milk that is available early in the feeding. When a baby consumes large amounts of foremilk and little of the fatty hindmilk, his stomach rapidly empties, dumping excess lactose into the bowel. This results in increased gas and colic symptoms.

Relief is achieved by getting the baby to empty one breast at each feeding so that he receives not only the foremilk but the fatty hindmilk, too. Allow the baby to nurse from the first breast until he spontaneously pulls away satisfied; do not interrupt the feeding at any point to switch the baby to the second breast. If this doesn't help, try limiting the baby to one side for one and a half to two hours before nursing on the other side. Some lactation professionals advise limiting the baby to the same breast for several feedings in a row until the colic subsides, but I feel that this is unnecessary. Keeping the baby at just one side per feeding should solve the problem.

Treatments and tests for colic. Because tests for colic are invasive, many doctors treat the problem without testing for it. They choose from three kinds of pharmaceutical drugs. First are antacids, which neutral-ize stomach acid without known side effects. Among these, Mylanta and Mylicon are best known for colic and are available over the counter. They contain simethicone, an anti-foaming agent intended to reduce bloating, discomfort, and pain caused by excess gas in the stomach or intestines. The drops are given right after feedings. Rarely do they seem to help.

Second among kinds of drugs for reflux are those that suppress acid production in the stomach. These include cimetidine (Tagamet), famotidine (Pepcid), nizatidine (Axid), ranitidine (Zantac), and the "acid blockers." Medications in the last group prevent any acid production at all. Among these, omeprazole (Prilosec) and lanseprazole (Prevacid) are approved for use in children, although others are sometimes prescribed. Since not all infants react in the same way to these drugs, you may have to try several before you find one that works well. It may take about two weeks before you can tell whether a particular drug works.

The third group of medications prescribed for reflux increase motility—that is, they improve the muscle tone of the digestive tract to keep food moving through it. These medications are more helpful in older babies who are eating solid foods; exclusively breastfed babies generally have fast digestion. Bethanechol (Urecholine), erythromycin, and metoclopramide (Reglan) are the motility drugs currently used in the United States. They can cause gastric cramping and diarrhea. Long-term use of metoclopramide in children (that is, over a period of weeks) hasn't been well studied; in fact, there are concerns about its long-term use in adults.

Some mothers turn not to pharmaceutical drugs to ease their babies' colic symptoms but to old-fashioned "gripe water," which has been marketed since the mid-nineteenth century and is today used around the world. There are many brands of gripe water, but they are similarly formulated; most contain different herbs, and some contain sodium bicarbonate. Although some mothers feel that gripe water has helped their fussy babies, a study published in the *New England Journal of Medicine* found it generally ineffective against colic symptoms.

A new approach to treating colicky babies uses "good" bacteria, or probiotics. In a study published in *Pediatrics* (Savino et al., 2007), exclusively breastfed infants with colic symptoms who were treated with *Lactobacillus reuteri* improved within seven days of the start of treatment. At the end of one month, they had reduced their average crying time by 95 percent. During the same period, colicky breastfed babies treated with simethicone reduced their crying time by only 7 percent. By changing the balance of bacteria in the intestinal tract, researchers speculate, probiotic supplementation may reduce the effects of both gastrointestinal infection and allergic disease. Other studies suggest that *L. reuteri* inhibits pain by reducing the sensitivity of nerves in the intestinal tract.

The probiotics used in the 2007 study were produced by BioGaia, a Swedish company. These drops have been purchased by Gerber and are now called Gerber Soothe Colic Drops. You can find more information about these drops in Appendix A, page 366.

Medical tests for reflux and other digestive disorders are rarely advised unless the baby shows signs of poor growth, severe choking, or lung disease. In such a case, the best test for severe reflux is the pH probe, in which a tube is put down the baby's throat to measure the acid level at the bottom of the esophagus. Less invasive is the barium swallow, in which the baby drinks a barium mixture, an X-ray is taken, and then the X-ray is examined for any blockage or narrowing of the stomach valves that may be causing or aggravating the condition. The X-ray, however, will not identify whether a baby's stomach contents are more acidic than normal or if the esophagus has been damaged by reflux. Damage to the esophagus is determined through a more invasive procedure, endoscopy with biopsy. All of these tests should be used cautiously; they do

Cereal for Colic?

Some doctors recommend thickening milk with cereal for babies who suffer with reflux or colic, on the theory that heavier food stays down better. But there is no proof that this helps; in fact, adding cereal to a baby's milk may slow the emptying of her stomach, increase episodes of reflux, and possibly cause choking. Regurgitated solids are more irritating than regurgitated human milk, and if bits of cereal are aspirated into a baby's lungs, they can cause pneumonia. Besides, cereal replaces rather than supplements breast milk in a baby's diet, and it can thus cause a decrease in the milk supply. Since many babies with severe reflux or colic have allergies, introducing cereal to them early can lead to fussing at the breast, refusal to nurse, and early weaning.

not always provide conclusive results, and they are stressful for both the baby and her parents.

When nothing works. Whether your baby has painful reflux or other colic symptoms, the extreme stress of caring for her may make you consider another feeding method in hopes that the symptoms will lessen. Keep in mind that these conditions usually improve without any such change. Switching to formula, in fact, might well make the problem worse instead of better. Continuing to breastfeed will provide important health benefits for both you and your baby and, most important, a strong bond that can help you both get through this difficult time.

Needless to say, a baby with colic or severe reflux may sleep poorly and fuss a great deal. Your baby may need to be held upright most of the time. She may deprive you of sleep and, by refusing the breast, make you feel rejected. The risks of postpartum depression and even child abuse are higher when a baby has severe reflux or colic. Since this can be a very challenging period even for the most stable family, it is important that you get emotional support, find practical help, and limit your commitments until the problem passes.

Coping Measures for Fussiness, Colic, and Reflux

1. Offer your breast—it is a source of comfort as well as nourishment for your baby.

2. Try a pacifier. Pacifiers are soothing to many babies who need a lot of extra sucking, who are fussy, or who have difficulty calming themselves. If your baby won't take a pacifier at first, try different kinds.

3. Be sure to burp your baby frequently while he nurses or sucks on a pacifier.

4. Try swaddling your baby tightly in a light blanket.

5. Soothe both yourself and the baby with a warm bath.

6. Most babies love motion. Try walking or using a baby pack, sling, or stroller. Rocking can also be comforting—borrow a rocking

chair if you don't already have one. Most babies are lulled to sleep by car rides.

7. White noise may calm a crying baby. Try helping him sleep by turning on a radio or a recording of a humming car or vacuum cleaner, or by placing an aquarium near the baby's bed. Or put on a white-noise CD (see Appendix A, page 366). White noise should be quiet, as recent studies have revealed hearing loss in infants exposed to loud white noise.

8. Consider sleeping with the baby, if you aren't doing so already.

9. Consider purchasing infant probiotics, specifically Gerber's Soothe Colic Drops, and give five drops once a day.

10. Take a short break from the baby each day. Your partner might play with him while you take a bath, go for a walk, or visit a friend.

11. Find another mother who has a fussy baby. There's nothing like a friend who really understands. You might also visit www.colicsupport.com, a website for parents with colicky babies.

Underfeeding

For any number of reasons, you may wonder if your baby is getting enough to eat. He may seem to be nursing all the time, or he may seem especially fussy. Most young infants want to nurse 8 to 12 times in each 24-hour period. Nursing this often is normal and seldom reflects a poor milk supply. You can't tell whether your baby is getting enough breast milk by offering him a supplemental bottle of water or formula after nursing. Most babies will take 1 to 2 ounces if it is offered, even when they have had enough milk from the breasts.

The baby is probably getting enough milk if

- he is nursing at least eight times in a 24-hour period,
- he is nursing for 10 to 45 minutes at each feeding and seems content after feedings,
- he has several periods of swallowing during each feeding,
- your breasts feel softer or lighter after the baby has nursed, and

- your baby is having bowel movements every day during the first month.

If any of these statements isn't true of your baby, have him weighed. Even if all are true, have your baby weighed if you need reassurance. The nurse in your pediatrician's office should be happy to do this for you.

Between the fifth day and the end of the third month after birth, a baby should gain an ounce every day. A weight gain of an ounce a day reflects an adequate milk intake. If your baby was weighed at any time after the fifth day, you can see whether he has gained enough by weighing him again now. If he hasn't been weighed since the fifth day, consider that by 10 to 14 days of age most babies have regained their birth weight. If your baby is two weeks old and weighs less than his birth weight, he probably needs more milk. If your baby is two weeks old and weighs more than his birth weight, he is probably getting plenty of milk, unless the baby is being supplemented. If you have any doubt about how much the baby is gaining, weigh him.

Inadequate weight gain usually occurs when a baby has had trouble latching on or nursing vigorously during the period of initial engorgement in the first week, or when nursing has been infrequent. Underfeeding often occurs among the group of mothers and babies described under "Babies Who May Not Get Enough," page 57. This problem can also occur when a newborn has a faulty suck (see "Sucking Problems," page 102), is tongue-tied, or has a high palate; when a mother has used a nipple shield over her nipple for nursing (see page 85); and, certainly, when a baby is sick. Some laxatives, when taken by the mother, can cause a baby to have excessive bowel movements and to lose weight or gain too slowly even if he is taking enough milk. A baby who gains weight slowly or not at all after gaining well at first may be suffering with painful reflux. Some babies with reflux limit their milk intake because of the discomfort of heartburn (see "Fussiness, Colic, and Reflux," page 204).

Usually a baby's failure to latch on or suck well during the early weeks quickly leads to low milk production. The solution is to build the milk supply by pumping after nursing, and to feed the baby the expressed milk along with any necessary formula.

Treatment Measures for Underfeeding

1. If possible, see a lactation professional. Your insurance provider should cover all the costs.

2. To estimate the amount of milk you are producing and to increase your milk supply, rent a clinical-grade breast pump. Any other pump may not be adequate for accurately estimating milk production and may be less helpful in increasing your milk supply.

3. Estimate your milk production by pumping your breasts instead of nursing. If you are pumping one breast at a time, pump each twice, for a total pumping time of 20 to 25 minutes. If you have a double-pump kit, use it for a total of 12 to 20 minutes. Feed this milk and any necessary formula to your baby. (See Chapter 5 for guidelines on expressing milk and Appendix B, page 370, to determine how much milk your baby needs at each feeding.)

   Exactly two hours after completing the first pumping, pump again. This time you may get less milk than in the first pumping. Multiply the number of ounces collected at this *second* pumping by 12. This will give you an estimate of how much milk you are producing over a 24-hour period; if you collected 1½ ounces, for example, you are producing about 18 ounces per day.

   Now you can compare the baby's daily milk requirement, as listed in Appendix B, with your milk production. For example, if you estimate that your baby needs 21.4 ounces per day and your milk production is 18 ounces per day, the baby needs about 3½ ounces of formula per day until your milk production increases.

   If you determine that you have enough milk for your baby and yet he has not been gaining well, it may be that he is not taking all of the milk available at some or many of his feedings. This can happen with newborns who were born prematurely, who tend to drift off to sleep while nursing, who have sucking difficulties, or who suffer with painful reflux. In such a case, you'll still want to take the steps that follow, feeding your baby expressed breast milk (rather than formula) after nursing until his feeding skill improves.

4. After you have estimated your milk production, go back to nursing your baby at least eight times in every 24 hours. This may mean waking him for feedings. Nurse him every two to two and a half hours during the day and evening (counting from the start of one nursing to the start of the next) and every three to four hours in the night, for 10 to 15 minutes on each breast. (I suggest limiting the nursing to this amount of time so that the entire nursing-pumping-supplementing session can be completed in 40 to 50 minutes.) Frequent short nursings are more effective in increasing milk production than infrequent lengthy ones. Be sure to observe the baby for swallowing. If the baby is sucking but not swallowing milk, gently compress your breast to get the baby to take more milk.

5. Pump your breasts right after each nursing to stimulate further milk production. If you're pumping one breast at a time, pump for 5 minutes on each side, and then pump each breast a second time for a few minutes. Pumping both breasts at once not only takes less time but increases milk production faster. Use a double-pump kit for 5 to 10 minutes after nursing.

6. Right after pumping, offer the baby whatever breast milk you've collected along with any necessary formula. If the baby needs supplemental formula, divide the total amount needed by the number of feedings the baby is getting each day (usually eight). For example, the baby needing 3½ ounces of formula could take a bit less than ½ ounce after each of his eight daily nursings. The goal is to offer about the same amount of milk and formula at each feeding so that he wants to nurse at regular intervals.

Many lactation consultants, fearing the bottle would interfere with the baby's ability at the breast, suggest that a baby be fed supplements with a nursing supplementer (see page 362), cup, eyedropper, or soft tube taped onto the parent's finger. If one of these methods is recommended to you and it works well, then continue with it. But if you find it too frustrating or time-consuming, use a bottle. After the first few days of nursing, using a bottle for supplemental feedings rarely causes latch-on or sucking problems.

7. To stimulate even greater milk production, try fenugreek capsules, blessed thistle capsules, or More Milk Plus capsules or tincture (see page 72). Go-Lacta is another herbal remedy for low milk supply and can be used with other herbs as well. There has been only one study on this herb that showed an increase in production, but some lactation consultants who recommend it in the United States are seeing good results (Estrella et al., 2000). (See page 363 for information on ordering Go-Lacta.)

8. Some mothers are told to drink a beer or two to help increase milk production. This is an old wives' tale; in fact, drinking beer can lessen milk production.

9. Weigh your baby every few days to be sure that he is gaining well. After each weighing, re-estimate his milk needs, since as he gains weight, his milk needs will increase. Re-estimate your milk production, too. Two hours after your last pumping, use the breast pump instead of nursing, and figure your milk production as explained in step 3. Hopefully your milk production will have increased enough that you can decrease or even eliminate any formula supplementation.

10. If you find that the herbs listed in step 7 do little to increase your milk production, consider using domperidone (see page 112).

11. Once your baby is gaining well, his nursing seems more vigorous, and he is receiving supplements only of your breast milk, try eliminating some of the supplement. For a few days, offer half of the milk that you are expressing to the baby, and freeze the rest. If the baby continues to gain well, keep pumping, but don't offer the baby any of the pumped milk. Once the baby is gaining an ounce a day without any supplement, you can gradually stop pumping. Continue to have your baby weighed weekly.

If treatment fails. Although the technique just described usually ensures a weight-gaining baby and higher milk production within several days, occasionally these measures won't work. Sometimes, when breast engorgement has been severe and little milk has been removed during the first week, the decline in milk production is difficult to reverse.

In unusual instances, a mother simply cannot produce enough milk. This sometimes happens to women who have had breast surgery, particularly when the surgical incision is around the areola (see "Nursing after Breast Surgery," page 119), or who have insufficient glandular (milk-producing) tissue, or "hypoplastic" breasts (see page 116). Mothers with polycystic ovary syndrome, or PCOS (see page 119), and mothers with retained placental fragments (see page 70) may also struggle with low milk supply.

In any of these situations, lack of support from family, friends, and health professionals can only make matters worse. But even with all of the best information and support, things sometimes don't turn out as we hope. If you have given nursing your best but finally end up having to bottle-feed, you have not failed as a mother. Be proud of your efforts to nurse, and concentrate on providing your baby with all of the cuddling and loving that you can.

Some mothers who can't produce enough milk have found that continuing to nurse with a nursing supplementer has been a rewarding, worthwhile experience. Others have found these devices to be cumbersome and frustrating.

Another option, particularly if the baby has become frustrated at the breast, is to first bottle-feed and then nurse. "Comfort nursing"—nursing after or between bottle-feedings, or during the night—may be a pleasant experience for both mother and baby.

Detailed information about formula and bottle-feeding can be found in *The Nursing Mother's Guide to Weaning* (see "Suggested Supplemental Reading," page 414).

EXPRESSING, STORING, AND FEEDING BREAST MILK

- Expression Methods
- Expressing Milk for Occasional Separations
- Expressing Milk Before Returning to Work
- Expressing Milk at Work
- Insurance Pumping
- Expressing Milk for a Baby Who Cannot Nurse
- Pumping Exclusively
- Increasing Your Milk Supply while Pumping
- Collecting and Storing Your Breast Milk
- Feeding Your Expressed Milk
- A Review of Breast Pump Models

T HERE ARE A VARIETY OF SITUATIONS in which mothers express milk for their babies. Some mothers, because of complications, need to express their milk full-time during the early days or weeks after birth; those who are struggling with latch-on difficulties or sore nipples, or whose babies are too premature or sick to breastfeed, may find themselves in this situation. Other mothers breastfeed full-time but need to do "insurance pumping" after nursings to maintain or increase milk production and to provide supplemental milk to their infants. Some mothers, for reasons of their own, exclusively express milk and bottle-feed it to their babies by choice. Some mothers express milk only for occasional separations. And, of course, many mothers who return to the workplace express their milk, not only to feed their babies when they are apart but also to maintain their production.

Expression Methods

Hand Expression

Although few mothers today consider regularly expressing their milk by hand, manual expression is a technique that every nursing mother should learn. If you need to express colostrum for a newborn, before mature milk production begins, you may well obtain more by using your hands than by using a pump, partly because the tiny amounts of colostrum produced in the hours following birth can get lost in the plastic parts of a pump. After milk production begins, hand expression can soften your breasts so the baby can latch on more easily. If you begin using a pump regularly, doing some hand expression after each pumping can be a good way to ensure complete drainage of the breast and maximize your milk production. And if pump parts get misplaced, batteries die, electricity goes out, your pump breaks, or you find yourself missing a feeding unexpectedly, hand expression may become a necessity.

When a mother is initiating lactation without a nursing baby, pumping and hand expression combined bring in higher volumes of milk than relying solely on a pump. Dr. Jane Morton of Stanford University has created a short video that shows how to use hand expression to collect more colostrum for a newborn who can't yet breastfeed. You can find this video at http://newborns.stanford.edu/Breastfeeding/HandExpression.html. With several practice sessions, most mothers can master manual expression. You might practice on the free side while nursing, after the baby stimulates the milk to let down. Place a towel in front of you to catch the spray as you get started. Or practice while standing in the shower.

To start, position the pads of your thumb and index finger 1 to 1½ inches behind the nipple directly across from each other. Gently press your fingers straight back toward your chest and then together. Relax your fingers, and then repeat these motions several times. Avoid sliding your fingers away from their original position. Once you have the motion down, rotate your fingers around the nipple to empty other areas of the breast.

When using hand expression, catch the milk in a cup or any other clean container.

The Hygeia milk expression cup

If you begin expressing milk when you're away from the baby, you will probably find that a few minutes of gentle breast massage will help the milk to let down. You can catch the milk in any clean container, but you might prefer a contoured cup specifically designed for the purpose (for purchasing information, see Appendix A, page 362). To get more milk, switch back and forth from one side to the other as soon as you notice the flow lessening. You may be able to save time by expressing milk from both breasts at once, into containers on a table in front of you. Once you have learned the technique, the whole process should take about 20 minutes.

Some mothers actually come to prefer hand expression to pumping. They feel that expressing milk by hand is quieter, more natural, and more convenient than using a pump.

Pumping

Mothers today are purchasing pumps in record numbers. This is mainly because so many women are returning to work or school within months of giving birth. But even many women who are planning to stay home with their babies see a pump as a necessity, for occasional separations or to allow their partners to participate in feedings.

The great variety of breast pumps available today makes choosing the right pump difficult. I divide pumps into four categories:

- clinical-grade (rental) pumps,
- personal-use pumps,

- single electric or battery-operated pumps, and
- hand-operated pumps.

The best pump for you depends partially on how much time you'll be spending away from your baby. If you'll be separated from the baby only occasionally, hand expression or an inexpensive battery- or manually operated pump may be most economical. If you'll be working away from home, say, one and a half days a week, an inexpensive pump may still suffice. If you'll be working full-time, or near full-time, you could find your supply dropping with an ineffective pump. You may want not only a higher-speed, stronger pump but one that will save you time by allowing you to express milk from both breasts at once.

When a full-time worker buys a pump according to price rather than quality, she often finds that her pump is so inefficient that it's useless. Its cycling—the speed at which the pump pulls and releases—is too slow, its suction pressure is too low, or both. She finds she cannot express very much milk. If she uses the pump regularly or often, her milk production may suffer.

The efficiency of a pump depends on two factors: its cycling speed and its suction pressure. The ideal cycling speed is 48 to 60 times per minute. The suction pressure of breast pumps is measured by the movement of mercury in a hydrostatic gauge. The pressure should reach at least 240 millimeters of mercury.

A mother who buys an inefficient pump may not notice the problem at first. Some mothers let down milk easily with nearly any pump in the early days, weeks, or even months, but often after a time a pump seems to lose efficiency. Usually, the efficiency of the pump hasn't changed, but the mother has come to need higher speed and suction.

Sometimes a mother assumes that if she can't pump much milk, she must not be producing much. She worries that she is underfeeding her baby, and she may work at increasing production, when in fact her baby is taking plenty of milk at the breast.

When a mother figures out, sooner or later, that her pump is inefficient, she often has to purchase a second, higher-grade pump, and so she ends up spending more than she would have if she had bought a good pump in the first place. Keep in mind that a high-quality pump is much cheaper than a couple of months' worth of baby formula.

A high price tag, however, is no guarantee that a pump is high-performing. As you will learn later in this chapter, the quality of pumps varies greatly within a particular price range. If you are sure you want to purchase a pump, start by determining the category of pump you need, and then identify a high-quality model within that category. This chapter will help you do just that. If you need extra help, a lactation professional can guide you to the best pump for your situation.

When's the right time to get a pump? Many women do so during pregnancy, but keep in mind that you won't be using your pump until after the baby is nursing well. (If you need a pump in the early days, because of breastfeeding complications, I strongly recommend renting a clinical-grade pump.) You can begin pumping after the first 7 to 14 days post partum, as your milk supply will most likely be well established by then. Pumping on a regular basis prior to this may cause an oversupply, which can lead to other problems like plugged milk ducts or colic symptoms if the baby is drinking from both breasts and taking in more of the low-fat foremilk than the fatty hindmilk.

Most mothers naturally have more milk during the night and in the morning, so I think that one of the best times to express extra milk is during the morning hours, right after nursing. Pumping in between nursings can be taking some of your baby's next feeding. When you pump in the morning after feeding the baby at the breast, you will most likely get just an ounce or two. But by doing this every day, or nearly every day, your freezer will fill up quickly.

Most young babies will need about 3 ounces per feeding in your absence. So when you pump, place the milk in the back of the refrigerator; when you get 3 ounces, combine the cold milk and then store it in the freezer. Older babies usually need 3 or 4 ounces per feeding. See page 250 for information on milk storage.

Just before the baby is a month old, you'll want to start giving bottle-feedings, of an ounce or so every few days, so that your baby will continue to accept the bottle.

Getting a Pump through Your Insurance Carrier

You may know that the Affordable Care Act (ACA) now mandates that mothers covered by private insurance are entitled to breastfeeding support and breastfeeding supplies, including breast pumps. This was signed into law in 2010, and most insurance plans began implementing this coverage on or after August 2012.

Getting a pump from your insurance company can be a bit complicated, but here is some information that can help you. While every plan is different, know that many insurance carriers are still establishing their coverage policies. Unfortunately, there is a great deal of variation in what sorts of pumps are covered, and how they are covered. Because the law's recommendations aren't very specific, coverage varies from insurance company to insurance company. Most plans require women to obtain the pumps from designated vendors, which may or may not offer the pump that a woman hopes for, and that means a mother usually can't simply buy a pump at retail and submit a receipt for reimbursement. Some plans cover only the purchase of cheap manual pumps that may not be effective enough, especially for mothers returning to the workplace. Also, know that there is no co-pay for your breast pump as long as you deal with an in-network provider. Your insurance company will either list these preferred contracted providers on their website, or you can call them for the list. Going out-of-network will usually result in out-of-pocket expenses and less recourse if you are unsatisfied.

Unfortunately, at this time, about a third of insurance plans are "grandfathered" out of having to comply with the ACA because they were purchased before the legislation went into effect. These plans don't have to follow the ACA rules and regulations or offer the same benefits, rights, and protections as new plans. But if the insurance carrier changes any language in its plan, it must then comply with the ACA.

When speaking with your insurance company, talk to them about what you want and need. Some companies offer a double collection electric pump within two months after giving birth, but may offer only a hand pump after two months post partum and up to a year after delivery. Be sure to ask your provider what your "ordering window" is—that is, when you are eligible to place your order and when the coverage ends. Mothers are eligible for a pump only every three years, but you may be eligible for a new collection kit or other parts.

Most insurance carriers refuse to cover clinical-grade rental pumps, which may be needed soon after birth to help mothers establish adequate milk flow because of a sick or premature baby or a breastfeeding complication, like low milk supply. If your insurance carrier does cover one, a written prescription from your baby's doctor and preauthorization is usually necessary. For mothers who need a hospital-grade pump, some insurance companies will cover a standard rental up to the value of the purchase price. In some of these cases, depending on how long the pump is needed, the insurance carrier could actually purchase the breast pump for the mother. The breast pumps must be purchased through a medical equipment company that the insurance company contracts with.

While you are pregnant, try to educate yourself about the many pumps on the market. Later in this chapter, I have included a thorough review of most of the pumps on the market, indicating which ones are commonly offered by insurance carriers, and which get good, mixed, or poor reviews by both mothers and lactation consultants (including myself). It is not too early to contact your insurance provider to see what pumps their durable medical equipment (DME) companies offer to nursing mothers before your baby comes. In this way, you will know which are higher-quality pumps.

Most insurance providers will require you to get your pump from an in-network DME company that they contract with. One recent review of insurance companies revealed that few of them allow mothers to upgrade to a better pump, even if the mother is willing to pay the difference. Some insurance companies without a contracted DME may be flexible if the pump you want isn't available, letting you choose another pump or, rarely, reimbursing your purchase from a retail store. Again, you need to ask for what you want! Because pump benefits vary from company to company, you will need to contact your insurance provider, using the number on the back of your insurance card. The National Women's Law Center can help you if your plan is denying you benefits, unless they are "grandfathered" out. They can be reached by phone at 866-745-5487 or by email at prevention@nwlc.org.

Unfortunately, coverage for lactation services and breast pumps does not cover all women who receive Medicaid or WIC benefits. Twenty-nine states are complying with the Affordable Care Act to provide services and equipment to nursing mothers, but that means that twenty-one states have opted out. You can see if your state's WIC program complies with the ACA at www.advisory.com/daily-briefing/resources/primers/medicaidmap.

Clinical-grade pumps. These piston-driven pumps, built for rental use, cycle automatically about 48 to 60 times per minute and have certain minimum suction pressures of approximately 240 millimeters of mercury. Clinical-grade pumps closely approximate the sucking action of an infant, and most drain the breasts gently as well as effectively. These pumps are available for rent at stations throughout the country.

Medical professionals and pump companies often refer to these pumps as hospital-grade, but usually all they mean is that a pump meets certain electrical and other standards that ensure a pump is safe for hospital use. Know that the designation *hospital-grade* has nothing to do with how well a pump works. I use the term *clinical-grade* to designate pumps of the highest quality.

Clinical-grade pumps are recommended for the following mothers and babies:

- Babies who fail to begin latching on to the breast and sustaining sucking within 24 hours after birth
- Mothers who have no signs of milk production 72 hours following birth
- Mothers who are pumping exclusively or nearly exclusively
- Premature or sick hospitalized newborns
- Babies with poor muscle tone, neurological problems, or birth defects such as cardiac abnormalities
- Mothers who are experiencing breastfeeding problems, such as severe sore nipples, that necessitate temporarily stopping breast-feeding
- Mothers attempting adoptive nursing or relactation
- Mothers estimating their milk supply
- Babies who are refusing the breast, because of colic or a nursing strike
- Mothers who are doing "insurance pumping" after nursings (see page 241)

Probably the finest breast pumps ever manufactured are the large, heavy, internal-piston pumps. To most lactation professionals, they are the gold standard for breast pumps. Unfortunately, most of these pumps are no longer being manufactured. Lighter-weight pumps, with the piston outside the motor case, are more available for rental in most areas but may not be quite as effective as internal-piston pumps.

Double collection kits, which can be purchased at the time of the rental, allow mothers to express milk from either one or both breasts at the same time. Double pumping can significantly cut the amount of time needed to empty both breasts and may stimulate greater milk production than pumping just one breast at a time.

You may be able to find local pump rental stations by calling the toll-free numbers provided by the pump manufacturers (see Appendix A, page 361). Rental rates vary tremendously, so shopping around can pay off. Rates for long-term, prepaid rental are usually lowest, but in general the cost of a pump rental is far less than the cost of formula-feeding. If your doctor prescribes the use of a clinical-grade pump, your insurance company may cover the cost of the rental depending on your situation.

The Special Supplemental Nutrition Program for Women, Infants, and Children, or WIC, lends external-piston clinical-grade pumps to some of its participants. A mother who qualifies for the program and who needs a pump because she has breastfeeding complications or a premature or sick baby, or because she is working or attending school, may be eligible for the loan of a portable electric pump. See Appendix A, page 359, for more information on WIC.

Some larger pump rental stations offer "grant pumps" to a certain number of mothers who can't afford to rent them. If you do not qualify for WIC services and yet don't have enough money to rent a clinical-grade pump, discussing your situation with local rental stations may be worth your while.

Using a clinical-grade pump is usually very simple. Place the flange carefully over the nipple so that the nipple is centered in the middle of the tunnel opening. (If the nipple is off center, it will rub uncomfortably against one side of the tunnel as you pump.) When pumping in the early weeks, many mothers find that a thin coat of lanolin applied around the base of the nipples decreases the friction between the nipples and the hard plastic of the flange.

Adjust the suction until it feels strong but not painful. Most mothers start out pumping with low suction and gradually turn up the suction until it feels strong but comfortable.

Personal-use electric pumps. These pumps generally cycle automatically. The best pumps in this category reach suction strengths of 240 millimeters of mercury and cycling speeds of at least 50 per minute. Many, but not all, personal-use pumps have separate controls for adjusting suction strength and speed, which many mothers prefer. Every personal-use double pump comes with a double milk collection kit. These pumps are recommended for

- mothers who have normal milk supplies but are separated from their infants nearly every day,

- mothers with normal milk supplies who are experiencing a breastfeeding complication at home (such as a preemie who is sleepy or has a weak suck), but who are still nursing their babies most of the time, and

- mothers who have initiated pumping with a clinical-grade pump, have an abundant milk supply, and pump exclusively.

Personal-use pumps are not designed for exclusive pumping, particularly in the early weeks. Women who are depending on a pump alone for milk removal usually get off to a better start with a more effective clinical-grade pump.

Many women borrow or are given personal-use pumps from friends or relatives or buy these pumps secondhand. As of this writing, only a few of the pumps in this category—the Hygeia EnJoye Pump (see page 267), PJ's Comfort Pump (see page 268), the Melodi Advanced Pump (see page 263), and the Nurture III Pump (see page 277)—are certified by the U.S. Food and Drug Administration (FDA) as "multiple-user pumps," which can be safely passed on if the new user buys a new collection kit. Other models in this category are designated as "single-user" pumps, which means they are not to be shared or resold. These pumps cannot be sterilized, so the risk of contamination from viruses transmitted through milk, such as HIV and cytomegalovirus (CMV), cannot be eliminated, even with

If you are using a breast pump at high altitudes—2,000 feet above sea level or higher—know that the pump will not generate as much suction as the manufacturer states. Pumps that normally have low pressures will be very ineffective at high altitudes.

the purchase of a new collection kit. Airborne viruses can get into the motors of these pumps and cause contamination for the next user. The used pumps that I check out for mothers often harbor mold.

It is important to understand, too, that most personal-use pumps have a limited life, so a used pump may not function as well as it did when it was new. Some manufacturers warn that after a year their pumps may not generate as much speed and vacuum as formerly. If you pump every day with a secondhand pump, you may find your milk supply faltering as the efficiency of the pump declines. And if a borrowed pump wears out after the end of the warranty period, you may feel obligated to purchase a new pump for the woman who lent you hers. So borrowing or purchasing a used pump may not be the bargain that it seems. If you own a pump that you used with a previous baby, you will want to check all of the pieces of the kit to be sure the pump will work well for you. Some lactation consultants offer pump "checkups."

Prices vary greatly within this category, as do warranty periods. Purchasing one of the better-quality pumps in this category may save money in the long run, especially if you are going back to work, you will have other children in the future, or both.

As with a clinical-grade pump, using a personal-use pump is fairly simple. Carefully center your nipples in the flange openings. Adjust the speed to about 50 cycles per minute. Start with minimal suction strength, and slowly increase the suction until it feels strong but comfortable.

Single electric and battery-operated pumps. Other pumps that run on batteries or electricity from a wall socket, or both, come in a huge array of styles and models. These pumps are used to express milk from only one breast at a time, which doubles the time it takes to drain both sides. One of these pumps is semi-automatic; that is, the suction is created and released by the user's finger. Other pumps in this category are fully automatic. Fully automatic pumps may remove milk more effectively than semi-automatic ones, but some of the fully automatic pumps in this category cycle much more slowly than the 50 times per minutes ideal for stimulating let-down and emptying the breast completely. Many have poor suction—less than 240 millimeters of mercury—which may also lessen the amount of milk a mother can collect.

Over time, the let-down reflex stops responding well to slow-cycling, low-suctioning pumps—typically the less expensive ones—and this can lead to poor drainage of the breasts and, ultimately, low milk production. As lactation continues, apparently, the breast requires stimulation and drainage that is more similar to that provided by the nursing baby.

In general, these pumps are best for mothers who pump only on occasion. I recommend them only for mothers who have adequate milk production and need to pump no more than five times a week.

To use one of these pumps, center your nipple in the flange opening. If there is a speed setting, try to reach about 50 cycles per minute. Adjust the suction to a strong but comfortable level.

Hand-operated pumps. The final group of pumps comprises those that are hand operated. These pumps are portable and relatively inexpensive; the best are also comfortable and easy to use. Hand-operated pumps are recommended for mothers with adequate milk supplies who need to pump only occasionally, no more than a few times a week.

As with other types of pumps, you'll need to carefully center your nipple in the flange. You may also have to repeatedly squeeze and release a handle or pull and release a cylinder to create suction and control the cycling speed. Familiarize yourself with the manufacturer's directions, and practice to see which techniques work best for you.

Expressing Milk for Occasional Separations

If you anticipate that you and your baby will be separated from time to time, you will want to begin expressing milk, by hand or with a pump, once breastfeeding is well established. For most mothers this means sometime after the first two weeks when your baby is latching well at the breast. If you are planning to buy a pump, see my reviews in the categories of "Personal-Use Fully Automatic Double Electric Pumps," "Single Electric Pumps and Semi-Automatic Pumps," and "Hand-Operated Pumps," pages 263 to 283.

Babies will usually happily accept a bottle if it is introduced before they are a month old. They will usually continue to do so thereafter as long as the bottle is offered every two to three days.

If you are offering a bottle just to keep the baby familiar with the artificial nipple, you will need to feed only an ounce or so of milk at a time. Most mothers find they can pump this much after a morning nursing, when production is a bit higher than at other times.

Expressing Milk Before Returning to Work

If you are facing a return to work or school and so will be missing feedings, you will want to practice hand expression, select a very good pump, or both. If you will be getting a pump, you will probably want to purchase a personal-use double pump that is designed either for personal use or for multiple users. See my review of these pumps on pages 263 to 275.

Most mothers find comfort in having a backup supply of milk in the freezer when they return to work. This extra milk may come in handy whenever you cannot pump as much in one day as you would like or the baby takes more milk than usual.

If your only freezer is a compartment of your refrigerator, collecting just a couple of ounces daily will quickly fill the space. Depending on how much milk you're saving, you may want to search out available space in someone else's deep freezer, or even buy your own. Breast milk will keep for 3 months in the freezer compartment of a refrigerator (with a separate door) and 6 to 12 months in a deep freezer. See page 250 for more information on storing breast milk.

Offer a little of the milk you express to your baby. Offering a bottle frequently and regularly will keep your baby willing to take it if you return to work before he is able to drink well from a cup. Use the oldest milk in the freezer for these practice sessions so that none of your milk becomes outdated. Whenever you offer thawed breast milk to your baby, express some milk to replace what you've taken from your supply.

You will probably discover that you produce the most milk in the night and in the morning. This means that the morning will be a good time to collect extra milk for your baby. Expressing milk right after one, two, or even three of the first nursings of the day typically yields the most milk—for most mothers, 1 to 2 ounces. This milk will have a very high fat content, which will be a bonus for the baby when you are apart.

Mothers whose babies begin a long sleep stretch early in the evening sometimes express milk right before they retire for the night. If the baby doesn't always sleep for a long stretch, however, pumping between nursings may not be a good idea, as you might be taking half of the baby's next feeding.

Expressing Milk at Work

If you will be missing one or more feedings while you are away at work or school, you should plan to express your milk. This will help to prevent engorgement and, more important, to maintain your milk supply. The milk you express can be used later to feed your baby while you are away. If you leave your baby for longer than four to five hours three or more times a week and do not express your milk, particularly if your baby is less than eight to ten months old, your milk supply will probably diminish.

How often you should express milk depends on the age of your baby, how long you are apart, and how often the baby nurses while you are together. Babies under four months should nurse at least eight times in 24

How Does Your Flange Fit?

The early weeks at home provide an opportunity to see how well your pump works for you. One question that may arise is whether the flange—the part that fits over the nipple—is the right size for you. If it doesn't fit well, pumping may be uncomfortable, and you may not be able to express milk effectively.

Tight fit

Good fit

Standard flanges are 24 or 25 millimeters wide at the nipple opening. If your nipples are as wide as or wider than a nickel, these standard flanges will probably be too small. Even if your nipples are narrower than a nickel, they may swell in the tunnel of a flange until the fit is clearly too snug. While you're pumping, your nipples shouldn't rub against the side of the tunnel, and the areola, the dark portion around the nipple, should move a bit with each pull. Pumping should be comfortable; experiencing pain on the side of the nipple is another sign that the flange may be too small. Aside from being uncomfortable, an undersized flange may not allow for complete drainage of milk. If you are pumping regularly, incomplete drainage can lead to a drop in overall production.

Sometimes when a mother telephones me to ask whether she may need a different flange size, I suggest pumping again 20 minutes after a regular pumping. Collecting more than ½ ounce of milk in the second pumping may indicate that the flange fits poorly.

If you are using a Medela or Ameda pump, you can order large or extra-large flanges from the manufacturer (see Appendix A, page 360). Or have a lactation professional check the fit; she may have a larger flange available for sale.

hours; emptying the breast this often is necessary to maintain adequate milk production. If your baby is less than four months old, then, plan on expressing milk every two and a half to three hours while away.

Four- to seven-month-old babies typically nurse at least seven times a day. If your baby is this age, express milk often enough so that, with pumping and nursings, your breasts are emptied seven times in each 24 hours. If your five-month-old nurses frequently during the day and twice at night, you may not need to express milk while you work four hours a day, unless you prefer that your baby receive only breast milk when you are apart.

A baby who is eight months old or older may be nursing often or just a few times a day. The decision to express milk at this point depends not only on how much time you spend away from your baby, but also on whether he is eating a wide variety of solid foods and on how you feel about providing formula instead of breast milk.

It is important to also understand this: Extended periods of time without complete breast drainage lessen overall milk production. For most women, if the breasts aren't thoroughly drained seven times in a 24-hour period, milk production declines.

This decline in milk supply involves several factors. A lessening in breast stimulation, experts think, leads to lower prolactin levels, the hormone responsible for milk production. Additionally, full breasts that go undrained for long periods of time probably release substances that cause the milk-producing cells to slow or even cease production.

Some people mistakenly theorize that when a woman regularly goes for lengthy periods without nursing or expressing milk, the breasts become "trained" to produce sufficient amounts of milk when she does put the baby to breast. Unfortunately, this is not the case. Neglecting to express milk when apart from the baby leads to an overall lessening of the milk supply. A low milk supply generally leads to a delayed milk let-down, frustration at the breast for the baby, and in many instances premature weaning.

If you decide against expressing milk, your baby will need a commercially prepared formula for missed nursings during the first year.

Insurance Pumping

There are several situations in which it may be important to express milk after nursing a baby. This is called "insurance pumping." Mothers and babies in this category include

- babies making the transition to full-time breastfeeding (see page 143),
- babies born at 37 weeks' gestation or earlier or weighing less than 6 pounds (see page 136),
- babies who have unusual conformations in their mouths, such as a short frenulum, a high palate, or a cleft lip or palate or both (see pages 98 and 150),
- babies who are being fed with the help of a nipple shield (see page 85),
- mothers who by 72 hours following birth have had no signs of milk production (see page 70),
- mothers with low milk production (see page 107),
- mothers whose breasts remain engorged because the baby isn't thoroughly draining them (see page 68),
- mothers with nipples as large in diameter as a quarter, or larger (see page 104),
- mothers who have had previous breast surgery involving an incision around the nipple or areola (see page 119),
- mothers diagnosed with polycystic ovary syndrome (PCOS) (see page 119), and
- mothers with hypoplastic breasts (long, thin, widely spaced breasts that didn't get larger in pregnancy and that may differ markedly from each other in size; see page 116).

Mothers in the categories just listed are at risk for low milk production, and their babies are at risk for poor weight gain. In many of these cases, the babies may not be vigorous enough to stimulate and drain the breasts well and to bring in a full milk supply. This is often true with near-term babies and babies making the transition to full-time nursing. A mother may bring in a full milk supply, but if the baby nurses poorly, the supply may plummet. In other situations, the baby may suck well, but the breasts may need more stimulation and emptying than the baby can provide. Examples are mothers with large nipples and mothers who have had breast surgery. In these cases, pumping right after nursings can be necessary to bring in an abundant supply, as well as to insure that the baby receives plenty of milk.

Generally, double-pumping for 5 to 15 minutes with a clinical-grade pump right after nursing will drain the colostrum or mature milk remaining in the breasts. When a mother pumps after each nursing, not only does her milk supply usually increase, but her baby begins receiving more milk. One pediatrician put it this way: "Insurance pumping makes the breast perform more like a fire hydrant and less like a garden hose."

Newborns in the insurance-pumping categories need to be carefully monitored for signs of adequate milk intake. If your newborn loses 10 percent of her birth weight (see Appendix B, page 369), or if she fails to gain an ounce a day after five days of age, you'll need to feed her some or all of the milk that you collect by pumping. If you can't collect enough milk, she may also need supplemental formula. In these cases, working with a lactation professional can be very helpful.

When your baby is gaining weight normally without supplemental breast milk, you can slowly wean yourself off the pump. After doing so, continue to monitor the baby's weight for a short while.

Expressing Milk for a Baby Who Cannot Nurse

Some mothers must bring in a milk supply without a nursing baby. If your baby is unable to nurse because of a latch-on problem, prematurity, or illness, you will want to start pumping as soon as possible, ideally within hours of delivery, so your baby receives plenty of colostrum.

Colostrum is especially beneficial because it has such a high concentration of protective antibodies.

The nursing staff should provide you with a suitable pump and instructions for collecting and storing your milk. Most maternity units have a clinical-grade breast pump available; this is the type of pump you want when you must pump around the clock. (If the hospital uses the Medela Symphony breast pump, see page 244 for information on using this pump to bring in a full milk supply.) If your baby is being transferred to another hospital for care, ask the transport team about their procedures for storing and transporting your milk. If you will be following the baby to a special-care nursery in another city, try to get a pump to take along with you. See page 361 for information on renting a clinical-grade breast pump.

It is very important that you have the right size flanges for pumping. Some standard pump flanges are too small for many mothers. If your nipples are swelling in the tunnels, and especially if pumping is painful, the flanges may be too small. If they are, your breasts won't drain completely. For advice on choosing the correct flange size, see page 239.

Initially, you may be more comfortable if you apply a thin coat of lanolin around the base of the nipples before starting to pump (for sources of modified, hypoallergenic lanolin, see Appendix A, page 364). If pumping is painful even with lanolin, again, you may need larger flanges.

You may receive differing bits of advice on how often and how long to pump your breasts. Some hospital nurses suggest that women pump every three to four hours during the day and sleep all night. With such limited stimulation, most mothers would find either that they wouldn't bring in an abundant supply or that after a while it would dwindle. Keep in mind that your milk supply depends on the frequent stimulation of your breasts. You should plan on expressing milk as often as your baby would nurse, or at least eight times in 24 hours. Some mothers prefer to express their milk every three hours around the clock, whereas others would rather pump a little more often during the day so they can sleep for longer periods at night. Determine a reasonable schedule for yourself, but do not go more than five hours without pumping.

Studies now suggest that the effectiveness as well as the frequency of colostrum removal in the first three days is highly predictive of how much milk will be produced in the days to follow. Surprisingly, dependence on a pump alone during the first several days may be associated with lower milk production. Dr. Jane Morton and others at Stanford University have found that pumping alone may remove only a fraction of the available colostrum and milk. In this study, mothers who both hand-expressed colostrum and pumped with the Medela Symphony pump (with its original circuit board; see page 260) collected 80 percent more milk than women who used only the pump. For instructions on hand expression, see page 225. You can see Dr. Morton's technique in the video at http://newborns.stanford.edu/Breastfeeding/HandExpression.html.

If you are hand-expressing for a healthy full-term or near-term baby who is unable to latch on to the breast, you can collect the colostrum in a plastic spoon, which you can then use to feed the baby. If your baby is sick or very premature, ask the hospital staff about using a small container to collect and store colostrum for later use.

Once your milk is in, how much you produce will depend on how much you manage to express. Ideally, you should pump more milk than your baby requires. Building and maintaining a volume of at least 24 ounces per day (or, for twins, 40 to 48 ounces per day) will allow you to have extra milk on reserve should you experience a temporary decline in production—due to stress or illness, for example—during your baby's hospitalization. Having an abundant supply will also help your baby get milk more easily once he is able to latch on to the breast and suck.

You can maximize the amount you collect by massaging or pressing firm areas of the breast while you pump. To see Dr. Morton demonstrate the hands-on pumping technique, go to http://newborns.stanford.edu/Breastfeeding/MaxProduction.html.

It may be easier to massage and compress your breasts if you pump one side at a time. Alternatively, you can wear a hands-free bra, also known as a pumping bustier, which will hold the pump flanges in place (see page 276). A tight sports bra with the centers cut out can also allow you to massage and pump both breasts at once.

After pumping, you can collect even more milk by hand-expressing for a few minutes, alternating breasts several times.

With practice and experimentation, you will develop your own method for collecting the most milk possible. Most mothers find that once they are able to pump 3 to 4 ounces at a time, they can gradually eliminate the other measures to increase milk production.

Whenever possible, provide freshly expressed or refrigerated milk for your premature or sick baby. Freezing breast milk preserves many but not all of its protective substances. You can keep your milk for 24 to 48 hours in the refrigerator (ask the intensive-care nurses for a more precise limit) or for up to three months in the freezer.

Depending on your baby's maturity or general progress, you may find yourself expressing milk for several weeks. It is important that you eat well, get plenty to drink, and rest enough to maintain your own energy as well as your milk supply.

If you notice that your milk production is declining for a few days in a row, you will need to assess the situation and make whatever adjustments are necessary. The most common causes of decreasing milk production are infrequent expression—fewer than eight times in 24 hours—and an inefficient pump. Although a few mothers can maintain a good milk supply while expressing less often than this or while using a non-clinical-grade pump, most can't do so for longer than a few weeks. If you have been using a hand pump or an inexpensive battery-operated or plug-in pump, or even a personal-use pump, rent a clinical-grade pump. Most mothers find that a clinical-grade pump requires less effort to operate and works more efficiently. Using Dr. Morton's methods to increase milk production, as described in this section, may also help improve your overall production.

Occasionally you may notice that your milk production drops when you and your baby have a difficult day. Stress can temporarily decrease a mother's milk supply; this is normal and usually temporary. The following suggestions have proven helpful when this occurs:

- Pump regularly, every two to three hours.
- Take a short nap or a warm bath just before expressing.

- Apply moist heat to your breasts before expressing.
- Massage each breast as you pump, and perform hand expression right after each pumping.
- Ask someone to rub your back between the shoulder blades while you are pumping.
- If possible, hold the baby while you are pumping at the hospital, or keep a photo of your baby with your pump.
- Hold the baby skin-to-skin as much as possible.

Pumping Exclusively

For any of a variety of reasons, a woman may find herself pumping all of her baby's milk and feeding it by bottle instead of nursing. It may be that the baby has been unable to latch on to the breast, or even that the mother prefers to feed her baby this way. Many women have managed to produce enough milk to meet their babies' needs for a year or beyond while pumping exclusively.

Pumping full-time for a baby requires dedication and discipline. Unlike a baby, a pump does not signal for attention, and for most women pumping is more a chore than a pleasure. To feed your baby entirely or mostly on your own milk, however, is to give him an extra-special gift.

If you are exclusively pumping, frequent and effective expression during the first week after birth is critical for establishing an abundant milk supply. Read "Expressing Milk for a Baby Who Cannot Nurse" (page 242), and make sure you have a high-quality, comfortable pump. Starting out with a clinical-grade rental pump is the best way to bring in a full milk supply—about 24 ounces per day during the first month. Since clinical-grade pumps are expensive, women who use them rent them rather than buy them. If your income is low or modest, you may qualify for a rent-free clinical-grade pump through the WIC program (see page 359). In any case, long-term pump rental is much less costly than buying formula.

A double collection kit, for collecting milk from both breasts at once, makes pumping quicker and is usually more effective in establishing and maintaining milk production. Unless you are given a collection kit in the hospital, you will need to buy one when you rent a clinical-grade pump.

It is essential to pump often—every two to three hours during the day and at least once in the night, or at least eight times in each 24 hours. You must also spend enough time at each pumping to drain both breasts completely, since it is the frequent, thorough drainage of the breasts that signals them to increase milk production and keep it high. Some women can completely drain the breasts by pumping for 10 minutes or less, but others need a longer time. Until you're sure how much time you need, pump until the milk stops flowing and then a couple of minutes longer.

Pumping shouldn't hurt. A properly fitting pump flange allows for the pull and release of the nipple without the nipple's swelling against the side of the tunnel. If the tunnel is too narrow for your nipple, your breast won't drain completely and pumping may be painful. For help in determining whether you need a larger flange, see page 239.

Once you have established a generous milk supply—at least 24 ounces per day—you might invest in your own personal-use pump, such as Hygeia's EnJoye, Medela's Pump in Style, or the Calypso pump. Some mothers, however, are unable to maintain high production with these pumps and continue to require a clinical-grade rental model.

After the first month, most women are able to maintain their production level with seven pumpings in each 24 hours. With less frequent pumping than this, however, most women find that their supply drops below the baby's needs. A small proportion of women produce excessive milk while pumping only five or six times in each 24 hours. If you are an overproducer, you can freeze the extra milk for later use.

Mothers who are exclusively pumping especially appreciate products that allow hands-free pumping. See "Other Purchases You Might Consider," page 276.

Your milk supply will need to grow as your baby does. From the fifth day after birth until about three months, babies generally gain about 1 ounce per day. After three months of age, their weight gain typically slows to about ½ ounce per day. They require 20 to 24 ounces of milk per day in the first month, and their intake gradually increases thereafter

You can use a fully automatic breast pump with a double collection kit to pump breast milk more quickly and efficiently.

to 28 to 32 ounces per day. Their intake stays at about this level until other foods slowly begin to replace breast milk in the diet.

Bottle-fed babies often drink more than they need for normal growth, even when they're fed breast milk rather than formula. Since overfeeding a baby can lead to obesity later, you may want to keep track of how much milk your baby is taking. These guidelines may be helpful: During the first month, offer about 1 ounce per hour, or 3 ounces every two and a half to three hours. After the first month, offer as much as 1½ ounces per hour, or 4½ ounces every three hours. If your baby seems to want more milk than this, try to keep in mind that babies often fuss when they are overstimulated, tired, or uncomfortable. A breastfeeding mother may put her baby to the breast hourly when he is tired or cranky, but he doesn't get a large meal at each comfort feeding. Carrying your baby or offering a pacifier between feedings may help in calming him. (If your baby is very fussy, see "Fussiness, Colic, and Reflux," page 204.) Learning how to do "paced" bottle-feeding can also help your baby take a more normal volume of milk by bottle. (See page 257 for information.)

If you're pumping out of necessity rather than choice, it may be helpful to know that many babies become able and willing to take the breast despite weeks or even months of bottle-feeding. If your baby has been unable to latch on and suck well, it is still worthwhile to try nursing periodically. A lactation professional may be able to help you.

Increasing Your Milk Supply while Pumping

Some women who exclusively or frequently pump struggle with low milk production. If your production is lower than the norms specified here, you can take measures to increase it.

1. Be sure that you are not pregnant or using estrogen-containing birth control (combination birth control pills or the vaginal ring with estrogen), which typically lessen milk production. The progestin-only "mini-pill" is usually fine.

2. Consider using a clinical-grade pump and a double-pump kit, if you are not doing so already.

3. Pump or nurse *at least* eight times a day—more if you can manage. Distribute the pumping or nursing sessions more or less evenly during the baby's waking hours. If your baby sleeps a long stretch at night, pump just before you go to bed or very early in the morning. If you work away from home, nurse or pump right before leaving the baby and as soon as you return.

4. If you're not sure whether your pump is draining your breasts completely, try pumping 15 to 20 minutes after a prior pumping. If you get ½ ounce or more at the second pumping, the collection kit, or even the pump itself, may be doing an inadequate job.

5. To be sure your pump is working efficiently, give it a checkup. Check the tubing, connections, rubber diaphragms, and filters. If the diaphragms get small tears, the pump will not work efficiently. If the filters get wet, the suction will stop entirely. A lactation professional may be able to check the pump's suction pressure, which should reach 240 millimeters of mercury. Some pumps are simply not capable of reaching these pressures.

6. Be sure the pump's nipple flanges fit you right (see page 239).

7. Pump at the highest suction possible without discomfort, and at a speed of about 50 times a minute. If your pump doesn't have a speed control labeled with the number of cycles per minute, count the cycles. Pumping too fast or too slowly can reduce the volume of milk expressed.

8. Practice "hands-on pumping," as described on page 244.

9. Consider using Pumpin' Pal Super Shields (see page 276), which might help you express more milk, especially if your pump has adequate suction.

10. Consider taking herbal products that stimulate milk production, such as fenugreek or blessed thistle capsules, More Milk Plus tincture or capsules, or Go-Lacta (see page 72).

11. If your periods have resumed and you find that your milk production dips when you are mid-cycle until your period begins, consider taking 500 to 1,000 milligrams of calcium and 250 to 500 milligrams of magnesium daily. Take this from the time of ovulation until the day of your heaviest flow.

Collecting and Storing Your Breast Milk

Regardless of whether you have a healthy baby or one who is premature or sick in the hospital, you will always want to take special care when expressing and storing your milk. Wash your hands before handling your breasts or any of the pump equipment. All pump parts that come in contact with the milk or your breasts should be thoroughly washed after each use, with hot soapy water and separately from family eating utensils and food preparation equipment. Use a bottle brush, one with a smaller brush on the opposite end, to reach all the nooks and crannies of the pump parts. (Some mothers buy a second collection kit so they can do the washing at their convenience.) Your daily bath or shower will cleanse your breasts sufficiently.

You can store your milk in plastic or glass feeding bottles or in plastic bags made for milk storage. Plastic bags take up less space in the freezer than bottles do, and you may be able to express your milk directly into the bags. Some mothers use disposable bottle liners, but these can break when the milk freezes and leak when it thaws. Bags designed for storing breast milk are made of thicker plastic, come sterilized, and have a place for writing the date. The main disadvantage of milk storage bags is that they are not reusable. Also, you cannot add fresh milk to a bag of frozen milk or feed the milk to the baby directly from a defrosted bag. The bags are more prone to leakage than bottles, but you can minimize this problem by putting the filled bags into freezer-weight food storage bags. For information on popular brands of milk storage bags, see Appendix A, page 365.

Some time ago, it was discovered that clear plastic baby bottles made of polycarbonate contain the chemical bisphenol-A (BPA), and that the BPA can leach into milk or other liquid in the bottle. Although most data concerning the safety of BPA come from animal studies, many scientists believe that the chemical can cause behavioral and developmental problems in children. Both the United States and Canada have outlawed the sale of baby bottles containing BPA. Flexible, opaque polypropylene bottles are BPA-free, as are glass bottles. Nearly all bottles and pump parts are now BPA-free.

Unless you are collecting 1- to 2-ounce bottles for practice feedings, store your milk in quantities of 3 to 4 ounces. Place your milk in the back of the refrigerator, at 34 to 40 degrees F., if you plan on using the milk within 72 hours. Freshly refrigerated milk is better for your baby, as it retains more of its live cells than frozen milk. If you wish to add more milk to some that is already bottled, chill the new milk in the refrigerator for about half an hour before adding it.

Many breastfeeding specialists say that milk can be safely refrigerated for up to eight days. Lois Arnold, former executive director of the Human Milk Banking Association of North America and currently the program coordinator for the National Commission on Donor Milk Banking, disagrees. The eight-day rule, she explains, fails to take into account that some mothers' milk may have high levels of bacteria, perhaps because of bacteria on the skin, inadequate cleaning of pump parts, or the use of contaminated water for cleaning equipment. Because you can't be sure that your milk doesn't have high bacterial levels, I recommend keeping it in the refrigerator for no longer than 72 hours. If you will not be using your expressed milk within this time, store it in the freezer compartment of a refrigerator (with a separate door) or in a freestanding freezer. Even milk that has been refrigerated for three days can be safely moved into a freezer.

Lack of refrigeration should not be a problem if you'll be expressing milk when you return to work. One small study found that freshly expressed milk could be kept at room temperature (66 to 72 degrees F.) for up to ten hours without spoiling. However, I recommend keeping your milk chilled in a small cooler with freezer packs if a refrigerator is not available.

Breast milk looks different from dairy milk, especially after storage in the refrigerator or freezer. Your fresh milk may be yellow, white, bluish, or even greenish, depending on what you have eaten and what medicines or vitamins you have taken. Frozen breast milk is usually yellow. Your milk will naturally separate in the refrigerator; the fat will rise to the top. After warming the milk, gently swirl it to mix the layers.

Fresh or thawed breast milk typically has a mild, slightly sweet smell. Occasionally a mother finds that her expressed milk has an unpleasant smell or taste. Certain vitamin or mineral supplements can cause this; so can steroidal nasal sprays. In either case, the affected milk is harmless.

Breast milk can take on a soapy smell if the fat has broken down, freeing fatty acids. Apparently, some women have an excess of lipase, the enzyme that breaks down the fat in milk. Usually they notice the soapy smell after the milk has been refrigerated or frozen, but in some cases the smell develops immediately after expression. Most babies will take such milk without complaint, but the peculiar odor and taste can usually be lessened or eliminated either by chilling the milk before freezing it or by putting it directly into the freezer, and then thawing it in the refrigerator before warming it in a hot-water bath. If these methods fail for you, you can inactivate the enzyme by scalding the milk on the stove—that is, by bringing the milk almost to a boil—and then immediately refrigerating or freezing it. Do not let the milk boil; doing so would destroy its anti-infective properties.

Although freezing destroys the white blood cells found in breast milk, it preserves the many other antimicrobial properties and inhibits the growth of bacteria. Freezing does not affect the nutritional composition of breast milk.

You can safely store your milk in the freezer compartment of a refrigerator for three to six months, provided that the freezer compartment is separate from, not inside, the refrigerator, and that the temperature stays at –4 degrees F. Store the milk toward the back of the freezer, away from the door. If the freezer automatically defrosts, keep the milk away from the walls.

Because the entire amount must be used once breast milk is thawed, you will want to store small amounts, probably 3 to 4 ounces. Regardless of what kind of container you use, leave some room at the top to allow for expansion and to avoid leakage. If you want to add fresh milk to some that is frozen, chill the fresh milk first to keep the top layer of frozen milk from thawing.

Date your containers so that you use the oldest milk first. While bottles are often recommended, you may find that bags made especially for breast milk will take up less space. Using other types of bags is not recommended due to leakage problems. If you will be taking the milk to day care, write the baby's name on the bags as well. Placing the bags in a plastic container will also help keep them safe from breakage.

Better yet, store the milk in a freestanding deep freezer, where the milk will be good for 12 months when the temperature is –4 degrees F. If you don't have a freestanding freezer and you are running out of space in the freezer section of the refrigerator, you might invest in a small one or find a friend or relative who has one that you can store your milk in.

Collecting Milk for a Premature or Sick Baby

If you are expressing milk for a premature or sick baby, you should not only wash the pump parts in hot, soapy water, you should also sterilize them every day. You can boil them in water for 15 minutes or run them through a dishwasher's sanitizing cycle, or you can sterilize them in special bags in a microwave oven: Place all of the parts that come in contact with milk in one of the bags with 4 ounces of water, and microwave for the time recommended on the bag, usually between 1 and 5 minutes. For more information about Medela's Quick Clean Micro-Steam Bags, see Appendix A, page 365.

After collecting your milk, pour it into a sterile container; ask the hospital nursery staff what type they prefer. To avoid wasting milk, ask your baby's nurses how much to put in each container. Freshly refrigerated milk is better for your baby, as it retains more of its live cells than frozen milk, so try to provide fresh milk for your baby whenever possible. Milk for a premature or sick baby can be safely stored in the refrigerator for up to 48 hours (ask the nursing staff for their specific limit).

When transporting your refrigerated or frozen milk to the hospital, pack the containers in ice, or surround them with refreezable ice packs, inside a small cooler. If you're traveling a long distance, keep your milk frozen with dry ice.

Milk for a premature or sick baby should not be frozen or refrigerated after it has been thawed or warmed. Whatever is left over after the feeding must be thrown out.

Feeding Your Expressed Milk

Take your milk out of the refrigerator shortly before your baby is due for a feeding. Gradually, over 5 to 10 minutes, warm the milk to room temperature in a container of warm water. Never warm or defrost milk in a microwave oven or on the stove. Microwaves do not heat evenly, and uneven heating can burn a baby's mouth. Bottles can explode in microwave ovens. In a microwave or on a stove, excess heat can destroy the immunological substances, proteins, and vitamins in breast milk.

When taking milk out of the freezer for feeding, choose the oldest milk; this way you're less likely to end up throwing away outdated milk later. Thaw the milk in any of three ways: Hold the container under warm running water; swirl it in a bowl of warm water; or let it thaw overnight in the refrigerator. Do not thaw milk by letting the bottle sit at room temperature.

When breast milk thaws, the fat separates and rises to the top. Gently shake the bottle to blend the fat back in with the rest of the milk. Use thawed milk within 24 hours. Do not refreeze it.

Mothers often ask whether they can reuse breast milk left over after a feeding. Although there have been no scientific studies on this question, most lactation professionals believe that warmed or defrosted milk can be refrigerated, reheated, and used for the next feeding so long as the baby isn't sick or premature and the milk has not been left out for longer than an hour.

Getting your baby used to a bottle is important if she will be fed by someone else while you are apart. It is best to wait until she is two to four weeks old before introducing a bottle. By this time nursing should be well established, so the bottle should not interfere with the baby's interest in the breast. Many babies refuse the bottle if it is first offered much after they are one month old.

Many kinds of bottles and nipples are on the market, and no one bottle or nipple is best for breastfed babies or more likely to be accepted over another. The best bottles are easy to clean and have accurate measuring indicators. Angled bottles are supposed to make it easier to keep the nipple filled, so the baby doesn't suck in air, but this is just as easy with straight bottles and actually unnecessary (see "Baby-Led or Paced Bottle-Feeding," page 257). Bottles molded into unusual shapes or split down the middle for self-feeding are nearly impossible to keep clean. Some bottles come with disposable liners, which are supposed to cause less air swallowing. They don't.

Most bottles come in two sizes: 4 ounces and 8 ounces. Four-ounce bottles make more sense for babies who are taking only 2 to 4 ounces at a feeding. You can buy 8-ounce bottles later, if your baby begins drinking 4 to 5 ounces at a feeding.

Nipples are made of latex or silicone. Silicone nipples are definitely preferable. Latex has a taste and odor and deteriorates faster than silicone. Latex also tends to break down in the dishwasher and so should be washed by hand. Silicone nipples *can* be washed in the dishwasher.

To introduce a bottle, manually express or pump your milk instead of nursing, and then, if possible, have your partner or someone else feed the milk to the baby. If you do this about three times a week until you go back to work, your baby should continue to accept a bottle. Offering a bottle periodically will also give you the opportunity to practice manual expression or become proficient with your pump.

Parents who stop offering a bottle once the baby has taken it sometimes find themselves struggling with the baby and bottle weeks later. Giving the baby 1 or 2 ounces of breast milk by bottle every few days is very important if you want to avoid problems later.

Should your baby refuse to drink from a bottle, keep trying. The following suggestions may help:

- To avoid wasting your milk, practice with just 1 ounce in the bottle.

- Don't substitute formula for your milk in these practice sessions. Most babies prefer sweet-tasting breast milk to formula.

- Try a variety of bottle nipples. Look for one with a faster flow. Try a tasteless silicone nipple instead of a latex one. Different mothers swear by different brands, including Avent, Playtex, Mimijumi, and Dr. Brown's.

- Try offering the bottle while walking with the baby. Hold the baby facing away from you, and bounce her gently as you walk. This will be easier if you put the baby in a front-facing carrier.

- Try nursing the baby for just a few minutes, and then unlatching her and slipping the bottle into her mouth. If she objects, try again after a few minutes more of nursing.

A baby may more easily accept the bottle if you hold her facing outward and walk.

- Have someone else try; frequently a baby is more confused and upset by a bottle when her mother tries to persuade her.

- As long as the baby is refusing the bottle, offer it a couple of times each day, both when the baby seems hungry and when she is not.

- Do not allow these sessions to become too upsetting for the baby or for you. Trying to force a baby to take a bottle is distressing for everyone and rarely successful. Also, "starving" the baby until she accepts a bottle is somewhat abusive and rarely effective.

Although you want to know before you are apart that your baby will drink from a bottle, the baby who won't take a bottle from Mom may do well when the caregiver offers it. At the age of three months, my daughter, Kate, screamed bloody murder whenever I approached with a bottle, but her caregiver had no problems feeding her when I was away.

The baby who refuses a bottle may do surprisingly well with an ordinary, unspouted cup, particularly if she is nearing six months or older. A sippy cup may be too much like a bottle for a baby who is continuing to refuse one.

Baby-Led or Paced Bottle-Feeding

When you are feeding your baby your milk by bottle, always hold him in your arms. Let him control the feeding in the ways he does when you nurse him: Wait for him to open his mouth instead of pushing in the nipple. Be patient when he pauses in sucking; don't stimulate him to suck continuously. Even if there is breast milk left in the bottle, let your baby stop drinking when he signals that he has had enough.

A full bottle-feeding should take 7 to 15 minutes. If the feeding takes longer, the nipple flow may be too slow. If the baby chokes frequently, the nipple flow is too fast.

Breastfed babies, in most instances, control the flow of breast milk as they nurse. When you're breastfeeding, the milk may spray as it lets down, and the baby may let go of the breast to prevent himself from choking. After the first let-down, the baby then controls the flow of milk by sucking and pausing when needed. In contrast, some babies fed from a bottle, particularly those younger than four months, struggle to keep up with the rapid flow of milk. If your baby seems to be gulping down the milk as fast as he can, you may think he is very hungry, but actually he may be swallowing quickly just to avoid choking. You may see signs that the baby is feeling stressed: He may tense up, and his eyes may open wide. Milk may leak from the corners of his mouth. He may try to pull away from the bottle or "shut down," pretending to fall asleep in an attempt to end the feeding. A baby who manages to chug his milk from a bottle may end up taking more than he needs.

You (or whoever is feeding the baby) can avoid this problem by making sure that the baby is comfortable, that he can pause to take a breath between swallows, and that he can end the feeding himself when he has had enough. This is known as "baby-led" or "paced" bottle-feeding. Use a slow-flow nipple, and sit the baby almost upright. Touch the bottle nipple to the baby's lips to stimulate him to open his mouth wide, as he does when he seeks out the breast. Then place the nipple in his mouth. Hold the bottle horizontally to slow the flow of milk through the nipple. There will be air in the nipple, but try not to worry about the baby swallowing it; you can burp him periodically. If he is sucking without pause but showing facial signals of stress, lower the bottle while keeping it in his mouth. This will give the baby the chance to rest and to begin sucking again when he is ready. When the baby stops sucking, do not jiggle the nipple in his mouth to get him to resume. Assume that he has had enough even if there is still milk in the bottle. You can view Jessica Barton's video on "Paced Bottle-Feeding for the Breast-Fed Baby" at www.youtube.com/watch?v=UH4T70OSzGs.

Some final words on bottle-feeding: Never prop a bottle for a young baby or allow an older baby to bottle-feed himself. A baby needs an adult in close contact not only to monitor the amount of milk taken but also to provide the pleasure of her arms and attention.

A Review of Breast Pump Models

Clinical-Grade Pumps

Clinical-grade pumps are referred to by many as hospital-grade pumps, but this term is somewhat inaccurate. "Hospital-grade" simply refers to the electrical standard of breast pumps, not their quality. This group of pumps includes the pumps that are generally mostly "piston" rather than "diaphragm" pumps available through rental stations. These pumps are intended for mothers who need an excellent pump for exclusive or nearly exclusive pump-

Clinical-grade pump

ing, often due to a breastfeeding complication or a baby who is yet to latch on well. Internal-piston pumps are generally more effective than external-piston pumps.

Medela Classic Electric Pump. A sturdy machine weighing over 20 pounds, this internal-piston pump is no longer being manufactured but is still available through some rental stations. If you can find this great pump, it cycles at about 50 times per minute and generates suction of at least 240 millimeters of mercury. When you rent the pump, you must purchase a milk collection kit, at a cost of about $60. To locate a rental station near you, call Medela at 800-435-8316 or check the website at www.medela.com.

Ameda SMB and Lact-E pumps. These automatic pumps are heavy, internal-piston machines; the SMB weighs more than 20 pounds, the Lact-E about 12 pounds. Both have ideal speed and suction strength. Like the Medela Classic, these pumps are no longer being manufactured, but they are still available through some rental stations. When you rent either pump, you must purchase a milk collection kit, at a cost of about $60. To locate a rental station near you, call 877-992-6332 or check the website at www.ameda.com.

Ameda Platinum Breast Pump. The Ameda Platinum is a wonderful internal-piston pump similar in many ways to the older large-piston pumps that are no longer being manufactured. Weighing just under 10 pounds, it is used in hospitals and available at rental stations. The speed and suction levels are

Ameda Platinum Breast Pump

displayed on the front of the pump to help mothers learn what speeds and suction rates are most effective for breast drainage in the least amount of time. Speeds that increase to as high as 80 cycles per minute help with milk ejection, and a suction that reaches an effective 240 millimeters of mercury helps with breast drainage. The pump speed can be lowered after milk let-down occurs for deeper suctioning and more complete emptying. Ameda's collection kit is a closed system, meaning that mothers won't need to worry about milk, condensation, and mold getting into the tubing and pump. When you rent the pump, you must purchase a milk collection kit, at a cost of $50 to $60. To locate a rental station near you, call 877-992-6332.

Medela Symphony Pump. The Symphony is a fully automatic pump with a two-phase sucking pattern controlled by an electronic circuit board. The first phase, lasting 2 minutes, has rapid cycling; the second phase has slower cycling and higher suction. If the milk lets down before the first phase is up, the mother presses a button to switch to the slower phase. It is not possible to adjust suction and speed independently, as can be done with other pumps. Still, many women report that the Symphony is gentler and more comfortable to use than other clinical-grade pumps. This may be important if you are pumping because of sore, injured nipples.

Medela Symphony Pump

Medela's own research has shown that with its original circuit board, the Symphony pump is ineffective in bringing in a full milk supply for mothers who are pumping exclusively for premature infants. Although the suction strength and cycling speeds reach ideal levels, mothers of preemies who relied solely on this pump to bring in a full milk supply averaged only 14 ounces of milk per 24 hours at 14 days post partum. Because many hospitals provide Symphony pumps for mothers expressing milk for their non-nursing babies, Medela and Dr. Paula Meier designed a new circuit board, the Preemie +/Standard 2.0, that can replace the original circuit board so the pump will more closely mimic a baby's sucking pattern, with more irregular, rapid sucks and longer pauses. Mothers using the Symphony with the new circuit board, studies show, have collected more colostrum in a shorter period of time. (Once the mother collects 20 milliliters of colostrum at three pumpings in a row, the old circuit board is returned to the pump.) Unfortunately, not all hospitals have bought the new circuit boards for their Symphony pumps.

Another study found that mothers who used the Symphony with its original circuit board were able to obtain much more milk if they used hand expression after pumping, especially in the early days after delivery. If you will be exclusively pumping and the hospital pump is a Symphony without the new circuit board, I recommend you either spend time hand-expressing after pumping or rent another clinical-grade pump.

Rental rates for the Symphony may be higher, about $75 per month, than for most other rental pumps. As with other rental pumps, you must buy a collection kit. The pump comes with a rechargeable battery. To locate a rental station near you, call Medela at 800-435-8316 or check the website at www.medela.com.

Medela Lactina and Lactina Select pumps.

Weighing just 4 pounds, these external-piston pumps are capable of strong suction. The Lactina Select has a variable speed control, which many mothers prefer. With either pump, a milk collection kit must be purchased. To locate a rental station near you, call Medela at 800-435-8316 or visit the website at www.medela.com.

Medela Lactina Pump

Ameda Elite Pump.

Intended for rental use, the fully automatic external-piston Elite weighs only 7 pounds, and mothers can vary the rate and the strength of suction with separate dials. For women who will be pumping where there is no electric outlet, one model comes with a built-in battery pack. The Elite reaches a suction strength of only 220 millimeters of

Ameda Elite Pump

mercury with double pumping, less than other clinical-grade pumps, and this may affect the pump's efficiency. Again, you will need to purchase a milk collection kit to use with the pump. Long-term rental rates of $30 to $60 per month are available through most rental stations. To locate a rental station near you, call 877-992-6332.

Ardo Carum Pump. This Swiss-made piston pump, new to the U.S. market, is available through Ardo's rental stations. It has a sleek, lightweight design and a quiet motor. A range of vacuums and speeds are available, all independent of one another, so that mothers can choose their own pumping patterns with both stimulation and expression modes. It has a

Ardo Carum Pump

large color display to help mothers learn what settings work best for them. It is also available in a battery-powered version. Milk cannot get into the tubings. In my opinion the Carum is one of the best pumps on the market today. To locate a rental station, visit www.ardo-usa.com.

Hygeia EnDeare Pump. The EnDeare, an external-piston pump, is similar to Medela's Lactina but has smoother suctioning, which has been described as close to that of the Classic, SMB, and Lact-E pumps. The pump reaches 60 cycles per minute and suction levels of 250 millimeters of mercury, and there are separate dials for suction strength and pumping speed. The pump also includes an internal rechargeable battery pack for pumping when away from an outlet. There is even a button for recording a baby's sounds, which can be played back to help with the let-down response. A double collection kit must be purchased, but at about $40 it is less expensive than those used with other pumps. To locate a rental station near you, call 888-786-7466 or visit the website at www.hygeiababy.com.

Melodi Advanced Pump. The Melodi pump is a very small, sleek, well-built double electric pump. This 1½-pound pump is offered by some hospitals and birth centers and through WIC. This pump is very different from other

Melodi Advanced Pump

pumps. Instead of a speed control, it has a pattern of sucking six times in a row with a long pause, mimicking a baby's sucking and resting pattern. The pump offers both a faster stimulation pattern and a longer sucking pattern for milk expression. The pump suction levels reach a strong 250 millimeters of mercury. While there is a standard flange size that will fit most mothers, the company also offers larger sizes, as well as silicone inserts. The Melodi is a closed-system pump that does not allow milk to enter the tubing; it also has a hydrophobic filter to prevent airborne viruses and bacteria from entering the pump. The pump runs on AC, and the internal battery holds a charge for up to six running hours. The pump is sold by Lucina Care for $800 and is available through some rental stations. Their excellent customer service can be reached at 888-809-9750.

Melodi Advanced One Pump. The Advanced One is the same pump as the Advanced but with a smaller display screen and without the hydrophobic filter on top. The pump runs on AC power. This is the pump sent out to insurance customers from Lucina for rental. Very few insurance carriers offer clinical-grade pumps, but TriCare and Humana both offer the Melodi pump with a prescription from a doctor for mothers with sick or premature babies or those newborns with oral feeding problems. Once the pump is rented for ten months, it then becomes a purchase for the mother. The pump is sold by Lucina Care for $700, and their customer service can be reached at 888-809-9750.

Personal-Use Fully Automatic Double Electric Pumps

Personal-use fully automatic double electric pumps are generally purchased for mothers who need to pump often, such as mothers who are returning to work or school. Some of these pumps, or downsized versions, are offered by insurance carriers through the Affordable Care Act. (See page 230 for information on getting a pump through the Affordable Care Act. See page 275 for pumps commonly offered through the durable medical equipment companies of many insurance companies).

Medela Pump in Style Advanced Pump.
The very popular Pump in Style was the first
fully automatic pump offered for sale to nursing women. The Pump in Style Advanced has a
dual cycling pattern—rapid during the first 2
minutes to stimulate let-down, and then slower
and stronger for expression—but it lacks separate controls for speed and suction. Designed
for the working mother, this pump weighs
about 4 pounds and comes with a choice of mi-

Medela Pump in Style
Advanced Pump

crofiber bags. Included is a collection kit that allows the user to pump
one or both breasts at a time. The flange size is 24 millimeters, which
one study suggests is too small for about 75 percent of mothers. Other
sizes of flanges are available. The pump comes with a one-year warranty
and a battery pack to use when no electric outlet is available.

Like some other Medela pumps, the Pump in Style can get condensation, mold, and milk in the tubing. If you notice condensation in the
tubing, you need to run the pump with the tubing attached after expressing to dry the tubing and prevent mold formation. If you have a
strong let-down response, you may get milk in the tubing; if this happens, you may have to purchase new tubing.

The Pump in Style Advanced comes with the pump motor built into
a backpack or shoulder bag for a suggested retail price of $300, or with
the pump motor removable from a shoulder bag (the Metro Bag) for
$350. Each of these models comes with an insulated milk cooler, freezer
pack, and bottles. The models are available from some Medela rental
stations and from stores such as Babies "R" Us, Target, and Bed Bath &
Beyond. For more information, call Medela at 800-435-8316 or check
the website at www.medela.com.

Medela FreeStyle Pump. This latest pump from Medela is intended
for hands-free, two-sided pumping. The tiny 1-pound pump fits in the
palm of your hand. Like most of the other Medela pumps, this one offers
two phases, rapid cycling to stimulate milk let-down and then slower
cyclingwith higher suction for expression. The vacuum pressure reaches

a strong 250 millimeters of mercury, although some mothers report that the suction is not as strong as the Pump in Style. An internal lithium battery allows for three hours of pumping per charge, and the pump comes with an attractive tote bag.

Medela FreeStyle Pump

Reviews of this pump, by both mothers and lactation professionals, are quite mixed. Although cute and portable, the pump is very noisy. Setting up the system for hands-free pumping, some mothers say, is complicated and difficult. There are also some reports that the pump does not suction well and that the motor doesn't hold up.

The FreeStyle pump retails for $400 and has a one-year warranty. The pump is available from some Medela rental stations and from stores such as Babies "R" Us, Target, and Bed Bath & Beyond. For more information, call Medela at 800-435-8316 or check the website at www.medela.com.

Ardo Calypso-to-Go Pump. This new pump from Switzerland is quiet and effective. The actual pump is small, weighing only 1 pound. The pump runs on AC power or six AA batteries and has push-button controls on the base for both speed and suction. The speed ranges from 30 to 60 cycles per minute, and the suction reaches a high of 240 millimeters of mercury, ideal for frequent pumping. The pump includes a nice tote bag, with an additional cooler bag that can hold six extra bottles. The company also offers three sizes of flanges, a standard size of 26 millimeters and two larger sizes of 28 millimeters and 31 millimeters for larger nipples. There is also a soft silicone "optiflow" insert for more comfortable pumping. Another great feature is that it is a closed system, meaning you won't have to deal with condensation, milk, or mold in the tubings. In addition, Ardo is the only pump

Ardo Calypso-to-Go Pump

manufacturer to offer a full, no-quibble guarantee for the pump's full 400-hour operating life, irrespective of the date of purchase. The pump is available from www.ardo-usa.com and costs about $260.

Ardo Calypso Double Pump. This pump is the same pump as the Calypso-to-Go, with three sizes of flanges and the "optiflow" insert. It also has a closed system, keeping milk out of the tubings and pump. The only difference is that this model does not include the tote bag and cooler with extra bottles. The pump is available from www.ardo-usa.com and costs about $200.

Melodi Prime Pump. The Melodi Prime is the single-user version of the Melodi Advanced (see page 262). It runs on AC power or four AA batteries. Instead of a speed control, it has a pattern of sucking six times in a row with a long pause, mimicking a baby's sucking and resting pattern. The pump offers both a faster stimulation pattern and a longer sucking pattern for milk expression. The pump suction levels reach a strong 250 millimeters of mercury. While the standard flange size will fit most mothers, the company also offers larger sizes, as well as silicone inserts. The Melodi is a closed-system pump, so it will not allow milk to enter the tubing. The pump is sold by Lucina Care or other distributors for $250. Their customer service can be reached at 888-809-9750.

Ameda Purely Yours Pump. This is another fully automatic pump developed for single users. With this pump you can separately control the speed—which reaches 60 cycles per minute—and the strength of suction. You can also pump either one or both breasts at a time, although the maximum suction is low, around 210 millimeters of mercury, when the pump is used with the double collection kit. If set up to pump just one breast at a time, the suction improves significantly. When an electric outlet is unavailable, you can operate the pump with six AA batteries or an optional car

Ameda Purely Yours Pump

adapter. Mothers who use Purely Yours have reported no problems with condensation or milk in the tubing.

The pump is available packaged with various related equipment. The basic package, which includes the collection kit and tote, costs $200 but can usually be found for less online and at big-box stores. The backpack, which includes a car adapter, cooler pack, and four 4-ounce bottles, costs about $290 but can also usually be found for less. The newest package, the Purely Yours Ultra, comes with a stylish messenger bag, car adapter, milk cooler, and a wide variety of flanges to accommodate various nipple sizes, all for the suggested retail price of $300. With a one-year warranty, the pump is available from Ameda rental stations, other retailers, and the manufacturer. For more information, call 877-992-6332 or check the website at www.ameda.com.

Hygeia EnJoye Pump. This small pump has an internal-piston and works much like a clinical-grade pump. The suction reaches 250 mil-limeters of mercury, the speed can reach 60 cycles per minute, and there are separate dials for speed and suction. The breast flange comes with a larger nipple tunnel (27 millimeters) than those of many other pumps. It is not a closed system, so it is possible to get condensation and milk into the tubing, but not the

Hygeia EnJoye Pump

pump. EnJoye also has an innovative feature: You can record your baby's voice or any other sounds to play while you are expressing. The U.S. Food and Drug Administration (FDA) has certified EnJoye as a multiple-user pump, so mothers can share it without risk, provided they use separate collection kits.

The EnJoye retails for $280 with a collection kit and power cord, $300 with an added backpack or messenger bag and external battery pack, and $340 with the collection kit, backpack or bag, and an internal, four-hour lithium battery. The pump is available from the manufacturer, some retailers, and online. For more information, call 888-786-7466 or check the website at www.hygeiababy.com.

PJ's Comfort Pump. Manufactured by Limerick, this fully automatic pump weighs just 1½ pounds and has soft silicone flanges that compress and release the areola and nipples. The nipple tunnels may be a bit small for mothers with large nipples. With either single or double pumping, the pump starts on a rapid cycling and low vacuum, with a compression of a low 15 millimeters of mercury. The suction can be increased to up to 250 milligrams of mercury. Cycling is independent of vacuum, but as the vacuum increases, the cycling slows down. With higher vacuums, the flanges actually squeeze down on both the areolas and the nipples, which could be uncomfortable for some mothers. This pump gets mixed reviews from mothers. The FDA classifies PJ's as a multiple-user pump, so mothers can share it, provided they use separate collection kits. The pump is available from the manufacturer for $525 without a carrying case or cooler or for slightly more with these accessories. This company offers a three-year warranty for the pump. For more information, call 877-546-3742 toll free or check the website at www.limerickinc.com.

PJ's Comfort Pump

PJ's Bliss Pump. Also manufactured by Limerick, this fully automatic pump is similar to PJ's Comfort Pump, but it has a smaller motor and is intended for single users, not as a rental pump. With either single or double pumping, the pump starts on a rapid cycling and low vacuum, with a compression of a low 15 millimeters of mercury. The suction can be increased to up to 250 millimeters of mercury. Cycling is independent of vacuum, but as the vacuum increases, the cycling slows down. The pumping kit is the same as PJ's Comfort Pump, so it also squeezes down on both the areola and nipples, especially with higher vacuums. The FDA classifies PJ's as a multiple-user pump, so mothers can share it, provided they use separate collection kits. The pump costs $260 and is warrantied for one year. For more information, call 877-546-3742 or check the website at www.limerickinc.com.

Philips Avent Comfort Double Pump. This lightweight pump offers two phases, a faster sucking pattern for milk let-down and a slower one for milk expression. The pump offers three suction levels, with the highest reaching a strong 240 millimeters of mercury. This pump has a closed system, meaning milk won't get into the tubings. The pump works

Philips Avent Comfort Double Pump

on AC power only and does not allow for single pumping. Included is a carrying bag, but it comes with only two bottles, and bottles from other companies do not fit this pump, nor is it possible to pump into milk bags. Some mothers complain about the motor breaking down, and it is quite noisy. In addition, the soft insert for more comfortable pumping may be too small or short for many mothers. The listed price for this pump is $200, but it can be purchased more inexpensively online or from big-box stores. For more information, call 800-54-AVENT or visit the website at www.philips.com.

Lansinoh Signature Pro Double Electric Pump. This double electric pump offers three different pumping patterns, as well as adjustable suction levels that reach as high as 250 millimeters of mercury. It comes with a 25-millimeter flange, which may be a bit small for mothers with large nipples. Larger flanges (30.5 millimeters) to accommodate mothers with larger nipples can be ordered from Lansinoh or purchased from Babies "R" Us. The bottles used with the pump are specific to Lansinoh. The pump has an LED display for timing, speed, and suction. The pump works with either AC power or batteries. It has a closed system, meaning milk won't get into the tubing or the pump. This pump has a nice carrying case and is priced at a reasonable $150. Retailers include Wal-Mart, Target, and Babies "R" Us. Lanisnoh's customer service can be reached at 800-292-4794.

Lansinoh Signature Pro Double Electric Pump

Rumble Tuff Serene Express Duo Electric Breast Pump. This small double electric pump is a fairly inexpensive personal-use pump that works surprisingly well. It has three different cycle patterns and reaches good suction levels of 250 millimeters of mercury. Mothers seem to be able to get a good deal

Rumble Tuff Serene Express Duo Electric Breast Pump

of milk compared with other personal-use pumps. It is a closed system, meaning that milk will not get into the tubes as with many other electric pumps. It has a flange that will fit most mothers' nipples, as well an optional silicone insert. It runs on AC power or with four AA batteries. It also has a timer and memory function. It can be converted to a manual pump as well. This pump is assembled a bit differently from many other pumps, but it is easy to master by following the instructions provided. Because it is not possible to pump directly into milk bags, you may need extra bottles when you are pumping away from the baby. When the pump first came out it was a bit noisy, as many small pumps are, but that has been remedied by the manufacturer and it is now quieter. The pump sells for about $170 at www.rumbletuff.com and other online stores. Rumble Tuff's customer service is available at 855-228-8388.

The First Years Breastflow Memory Pump. This pump from The First Years is relatively quiet and runs on AC or a rechargeable battery. It includes a touch screen for starting the pump, timing pumpings, and increasing the speed and suction. The memory button remembers the settings from the previous pumping. This pump offers three low speeds and eight suction levels that reach only a weak 180 millimeters of mercury. Some mothers also complain that the soft silicone flanges are uncomfortable and difficult to position

The First Years Breastflow Memory Pump

with the unusual handlebar that holds the flanges and bottles together for one-handed pumping. This pump includes a tote bag and a cooler tote but no additional bottles, and the bottles are not standard-sized. The price for this pump is $180, and it is available online or at most big-box stores. Customer service can be reached at 800-704-8697, or you can visit the website at www.thefirstyears.com.

The First Years Quiet Expressions Double Breast Pump. This pump is similar to the First Years Breastflow Memory Pump with a few exceptions. Most notably, there is only one speed on the pump. But like the Breastflow, this model has eight suction levels, reaching a low 180 millimeters of mercury. It works on both AC power and AA batteries. Some mothers complain that the soft silicone flanges are uncomfortable and difficult to position with the unusual handlebar that holds the flanges and bottles together for one-handed pumping. The pump offers only one size of silicone flanges, which may be too small for mothers with larger nipples. The price of the pump is $100, and it is available at some big-box stores and online at www.thefirstyears.com. For customer service, call 800-704-8697.

The First Years miPump Double Electric Breast Pump. This pump is a relatively quiet automatic pump that runs on AC power or four AA batteries from a rechargeable base. The highest of eight suction levels is a weak 180 millimeters of mercury, and the speed is only 40 cycles per minute. Some mothers complain that the soft silicone flanges are difficult to position and uncomfortable. As with the other First Years pumps, it has an unusual handlebar connecting two collection bottles but only one small-sized flange for one-handed pumping. The pump comes with a carrying case. The price of the pump is $80, and it is available at some big-box stores and online at www.thefirstyears.com. For customer service, call 800-704-8697.

Evenflo Deluxe Advanced Double Electric Pump. This pump runs on either AC power or with six AA batteries and has a closed system to keep milk, condensation, and mold out of the tubing. It comes with two sizes of soft inserts. It offers four different speeds and eight suction levels, but the suction does not reach very high levels, only about 170 millimeters of mercury. The speed slows when the suction increases. This pump can be used as a single pump as well as a double. When the pump is used as a single, the suction levels increase to a strong 240 millimeters of mercury. The pump costs about $180 and is available through big-box stores and online. Customer service can be reached at 800-233-5921.

Evenflo Deluxe Advanced Double Electric Pump

NUK Expressive Double Electric Pump. This pump works as a double or single pump. It has four speeds and eight suction levels, although the suction is low, at only 200 millimeters of mercury. There is also a memory button that recalls the settings from the previous pumping. It runs on AC power only. It is a closed system, so you won't get milk,

NUK Expressive Double Electric Pump

mold, or condensation in the tubing, and it comes with soft silicone inserts. The pump costs $150 and can be purchased both online and at big-box stores. Another model, available through Babies "R" Us, includes a cooler bag and costs $180. You can reach NUK at 888-NUK-1238.

Spectra S1 and S2 pumps. These two pumps are for either double or single pumping. Both offer a closed system that keeps milk out of the tubes and the pump. They are very lightweight, at only 2 pounds, and are quiet and effective. The pumps have

Spectra S1 and S2

an LCD display for both suction and speed modes. The underside of the handles light up for nighttime pumping. The Spectra S1 offers AC power as well as an internal rechargeable battery that will hold a charge for up to three hours of pumping time; the S2 runs on AC power only. The S1 pump retail for $300 and the Spectra S2 for $225. Visit www.spectrababyusa.com or call 855-44-MOMBABY.

Spectra Dew 350 pump. This 5-pound pump can be used as either a single or double pump. The pump does not get strong pressures, only 200 millimeters of mercury, unless used as a single pump or unless the filters are removed. This pump does not have a closed system, but there is a filter to keep milk from

Spectra Dew 350

entering the pump. The pump has a set speed of around 48 cycles per minute. The pump sells for $190. Visit www.spectrababyusa.com or call 855-44-MOMBABY.

Spectra M1 pump. This 1-pound pump can also be used as a single or double pump. It is a closed system. It has five speeds and gets high pressures of up to 250 millimeters of mercury. The plastic flanges will fit most mothers. The price of this pump is $160. Visit www.spectrababyusa.com or call 855-44-MOMBABY.

Spectra M1

Spectra 9+ pump. Weighing less than 1 pound, this tiny pump offers multiple pumping speeds of up to 60 cycles per minute. The pressure reaches high levels. The pump works on AC power and also has an internal rechargeable battery.

Spectra 9+

The price of this pump is about $230. Visit www.spectrababyusa.com or call 855-44-MOMBABY.

Tommee Tippee Closer to Nature Double Electric Breast Pump System. This pump can be used for both single and double pumping, and it runs on either AC power or an internal battery. The pump is a bit noisy, but it reaches high suction levels. There are no speed controls, but there are five levels of pumping. While the speed stays the same, the suction increases with each level, reaching a very high 270 millimeters of mercury. The pump comes with a nice insu-

Tommee Tippee Closer to Nature Double Electric Breast Pump System

lated tote with a cooler bag and extra pumping bottles (not standard-sized), plus 2- and 4-ounce storage bottles. The flanges have soft inserts for more comfortable pumping. It has a closed system, so milk won't get into the tubing. The pump costs $200 and is available online.

Dr. Brown's Double Electric Breast Pump. This double electric pump comes in a nice carrying bag and includes a cooler bag and two Dr. Brown "Natural Flow" bottles. This pump works on AC power only, and it is noisy. It allows for adjusting speed as well as suction. The soft comfort flanges have very small openings and will not fit many mothers' nipples. The suction is quite low, and mothers complain that they are unable to get much milk using this pump. In addition, numerous parts must be assembled before each use. The list price is $250, but it can be found for much less at big-box and online stores. Customer service is excellent and can be reached at 800-778-9001.

Dr. Brown's Double Electric Breast Pump

Common Personal-Use Pumps Offered by Insurance Carriers

Medela Pump in Style Advanced Breast Pump Starter Set and Medela Pump in Style Advanced Tote or Backpack. The "Starter Set" model is the same pump as the Pump in Style Advanced Tote or Backpack (see page 264). Like the models sold in stores or online, this pump offers two-phase expression and strong suctions of up to 240 millimeters of mercury. The flange size is 24 millimeters, which one study suggests is too small for about 75 percent of mothers, but larger sizes are available. As with other Medela pumps, milk can get into the tubing and the pump.

Medela Pump in Style Advanced Breast Pump Starter Set

Medela Personal Double Pump. While this pump does not have the two-phase expression as in most other Medela pumps, it does have three speed settings, up to 60 cycles per minute, which can be used instead of the two phases. The pump has good suction. The flange size is 24 millimeters, which one study suggests is too small for about 75 percent of mothers, but larger sizes are available. As with other Medela pumps, milk can get into the tubing and the pump.

Medela Personal Double Pump

Hygeia EnJoye Q Pump. The Hygeia EnJoye Q pump is the same as the Hygeia EnJoye (see page 267) with two exceptions: It does not have a handle or a button that can record your baby's voice.

Other personal-use pumps commonly available from insurance companies are the **Ameda Purely Yours** (page 266), **Hygeia EnJoye** (page 267); **Lansinoh Signature Pro** (page 269), **Melodi Prime** (page 266), and **Rumble Tuff Serene Express Duo** (page 270).

Note that some insurance companies offer higher-grade pumps with a co-pay.

Other Purchases You Might Consider

If you will be pumping your milk often, you might consider whether you'd like to be able to pump with your hands free. Some women, particularly those who are exclusively pumping or who want to multitask while pumping at work, find breastfeeding "bustiers" helpful. These commercially available zippered bras (see Appendix A, page 360) can hold the pump flanges in place while you talk on the phone, work on a computer, or read a book to an older child. Or you may prefer to use a tight-fitting sports bra with small circles cut out at the nipples (you can slip nursing pads into the holes each time you finish pumping).

You might also consider investing in special flanges for more comfortable pumping. The angled, elliptical Pumpin' Pal Super Shields can be inserted into regular pump flanges to allow you to sit back while pumping. Many mothers report that the flanges gently milk the breast instead of simply pulling on the nipple and areola, and some mothers say they can tolerate higher suction with Super Shields and therefore collect more milk in less time. A few mothers claim that while using the flanges, they suffer fewer incidents of plugged milk ducts. A neck strap allows for pumping hands-free. Especially helpful for mothers who pump regularly or often, Super Shields work with Medela, Ameda, Lansinoh, Hygeia, Philips Avent, Nurture III, and certain other pumps. See Appendix A, page 360, for ordering information.

Single Electric Pumps and Semi-Automatic Pumps

Single pumps are less popular with nursing mothers because they take twice the time to express both breasts. On the other hand, they are typically less expensive. Semi-automatic pumps require the mother to use her finger or thumb to create and release the suction.

Medela Swing Pump. Operable either by battery or by electricity from a wall socket, this pump is designed for pumping one breast at a time. Like most other Medela pumps, the Swing has two phases: fast cycling and light suction to stimulate let-down, and slower cycling

Medela Swing Pump

and stronger suction for expression. The adjustable suction reaches high levels. With a suggested retail price of $170, this pump is available from some Medela rental stations and also from stores such as Babies "R" Us, Target, and Bed Bath & Beyond. For more information, call Medela at 800-435-8316 or check the website at www.medela.com.

Nurture III Pump. The semi-automatic Nurture III, about the size of a small aquarium pump, operates with electricity from a wall socket. The pump has variable suction strength and speed (determined by how long you cover a vent with your finger), single- or double-pumping capability, and a five-year warranty. The

Nurture III Pump

Nurture III costs $130 or, with a tote bag, freezer pack, extra bottles, and instructional DVD, $160. Mothers with low incomes can get either model for $50 less. Order through the website at www.baileymed.com or call 800-413-3216.

Philips Avent Comfort Single Electric Pump. The Avent Comfort Single is similar to the Avent Comfort Double (see page 269) but works for single-sided pumping only. The pump operates with electricity from a wall socket or from four AA batteries and is a bit noisy. The pump offers two speeds and three suction levels, reaching 240 millimeters of mercury. A soft cover over the hard plastic flange increases the suction strength and massages the areola, although the insert works best for mothers with smaller or shorter nipples. Several parts must be assembled before each use. The manufacturer's suggested retail price is $130, but the pump can be ordered online from a variety of retailers for less. The pump comes with a one-year warranty for defects. For more information, check the website at www.philips.com or call 800-54-AVENT.

Evenflo Single Electric Pump. Powered by AC power or three AA batteries, this fully automatic pump cycles at about 57 times per minute and reaches suctions of 250 millimeters of mercury. A dual model is simply two single pumps, which are

Evenflo Single Electric Pump

held one to each breast. Both models are available in discount stores, for about $45 for the single pump and $70 for the double pump. For more information, visit the website at www.evenflo.com or call 800-233-5921.

Rumble Tuff Easy Express Single Electric Breast Pump. This small single electric pump is fairly similar to the Rumble Tuff Serene Express Duo Electric Pump (see page 270) with the exception that it expresses milk from just one breast at a time. It can be converted to a manual pump as well. Like the Duo Electric, it has three different cycle patterns and reaches good suction levels of 250 millimeters of mercury. It also has a timer and memory function. It has a flange size that will fit most mothers' nipples, as well as an optional silicone insert. It runs on either AC power or four AA batteries. It also includes a timer and memory function. This pump is assembled a bit differently from many other pumps, but it is easy to master by following the instructions provided. Because it is not possible to pump directly into milk bags, you may need extra bottles when you are pumping away from the baby. When the pump first came out it was a bit noisy, as many small pumps are, but that has been remedied by the company and it is now quieter. The pump sells for about $85 at www.rumbletuff.com and other online stores. Rumble Tuff's customer service is available at 855-228-8388.

Ardo Calypso Single Electric Pump. This pump is exactly the same as the Calypso-to-Go (see page 265) and the Calypso Double (see page 266) except that it expresses milk from just one side at a time. It comes with just one flange size. It also has a closed system, keeping milk out of the tubing and pump. The pump is available from www.ardo-usa.com and costs about $160.

NUK Expressive Single Electric Pump. This pump runs on either AC power or three AA batteries. It has a very hard silicone flange and reaches a weak 190 millimeters of mercury. If the pump tips in any direction, it turns off. This pump can be purchased for $50 from online and big-box stores. You can reach NUK at 888-NUK-1238.

NUK Expressive Single Electric Pump

Tommee Tippee Closer to Nature Electric Single Breast Pump System. This pump runs on either AC power or four AA batteries. It has a closed system, so milk won't get into the tubing. The pump is a bit noisy, but it reaches high suction levels. The bottles are not a standard size. The flange has soft inserts for more comfortable pumping. There are no speed controls, but there are four levels of pumping. While the speed

Tommee Tippee Closer to Nature Electric Single Breast Pump System

stays the same, the suction increases with each level, reaching a low suction of only 210 millimeters of mercury. The pump costs $150 and can be purchased online.

Freemie Freedom Pump. This new pump uses special cups instead of flanges and bottles for milk expression and collection. The cups are held in place by a bra, making the pump hands-free. The pump reaches reasonable suction levels of about 220 millimeters of mercury. There are three cup sizes for small, medium, and large nipples: 25 millimeter, 28 millimeter, and 32 millimeter. The tubings go from the top of the cups to the breast pump. Some mothers report that they like the feel of the cups compared to typical pump flanges but that the cups are too large to be covered by most shirts—each cup holds up to a whopping 8 ounces of milk. Some mothers complain that because the cups are opaque, they can't see how much milk is being pumped. There are also complaints that the cups are difficult to pull apart for cleaning. Mothers with very large or very small breasts may have difficulty using this pump system. It is possible for milk to get into the tubing. The pump and cups are sold online and directly from www.freemie.com for about $160. The cups can also be ordered separately for $50, along with a conversion kit to be used with Medela, Philips, and Ameda pumps. Customer service can be reached at 916-339-7388.

Freemie Freedom Pump

Hand-Operated Pumps

Manual pumps are reasonable for mothers who are rarely apart from their babies. They are inexpensive, and some are more comfortable and less tiring to use than others.

"Bicycle horn" pumps. These old-style pumps are available for less than $10 in some drug-stores. A bulb is squeezed for suction, and the milk flows directly into it. Most authorities warn against using milk collected this way, since the

"Bicycle horn" pump

bulb is difficult to clean and may harbor harmful bacteria. In addition, many women find that these pumps work poorly and can be uncomfortable. When used improperly, they can cause trauma to the breast or the nipple. And, since they hold little milk, they must be emptied frequently.

Medela Harmony Pump. With a soft flange and a squeeze handle, this manual pump offers two basic settings, one to stimulate let-down and the other for after the milk starts flowing. In place of Medela's standard hard plastic flange is a soft, flexible silicone one; it tends to ripple and leak milk, and its nipple tunnel may be too small for some mothers. The Harmony is avail-

Medela Harmony Pump

able, with a 30-day warranty, for $40 from Medela pump rental stations and discount stores. For more information, call Medela at 800-435-8316 or check the website at www.medela.com.

Philips Avent Isis Manual Pump. This pump has been available for quite some time and is a favorite among some nursing mothers. When you squeeze the handle, a soft silicone cover over the hard plastic flange gently compresses the areola to stimulate milk flow, but the silicone insert may be too small or short for some mothers. The pump is available at ba-

Philips Avent Isis
Manual Pump

by-goods stores and from the manufacturer for about $45. To find a supplier or to order direct, visit www.philips.com or call 800-54-AVENT.

Lansinoh Manual Breast Pump. This squeeze-handle pump is like most others, but it has two sizes of silicone flanges for comfortable pumping. This pump does reach high suction levels. The pump is available in some drugstores and at Babies "R" Us, Wal-Mart, and Target for about $35, or at www.lansinoh.com. Lanisnoh's customer service can be reached at 800-292-4794.

Evenflo Manual Pump. Available for about $25 in many discount stores, this pump creates suction by use of a squeeze handle. There is a dial for adjusting vacuum strength and a soft silicone insert in the flange. For more information, check the website at www.evenflo.com or call 800-233-5921.

The First Years Easy Breastflow Manual Pump. This is another lightweight manual pump that is operated by squeezing the handle. The pump reaches high suction levels. Quiet and easy to clean, the pump comes with two 5-ounce bottles. It costs about $30 and can be ordered online at www.firstyears.com or purchased at some big-box stores. For more information, call 800-704-8697.

Ameda One-Hand Pump. With this pump you create suction by squeezing a hand grip. As the name implies, you can operate the pump with just one hand. The One-Hand is available for about $40 from Ameda, its rental stations, and some other retailers. For more information, call 877-992-6332 or check the website at www.ameda.com.

Ameda One-Hand Pump

Dr. Brown's Manual Breast Pump. This squeeze-handle pump is similar to others in this category with the exception of the soft flange that is placed around the nipple. The flange opening is very small, probably too small for most mothers, and the suction is rather low. The price is $35, but it can be purchased for less at drugstores and big-box stores, or online. Dr. Brown's customer service can be reached at 800-778-9001.

Rumble Tuff Sweet Essence Manual Breast Pump. This squeeze-handle pump is like most others in this category with a few exceptions.

First, it comes with a soft silicone flange insert. Also, with the handle in the higher slot, it provides a short, quick sucking pattern to stimulate let-down; changing to the lower slot position, it provides deeper, slower sucking at good pressures of 240 millimeters of mercury. On the top of the pump, there is a dial to turn the suction higher or lower. This pump sells for about $20 at www.rumbletuff.com other online stores. Rumble Tuff's customer service is available at 855-228-8388.

Rumble Tuff Sweet Assist Manual Breast Pump. This squeeze-handle pump is like many others in this category with a few exceptions. The squeeze handle can be held in any position away from the pump, which may mean more comfortable hand motions. It comes with a soft silicone flange insert. Like the Sweet Essence pump, this model has a higher slot to provide a short, quick sucking pattern to stimulate let-

Rumble Tuff Sweet Assist Manual Breast Pump

down, and then a lower slot to provide deeper, slower sucking at good pressures of 240 millimeters of pressure. On the top of the pump, there is a dial to turn the suction higher or lower. This pump sells for about $25 at www.rumbletuff.com and other online stores. Rumble Tuff's customer service is available at 855-228-8388.

Lucina Melodi Advanced Manual Breast Pump. This squeeze-handle pump is similar to others in this category. The handle can be used by either right- or left-handed mothers. The pump is sold by Lucina Care for $20; their excellent customer service can be reached at 888-809-9750.

NUK Expressive Manual Pump. This squeeze-handle pump is like most others. It has a hard flange with a soft insert. The pump offers rapid suction with fast squeezing of the handle, and deeper suction with slower squeezing of the handle. This pump can be purchased for about $30 from online and big-box stores. You can reach NUK at 888-NUK-1238.

Hygeia EnHande One-Hand Manual Breast Pump. This is another squeeze-handle pump. This pump costs $35 and can be ordered from Hygeia at 888-786-7466 or from retailers who carry Hygeia products.

Hygeia Two-Handed Manual Breast Pump. This pump requires both hands to hold the flange against the breast and pull the plunger back and forth to create and release the suction. It can be more tiring to use than typical squeeze-handle pumps. This pump costs $20 and can be ordered from Hygeia at 888-786-7466 or from retailers who carry Hygeia products.

Hygeia Two-Handed Manual Breast Pump

PJ's Manual Breast Pump. This squeeze-handle pump is similar to most others with the exception of the flange. This flange squeezes down on both the areola and nipple. The pump costs $40 and is available through Limerick. For more information, call 877-546-3742 or check the website at www.limerickinc.com.

Spectra Handy Plus Manual Pump. This squeeze-handle pump is similar to most other manual pumps. It includes a silicone insert for more comfortable pumping, but the insert may make pumping more comfortable for mothers with larger nipples. This pump sells for $30 and can be ordered from Spectra at 855-766-4719.

Tommee Tippee Closer to Nature Manual Breast Pump System. This squeeze-handle pump is similar to most other manual pumps. The bottles are not a standard size. The flange has soft inserts for more comfortable pumping, but it is too small for even the smallest nipple. The pump can be purchased for $47 online.

Freemie Equality Hand Pump. This pump uses the unique breast cup that is also available with the Freemie Freedom Pump (see page 279). This manual pump can be used to pump one or both breasts at the same time. The pump does get high pressures but can be a bit tiring to use. The pump is sold online and through www.freemie.com for about $70. Customer service can be reached at 916-339-7388.

The Freemie Equality Hand Pump

TRAVELING TOGETHER, BEING APART

TODAY'S NURSING MOTHER IS OUT AND ABOUT, taking care of business, enjoying the company of friends, returning to work or school, taking time out for fun. In many ways, nursing simplifies life considerably. With the increasing acceptance and popularity of breastfeeding, more and more mothers are able to nurse their babies while participating in a wide variety of activities.

TAKING THE BABY ALONG

Your nursing baby can go with you almost anywhere—and with a lot less hassle than you would face if you were fussing with formula and bottles.

You may feel comfortable nursing in the presence of family or friends you are visiting, or you may be a bit uneasy. You can always retreat to the bedroom, of course, but that's not much fun. Learning to nurse discreetly and without embarrassment will put most people at ease. You might want to practice ahead of time getting the baby on your breast with a blanket or shawl draped over your shoulder and the baby's head. If you wear a shirt or a sweater you can pull up, or if you unbutton your blouse from the bottom, you will expose less of yourself. Most maternity shops carry a line of attractive tops and dresses designed for discreet nursing. Try nursing in front of your partner or in front of a mirror so you'll know what others will see. There are also nursing covers available for purchase that cover the baby but allow you to look down at him while feeding.

If you are going out for the day or spending a few hours in town, you may want to nurse just before you leave. A couple of diapers and a few moist wipes in a zipper-top bag, and you're off. If you are using a cloth baby carrier, you may find it easier to put it on before you go.

After a couple of hours out, look around for a comfortable place to sit with your baby. Many mothers feel comfortable nursing in public places and are hardly noticed when they do so. Some stores and restaurants have dressing rooms or pleasant restrooms where you may prefer to feed the baby.

Many first-time mothers worry about being asked to cover up or leave when they are nursing out of the house. You may have heard of others who have been harassed when they nursed their children in public. But know that most states have laws protecting the rights of nursing mothers in public. As of this writing, only two states, West Virginia and Idaho, have no laws protecting a mother's right to nurse in public. The other states have protection laws that vary in their language. You can find your state's laws at www.nursingfreedom.org.

Mothers appreciate the ease of taking long trips with their nursing babies. Most young infants travel well in a car. (Of course, the baby should always ride in a car seat approved for safety, no matter how short the trip.) You will want to stop every few hours for nursing and a diaper change. As the baby's car seat faces backward, you may be able to manage nursing while sitting in the back seat next to her.

The older baby may be less happy in the car seat for long periods. Whenever possible try to start long stretches in the car just before naptime. Try hanging some of the baby's toys on her car seat or keeping a bag of toys and other fun things in the back seat.

If you are planning to fly, you might try to reserve bulkhead seating; this will give you extra space. Try to choose a flight that is lightly booked. This way you are more likely to get an empty seat next to you for more room and privacy. Nursing during takeoff and landing will help the baby's ears adjust to the changing air pressure. If you must fly when the baby has a cold, give her a safe decongestant an hour before takeoff.

BEING APART

Occasional Separations

Any number of situations may come up in which you must be separated from your baby—an evening out, a family or career obligation, or a stay in the hospital.

When you plan to be away from the baby for just a few hours, you can manually express or pump some milk for him ahead of time (see Chapter 5). If you will be separated from the baby for a day or longer, you may be able to store enough milk for him ahead of time. If not, you can substitute a commercially prepared formula. While you are away, try to pump at least once every three hours. A clinical-grade rental pump or a near-clinical-grade personal pump may be more convenient than other kinds, and also most effective for keeping up your milk supply. If possible, keep the milk you pump cold while you are apart so that it can be frozen and used later.

If you will be flying with expressed breast milk, either with or without the baby, you may wonder about getting through airport security. Mothers are now permitted to bring any amount of milk on flights, as long as it is declared for inspection at the security checkpoints.

Hospitalization of a nursing mother rarely necessitates weaning, even though some doctors advise it. Some hospitals have electric breast pumps available for nursing mothers. If your hospital doesn't, you can rent a pump and take it with you, or have one brought in. You may be able to arrange for the baby to be brought in for nursing visits, or even for the baby to stay with you (providing that you, a family member, or a friend can care for him). Try to express your milk frequently to maintain your milk supply. Ask the nursing staff to refrigerate your milk so that it can be taken home for your baby. After surgery, mothers can safely nurse or express milk and save it for the baby, as once you are awake from anesthesia, there is not enough left in your body to be a problem for the baby. See Appendix D, page 377, for more information on anesthesia.

Questions may arise about the safety of medications you need to take in the hospital. Although most medications pass through into the breast milk, the majority are safe for nursing babies. Occasionally, a doctor may be unsure whether a given medication is safe for a baby and so recommends weaning when the question arises. You can check the safety of the drug yourself in Appendix D. If a drug is not considered safe for a nursing baby, you can continue to pump your milk, discarding it until the medication is no longer required.

RETURNING TO WORK OR SCHOOL

Not so long ago, a new mother planning to return to work might never have considered nursing her baby or would have decided to wean near the end of her maternity leave. Today, with the growing number of working women and the increasing awareness of the many benefits breastfeeding offers, more and more mothers are choosing to nurse their babies while continuing with their careers.

Your extra efforts to continue nursing are well worth your while. The cost of formula aside, breastfed babies are generally healthier. The less your baby is sick, the less time you must spend away from work or school. Nursing also saves you time and energy, which is especially important when you are combining the responsibilities of employment and family. Perhaps most important, nursing helps you maintain the close, loving relationship you have with your baby. Many mothers who work outside the home or attend school feel that breastfeeding offers emotional compensation for the hours that must be spent apart. The security of your breast comforts the baby and helps make the time you are together special and rewarding for both of you.

Work Options

Although there may be no question in your mind that you will be returning to work or school after your baby is born, you are lucky if you have some flexibility in determining the length of your maternity leave. Your time at home after giving birth is important for both you and the baby: It is the time in which you will get to know each other and form a special bond. It will also be a time for you to rest and recover from the physical stress of the birth process. Some women need a little while, and some need a long while, before they are ready to add the demands of work or school. Breastfeeding experts have noted that mothers who stay home for 16 weeks or longer experience fewer difficulties maintaining their milk supply once back at work.

Because you cannot know just how you will feel after you deliver, explore what options may be open to you ahead of time. Depending on your financial situation and your work demands, you may be able to arrange for an extended leave, beyond the usual six to eight weeks. In 1993, the United States enacted the Family Medical Leave Act (FMLA), which requires employers with 50 or more employees to allow 12 weeks unpaid leave each year for any employee who needs to care for a dependent. Taking unpaid leave may be helpful to you, or it may not be financially feasible. You may be able instead to arrange to work at home, return to work part-time, or share your job with another person. Each of these options has worked well for many mothers. If you are a student, perhaps you can take fewer classes for a term or take some classes online.

Part-time work offers many advantages to the nursing mother. Fewer hours apart means fewer missed feedings, lower child-care costs, and generally less stress for both mother and baby.

An employer also benefits by agreeing to shorter hours. Replacing an employee is time-consuming and costly, especially if she has special skills that are an asset to the organization. Besides, many employers find part-time employees to be just as productive as those who work full-time, if not more so. Part-timers tend to stay out sick less often, and they generally waste less time when they are at work.

You might agree to come in for fewer hours each day, or have fewer full-hour days. Both arrangements have advantages and drawbacks for the nursing mother.

Still, a somewhat flexible arrangement may be possible. With a "flex-time" schedule, you might work eight hours a day but remain free to start earlier or later than normal. This system could allow you to spend a leisurely morning with the baby and perhaps get a few chores done. If your partner also has a flexible schedule, you might be able to minimize the number of hours that the baby must be left with someone else.

Some mothers arrange to take their babies to work with them. Although this is not possible for most women, it can be managed in some work settings. Another option is childcare at the work site. Some employers and employees have found this to be an ideal arrangement. If you work with other parents of infants or small children, you might together explore this possibility.

Another possibility is having the baby brought to you for nursings, or going to the baby yourself during your lunch hour. Usually, the major obstacle in having the baby come to your workplace is finding someone willing and able to bring her. If instead you'll go to the baby, you will want to find childcare as close as possible to your workplace. If you have a full hour for lunch and your baby is nearby, you may have enough time to leisurely manage travel, nursing, and eating.

Choosing a Caregiver

Finding just the right person to care for your baby can make all the difference in your state of mind while you are away. If you will be shopping for a caregiver, be sure to start early so you can take your time. You may prefer someone who will care for your baby alone, or you may be willing to share the caregiver's services with others. Finding a caregiver who lives close to your workplace or school will help you minimize the time you and your baby are apart even if you decide against nursing during your lunch breaks.

You may be fortunate enough to have a partner or another relative who is able and eager to provide childcare. Childcare with a loving relative can make the separation easier on both mother and baby and is usually inexpensive, if not free. Working out differences in philosophy about napping, feeding, and the like, however, may be more difficult with a family member.

Some families decide to hire a nanny. This is usually the most expensive option for childcare, but it also has some great benefits: The baby has one-on-one attention and is less exposed to infectious disease, and the nanny may offer more flexible scheduling and may also be willing to take on household duties besides infant care. Special arrangements may need to be made, however, if the nanny gets sick. Some nannies commute to the family home each day, while others live in. You can find a nanny through a local or Internet-based agency or through private advertisements and word of mouth. If you plan to hire someone without the help of an agent, you will want to not only interview the nanny but also check her references and perhaps order a criminal background check.

The U.S. Department of State authorizes agencies for au pairs, college-aged women who come to the United States from other countries to live with a family and care for the family's children for a year. Au pairs speak English, have at least 200 hours of child-care experience, and have received instruction in child safety and child development. The family provides meals, a private room, and $500 toward six semesters of college classes. The agency that sets up the relationship also monitors it. An au pair costs approximately $13,000 for the year, less than a typical nanny. For more information about the Au Pair Program, visit the website at www.iapa.org.

Family day care is the most popular child-care option, partially because it's usually less expensive than one-on-one care. For older babies and toddlers, family day care also offers the benefit of getting to know other children. In most states, family day-care providers are licensed, unless they are caring only for their own children and one other child, and are legally limited in the number of infants and older children they can care for. Family day-care providers aren't required to have had formal instruction in child development, and some states don't even require health and safety certifications. Like nannies, family day-care providers seldom offer alternative care when the provider gets ill or goes on vacation, although parents may be expected to pay for vacation time.

Lastly, there are day-care centers, which care for large numbers of children and are usually licensed by the state. Many day-care centers have numerous employees with education in childhood development. If one employee gets sick or goes on vacation, there is always another to fill in. There are disadvantages to day-care centers: The children generally get less one-on-one care than those with a nanny or au pair or in family day care; there may be much more sickness when large groups of children are kept together; and hours at a center are usually strict, so you may have to pay extra if you are late picking up your child. Also, some centers do not take infants. Often the best centers have waiting lists; you may need to get on one months before your baby is born.

Let each prospective caregiver know about your nursing relationship and your own particular style of baby care. Ask for the names and telephone numbers of other families whose children she has cared for in the past or is caring for now, and call the families to hear about their experiences with the caregiver. If she is caring for other children now, plan to meet with her at a time when they will be present and awake. This way you'll be able to not only see the environment but also observe her style, and judge whether she would give your baby enough individual love and attention. As you chat with the caregiver, try to find out if she can make a long-term commitment to your baby; having to find a replacement suddenly could be upsetting for both you and the baby.

Discuss arrangements for illness (either your baby's or hers) and vacations (your family's or hers), who would be called in an emergency, how much advance notice would be necessary if the baby were to be absent or late, and fees and when they would be due. Ask to look at any written agreements before you're expected to sign them. In making your final choice of who will care for your baby, trust your intuition. If something doesn't feel quite right, look elsewhere.

Consider having the baby spend several hours or a full day with the chosen caregiver a week or so before you go back to work or school. Such a "trial run" might be reassuring for you, or you may feel, as many mothers do, that the first separation should occur only when the situation demands it.

Planning Your Return to Work

If you will be missing one or more feedings while you are away at work or school, you should plan to express your milk. This will help prevent engorgement and, more important, maintain your milk supply. The milk you express can be used later to feed your baby while you are away.

See Chapter 5 for information on

- expression methods,
- types and brands of pumps,
- other purchases you may want to consider,
- pumping at home in preparation for your return to work or school,
- expressing milk in the workplace,
- increasing your milk supply,
- storing your expressed milk, and
- feeding your milk to the baby.

Besides finding a caregiver for your baby, choosing a pump, and learning to use it, your main task in planning a return to work is to identify a place to express your milk. For some mothers, this can be difficult.

Working out this problem ahead of time can help reduce the stress once you are back at work or school.

In 2010, the Affordable Care Act amended the Fair Labor Standards Act to require employers with 50 or more employees to provide a "reasonable" break time for employees who need to express breast milk for their nursing children. They are required to provide this until the baby turns one year old. Employers must also provide a place for the employee to express the milk, other than a bathroom. This area must be shielded from view and free from intrusion from co-workers and the public.

Employers are not required to pay an employee for any work time spent for expressing breast milk. However, employees who already receive compensated breaks may use that time to express milk.

State laws override this federal law if they provide greater protections to employees. For example, some states may mandate providing paid break time or providing break time beyond the baby's first birthday. As of this writing, 24 states, the District of Columbia, and Puerto Rico have additional laws regarding breastfeeding in the workplace. If you have additional questions about this law, visit www.usbreastfeeding.org.

Ideally, the place where you will pump will be quiet and private, with few distractions. Because many popular pumps operate with a battery pack, you may not need an electric outlet. A women's lounge with a comfortable chair (and preferably a sink and a refrigerator) or your own private office might be perfect. Other possibilities include a lighted storage closet, a conference room, or a borrowed office. If your workplace has a break room that both male and female employees use, you might be able to schedule your break at a time when you can have the privacy you need.

You may find that the only available place for you to express milk is a bathroom. It may be adequate as long as it is clean and has a chair, or room for one to be brought in.

If your job requires a good deal of travel, you can express milk in your car or in comfortable restrooms on your route.

If you are returning to school, you may be able to find a private place there as well. Locker rooms, empty classrooms, and health centers are all possibilities.

You may have an easier time identifying a pumping place if other mothers have worked this out before you. Otherwise, you may need to make a special trip to your workplace or school to search out a site that could work for you.

Once you're sure of your rights, discuss your need for a pumping place with your supervisor or human resources manager. Do so by letter or email if you fear your boss will be uncomfortable discussing your breasts in person or over the phone. You might consider including a letter from your doctor or your baby's doctor (you can find a letter to download and have your physician sign at www.workandpump.com/letter.htm). You might also refer your boss to two good sources of information about why employers should support nursing mothers in the workplace. One is the United States Breastfeeding Committee website, at www.usbreastfeeding.org; the other is the Office on Women's Health website, at www.womenshealth.gov. The latter site includes an excellent printable brochure called "The Business Case for Breastfeeding." Your boss may be more supportive knowing that by facilitating breastfeeding the company will be reducing medical costs, absenteeism, and employee turnover.

Your boss may want to know whether you'll be using work time to express your milk. Your regular breaks will probably be adequate. If you need extended breaks, you can deduct the time from your total hours or make it up at the end of the day.

You will also need a cool place to store your milk. Investigate whether a refrigerator is available. Note that breast milk is not considered by the U.S. Centers for Disease Control and Prevention (CDC) or the Occupational Safety and Health Administration (OSHA) to be a "biohazardous material," which would require storage in a refrigerator where no other food is kept. If it makes you or your co-workers more comfortable, of course, you can put your milk containers in an opaque sack or lunch bag.

If no refrigerator is available, you can plan to bring a small cooler with plastic ice packs inside. Milk stays cold for several hours in a cooler, which is also handy for transporting milk home or to the caregiver's.

Instructions for the Caregiver

Whether your baby goes to day care, has a nanny, or stays with a friend or family member, it is important for you to communicate exactly what you expect. Reviewing your expectations with your baby's caregiver before your return to work can help prevent misunderstandings and disappointments.

There may be many other matters that you wish to discuss, but when it comes to feedings, the first and most important rule should be that your baby always be held while being fed. Your baby may be capable of holding his own bottle, but he would miss out on important human contact if he were left to feed himself.

Your baby's caregiver will also need to know how to defrost and warm breast milk. You can write these instructions out so she won't forget them. Be sure to say what to do with milk that is left in the bottle.

Give the caregiver general guidelines on how often the baby should be fed and how much he will need at each feeding. When a baby fusses, it's easiest to respond first with a bottle. Without guidelines, a caregiver may feed a baby as much milk during an eight- to ten-hour period as he would normally take over an entire day! Explain that most breastfed babies need to be fed about every two to three hours and need no more than 1½ ounces per hour. This means, for example, that a typical baby needs about 3 ounces every two hours or 4½ ounces every three hours. You might also describe to your care provider how to feed your baby using "paced" bottle-feeding (see page 257).

Underfeeding can become a problem, too. A baby who enjoys sucking on his fingers or a pacifier much of the time may not give clear feeding cues and end up not taking enough milk during the time mother and baby are apart. The general rule of 3 ounces every two to two and a half hours should prevent this.

Ask the caregiver to plan feedings so that the baby is hungry when you return for him. This generally means that the baby's last bottle-feeding of the day should be two to three hours before you are expected. If the baby seems hungry after that, the caregiver might offer a partial feeding.

When you pick up the baby at the caregiver's house, you can leave milk, labeled with the date, in her refrigerator for the next day. Fresh refrigerated milk is best for the baby, since it retains more antibodies than frozen milk. If the milk will not be used during the following three days, it should be frozen.

A few caregivers express concern about the safety of handling breast milk; they apparently fear that diseases might be transmitted through it. You can assure your caregiver that, according to the CDC and OSHA, people handling and feeding breast milk need not wear rubber gloves nor store the milk in a refrigerator where no other foods are kept.

Refrigerated Milk

Use refrigerated milk within 72 hours. Take the milk out of the refrigerator just before the feeding. Over 5 to 10 minutes, warm the milk to room temperature in a container of warm water. Do not warm the milk in a microwave or on the stove. If the baby doesn't take all the milk at once, you can return the leftover milk to the refrigerator and use it at the next feeding.

Frozen Milk

Use milk within three months if it has been stored in the freezer compartment of a refrigerator. Milk stored in a deep freezer is good for six months or longer. Always use the oldest milk first. Thaw the milk either in the refrigerator, where it can remain for up to 24 hours, or in water just before feeding, gradually increasing the temperature to warm. Do not defrost the milk in a microwave or on the stove. Whatever milk the baby does not take must be discarded. Breast milk should not be refrozen.

Back at Work

Once you are back at work, you will discover what routines work best for you, your baby, and your milk supply. It will help if you can nurse as much as possible when you are with the baby and express milk frequently when you are apart. Some mothers keep their milk plentiful by encouraging their babies to nurse frequently during the evening and night. You may find that bringing the baby to bed with you, if she isn't already there, and nursing an hour or so before getting up works well. Nursing twice in the morning before you leave the baby is ideal. You can nurse again just before you leave home or when you arrive at the caregiver's. While you are at work, try to express milk about as often as you would be nursing at home. Ideally, if you will be missing three feedings, you should express milk three times. Your goal should be to drain both breasts as completely as possible, by either nursing or expressing milk, at least seven times in each 24 hours.

While some mothers need to concentrate on the task at hand while they are expressing milk, others take this time to simply relax, and some mothers use the time to get work done. For mothers who use a pump, pumping both breasts at once not only increases the amount of milk collected but cuts the time of expression in half. You can probably learn how to hold both flanges to your breasts using just one arm so you can use your free hand to massage your breasts, turn pages of a book or magazine, or hold the phone to your ear. You might also try a "pumping bra," which holds both flanges in place so that a mother can express her milk and have both hands free (see page 276 and Appendix A, page 360).

Label your milk with your baby's name and the date before storing it in a refrigerator or placing it in a cooler for transport.

Some mothers leak milk while they are at work. You may need to wear thick pads in your bra; keep an extra supply of them with you. Or try silicone nursing pads, which don't absorb milk but instead apply pressure to prevent leakage (see Appendix A, page 361). Some mothers prefer to use plastic breast shells to keep their clothes dry. Although they usually serve the purpose, these cups can also encourage further leaking. Finally, wearing printed blouses or keeping an extra jacket or sweater at work will help hide any wetness.

After work, you may want to nurse when you arrive at the caregiver's, before going home. Many mothers find this provides a welcome opportunity to relax and talk with the caregiver about the baby's day.

Some women find that they are unable to express as much milk as they would like, especially after three to four months post partum. At this point you may notice a drop in the amount you can pump, but this doesn't necessarily mean you can't meet your baby's needs. Many women overproduce in the first few months; after about four months, milk supply is determined by demand. If you had previously been pumping excess milk, you might now find yourself producing only as much as the baby drinks while you are away. This means that your body has adjusted to the baby's needs. Normal milk production is about 1½ ounces per hour, so if three hours have passed since you last pumped, you should get 4 to 5 ounces combined when you pump both breasts.

If your milk production is good but your caregiver is running out of the milk you save, find out just how much milk your baby is taking while you're away. A baby in day care for eight hours needs no more than 12 ounces of milk during that period. If you are able to nurse when you drop your baby off, or shortly before that, and again when you pick her up, she needs only about 8 ounces while you're gone. Your baby is being overfed if she is taking much more than this. If the caregiver complains that she needs more milk to feed your baby, say that your doctor recommends that the baby have no more than 1½ ounces per hour. You might have the baby's caregiver try a slow-flow bottle nipple so the baby can suck for a longer period of time without taking more milk. Although babies do not require fluids in addition to breast milk, you might suggest a bottle of water to soothe your baby when she has been recently fed but is fussy, especially if you are expected to arrive shortly.

Your caregiver may say that your baby needs more milk because she is getting bigger. In fact, researchers report that the amount of breast milk needed over a 24-hour period by an exclusively breastfed baby changes little between the ages of one and six months. As they get older, babies utilize breast milk more efficiently.

If a baby begins taking less milk at home because of longer sleep stretches at night, however, she may want to make up for it with more milk during the day, at least until she begins eating solid foods. In this case, try to nurse more often in the evening and early morning.

If you think that your milk supply truly is too low, be sure to read "Increasing Your Milk Supply while Pumping," in Chapter 5, page 249.

If you follow all of the other recommendations here and in Chapter 5 and still cannot express milk as often as necessary at work, you may find that the baby needs supplemental formula when you are away.

If you and your partner are both working, you may be too overwhelmed by chores to cuddle and enjoy the baby as much as you would like during your hours at home. Perhaps you can afford to pay someone to come every week or so to catch up on the housecleaning.

Combining nursing and working takes a great deal of time and energy. Aside from the responsibilities of your job, the baby, and the rest of your family, it is very important that you take time to care for yourself. Nursing mothers need to eat well. Although it may be tempting to skip breakfast or lunch, most women who do this find they have little energy to meet the many demands of the day. Get up a little earlier, if you must, to fix a nutritious breakfast. Bring snacks such as yogurt, cheese, nuts, and fruit to eat throughout the workday. Some mothers find that brewer's yeast gives them an energy boost and helps keep up the milk supply. To avoid constipation and plugged milk ducts, you will also need to drink plenty of fluids while you are at work. Finally, rest is essential. Most working and nursing mothers find that they must go to bed earlier than they once did. If you can, take an hour's nap just before dinner, and nap on your days at home with the baby.

THE REWARD PERIOD: FROM TWO THROUGH SIX MONTHS

- Caring for Yourself
- Making Love
- Nursing Your Baby
- Distractibility
- Night Waking
- Starting Solid Foods

T HE PERIOD BETWEEN THE BABY'S SECOND and sixth months is exciting and rewarding. With the newborn stage behind, most mothers feel relaxed and confident. The baby is more predictable, his needs easier to interpret. By three months, his crying lessens considerably. Day by day, the baby becomes more sociable and attuned to the people and things around him. Still, nursings are an important part of his day, intervals for nurture and nourishment at the breast.

Caring for Yourself

During this time, I hope, you are beginning to feel more like your usual self. Napping whenever possible is still important, especially if your baby is waking at night for feedings or if your energy seems low. Your intake of food and drink continues to be essential to your well-being. Neglecting your need for fluids could lead to constipation and, possibly, recurrent plugged milk ducts. Skipping meals or substituting "empty calorie" foods for more nutritious ones could result in fatigue. If you are overweight, limit your weight loss to 1 pound per week; crash dieting could decrease your milk supply. Most nursing mothers lose weight gradually without worrying about snacks or calories, but others find that eating three regular, satisfying meals and limiting high-calorie snacks and beverages, such as juices and soft drinks, helps them achieve their weekly goal.

If you have your cholesterol levels checked during these months, keep in mind that it's normal for some women to have very high levels of both "good" and "bad" cholesterol during pregnancy and lactation. Although your doctor may be unaware of this, levels as high as 200 and 325 milligrams per deciliter are normal for pregnant and nursing women and do not require treatment.

Making Love

After the birth of a baby most couples need time to readjust to each other sexually. You can probably resume intercourse by the sixth-week postpartum exam. In the meantime, you and your partner can enjoy physical loving such as cuddling, kissing, massage, and fondling. If your perineum feels fine and you want to have intercourse at three or four weeks post partum, there is no reason to wait. But you may not yet feel ready even when your doctor, nurse, or midwife gives you the go-ahead.

You may be worried that intercourse will be painful. If you have had an episiotomy, you may feel some initial tenderness and tightness, but your stitches should be completely healed after one month. Relaxing as much as possible will help make lovemaking more comfortable the first few times. A warm bath, a glass of wine, and extra time with foreplay may be helpful. You may also want to experiment with different positions, especially if you have had an episiotomy. Some women prefer to be on top so that they control the degree of penetration. Others find that a side-lying position feels best at first.

Most new mothers experience some vaginal dryness during lovemaking because of the hormonal changes that occur after giving birth. The vaginal secretions will increase again once regular ovulation resumes, but ovulation is generally delayed during nursing. Until your periods resume, a lubricant can make intercourse more comfortable and pleasurable. Use a generous amount of lubricating gel, such as K-Y, Astroglide, or a contraceptive gel, in and around your vagina (I don't recommend tablets or creams containing estrogen, which when absorbed can diminish milk production).

Your breasts need not be off limits when making love. Some women, however, find them less sensitive to stimulation during the nursing period; they may also feel tender during the early weeks, and later on just after nursing. Breast stimulation and orgasm may cause the milk to let down and leak or spray. If leaking milk is bothersome for you or your partner, you might nurse shortly before you make love, or wear a blouse, a bra, or a nightgown during lovemaking.

For some time after having a baby, many women find they have less interest in making love than formerly. There are a variety of reasons for this. Estrogen, which influences a woman's sex drive as well as the amount of vaginal secretions, is produced in lower levels after she gives birth. Sometimes having so much skin-to-skin contact with the baby all day dampens a woman's desire for more physical contact. A new mother may also fear another pregnancy—whether or not the recent one was planned. At the end of the day, too, a mother may be just too tired for lovemaking.

New fathers also suffer from overwork and night wakings. Like their partners, they may be too exhausted to make love, and they may also worry about having another baby too soon.

It is important that your intimacy as a couple continue. As with most other changes in life, talking over your feelings and making some adjustments will make this period easier.

Finding the time to make love can be difficult, especially when you are tired. You may need to plan times to be together when you are rested and when the baby is likely to be asleep. Making love early in the morning or when the baby is napping may work the best. Perhaps you can take a nap in the afternoon so you will have more energy for your partner in the evening. Having the baby sleep in another room may help you to feel more comfortable.

But if neither you nor your partner is much inclined to have frequent intercourse, your physical and emotional intimacy can continue without it. Passionate feelings will probably come more easily as the baby gets older. Remember, you have a lifetime ahead of you to share your love.

Contraception

If you are concerned about the possibility of getting pregnant again, talk over birth control options with your partner and your health-care provider. Foam, condoms, an IUD, a diaphragm, a cervical cap, a female condom, and surgical sterilization are all considered safe during nursing. If you used a diaphragm or cervical cap before your pregnancy, you will need a refitting now.

Many women want reliable and convenient birth control in hormonal form. Although "the pill" and other hormonal birth control products apparently do no direct harm to the nursing baby, pills containing estrogen, even in low doses, often reduce a mother's milk supply and may thereby lead to poor weight gain in the baby. The vaginal ring (NuvaRing), the contraceptive patch (Ortho Evra), and one hormonal injection product (Lunelle) also contain estrogen and so can diminish milk production. These products are best avoided during breastfeeding.

Fortunately, not all types of hormonal birth control interfere with milk production. The progestin-only pill, also known as the "mini-pill," usually has no effect on milk supply. Nor do progestin-only injections, which give three months' protection against pregnancy. All of these products are considered safe during breastfeeding. IUDs that contain small amounts of progesterone or progestin are also considered safe and should not have any effect on milk production.

Some health-care providers offer hormonal contraceptives just hours or days after birth. This practice may interfere with the onset of lactation and should be postponed for at least four to six weeks.

Whichever birth control method you use, its reliability is increased by the fact that you are breastfeeding. For now, in fact, breastfeeding may be the only birth control method you need. That breastfeeding affects fertility is a truth that has been largely ignored in an era when partial breastfeeding and early weaning have been the norm. But breastfeeding has provided more contraception worldwide than all other methods combined. Frequent nursing, especially during the first several months after birth, suppresses ovulation in most women. In fact, if a woman hasn't yet had a period since her pregnancy, exclusive breastfeeding provides her more than 98 percent protection against pregnancy in the first six months post partum (Kennedy, 1989). But when her periods resume, when the baby is receiving any food or drink besides breast milk, or when the baby reaches six months of age, the mother's chance of getting pregnant again increases. If you want to rely on breastfeeding-as-contraception (which medical texts call the lactational amenorrhea method, or LAM), nurse at least eight times in every 24 hours, with no more than six hours between nursings and a cumulative sucking time of at least 60 minutes per day. For best results, don't feed formula or solids or even use pacifiers.

Once your periods resume, you may prefer to track your natural menstrual cycle, abstaining from intercourse around the time of ovulation, instead of relying on birth control pills or devices. If you want to use "natural family planning," try to get personal instruction in it. Learn to keep track of all three basic body measures: basal body temperature, cervical mucus, and length of menstrual cycle.

Nursing Your Baby

As your baby quickly grows and develops, you will notice that her nursing pattern also changes. You can expect two more appetite spurts during this period, the first at about two and a half to three months and the second between four and a half and six months. As with the earlier appetite spurts, the baby will nurse more frequently for a few days to stimulate an increase in milk production. Most mothers produce 28 to 32 ounces of milk each day during this period, about a 30 percent increase over the first month.

By three or four months of age, many babies have dropped a feeding or two and are nursing seven or eight times a day. Nursing less often than seven times a day may result in decreased milk production and slowed weight gain for the baby. This most commonly occurs when a baby spends much of her day sucking on her fingers or on a pacifier, or when she begins sleeping long stretches at night but isn't nursed more often during the day. It can also happen when a working mother expresses milk infrequently while she is away. Your baby should continue gaining about 1 ounce a day until she is three months old. Between three and six months of age, a breastfed baby normally gains about ½ ounce each day.

During this period, some women begin to fear that their babies aren't "getting enough." You may find that your breasts feel less full, that you leak less or not at all, and that the sensations of the milk letting down are less intense than before. None of this necessarily means your supply is low or your baby isn't getting enough milk. If your baby is taking the breast at least seven times in 24 hours, has plenty of wet diapers and yellow bowel movements, and seems content after feedings, you probably have no cause for concern. Your breasts may feel less full simply because they have adjusted to your baby's needs and now produce only as much milk as she wants.

However, if your baby does not suck well or take the breast often enough, if you are using a birth control product containing estrogen, or if you are taking a medication that can interfere with milk production (such as a pseudoephedrine-containing decongestant like Sudafed or an antihistamine like Benadryl), your production may truly be low. The baby's weight gain is the best gauge of adequate milk production. A quick weight check at the doctor's office may help you feel more confident.

Some babies prefer to nurse from just one breast at each feeding. So long as the baby seems content and is continuing to gain enough weight, this is normal.

You may notice that your baby is nursing for shorter periods. She can now get a large quantity of milk quickly because both she and your breasts have become so efficient.

Most three- to six-month-old babies are chubby; some may be quite plump. Parents and sometimes even doctors may become concerned about the baby who gains weight above the norm. These babies slow their growth during the second half of the first year and typically begin to slim down during toddlerhood. It is not advisable to restrict the baby's nursing because of her weight.

Doctors have long charted babies' growth according to standards based on infants chosen without regard to what or how they were fed. Because formula-feeding alters a baby's normal growth pattern, old growth charts are inaccurate for breastfed babies. In 2006, the World Health Organization (WHO) released findings from a study of breastfed babies in Brazil, Ghana, India, Norway, Oman, and the United States. The children were exclusively breastfed for several months, and their growth and development were monitored for several years thereafter. In accordance with the findings, WHO introduced new universal growth standards for infants and children.

The study showed that healthy children from around the world grow within the same range for both height and weight. For the first time, we have charts showing how all children naturally grow, beginning during six months of exclusive breastfeeding. These charts are useful tools for monitoring children and identifying those who are under- or overfed or in some other way malnourished. The new charts show that breastfed babies tend to be slightly leaner and somewhat taller after the first six months than the old charts showed. Because some doctors still don't use the WHO charts, I have included the weight charts for your use in Appendix C (see page 371).

Distractibility

Between three and five months, a baby starts to become more aware of the world around her. When she can see clearly across the room and interact more with her family, she becomes easily distracted while nursing. At any new, sudden, or interesting sight or sound, she pulls away from the breast to look around. Older siblings are a common distraction. At around this age the baby may also start to play nursing games; she may stop sucking, for instance, to pat Mom's face and smile. Although these antics can be adorable, you may become frustrated if nursing sessions become longer and longer because the baby seems never to want to get down to the "business" of nursing.

This behavior does not mean the baby has lost interest in nursing. Of course, you'll want to rule out any contributing problem, such as a low milk supply or painful reflux. But if the baby is generally content, you needn't worry about her distractibility. It may help to nurse while lying down in a quiet, semidarkened room. Some mothers reserve for nursing sessions a special toy—a blanket or necklace that the baby likes to hold and stroke—to keep her from being distracted by other things.

After several weeks of interrupted feedings, your baby will no longer have to let go of the nipple to check out what's going on around her. Instead, she'll turn her head with the nipple still in her mouth.

Night Waking

Although some babies start sleeping in stretches of up to 10 hours as early as six weeks of age, most continue to wake at night until they are six to twelve months old or older. Most babies, especially those under six months of age, can be expected to wake up to nurse at least once each night, and as often as every three hours.

Night wakings may frustrate you, especially if your older child or a friend's baby slept long stretches at an early age. If you are tempted to give the baby formula or cereal in a bottle just before bedtime in the hope of encouraging him to "sleep through," keep in mind that night waking is normal for a baby this age. Besides, as many studies have shown, feeding cereal early has no effect on when a baby starts sleeping through the night. In fact, one recent study suggested that when parents supplement their babies' last nursing of the day with infant formula, babies sleep even less at night.

Babies who sleep long stretches during the first few months typically begin waking again around three to four months of age. Perhaps teething is to blame. Other signs of teething may include general fussiness, drooling, changes in nursing patterns, biting, and finger sucking. Giving the baby a cold washcloth or a chilled water-filled teething ring to bite on may make her more comfortable. For babies who are at least six months old, some doctors recommend the use of gum gels, acetaminophen drops (Infants' Tylenol), or ibuprofen drops (Infants' Motrin, Infants' Advil) for teething pain. Amber necklaces are used in some European countries for teething pain and are gaining popularity here. Worn against the baby's skin, the amber beads are thought to have an anti-inflammatory effect. Although scientific evidence is lacking, many parents swear that amber beads ease teething pain. At night, they can be wrapped around the baby's ankle and covered with a sock.

A baby may also wake more at night when daytime nursings decline, because Mom is away during the day, because he gets distracted during daytime feedings, or because he spends too much time sucking his fingers or a pacifier. To encourage your baby to get more of his milk during the day and evening, try offering the breast in a quiet, darkened room, nurse whenever he begins sucking his fingers, and limit or eliminate the use of a pacifier.

Waking every one to two hours all night long is *not* normal for a baby this age. If your baby starts waking very frequently, perhaps teething, an ear infection, or another illness is to blame. If he has recently had a cold or an ear infection, his ears may be the problem now, even if he has no fever and isn't pulling on them. If the baby has never been a good sleeper, reflux or a low milk supply might be causing the problem. For more information, see "Fussiness, Colic, and Reflux," page 204.

If your baby wakes frequently at night, for whatever reason, taking him into your bed for all or part of the night may make nursing easier and lessen your own sleep disruptions. For information on bed sharing, see "Sleeping with Your Baby," page 171.

For additional information on babies and sleep, I recommend the book *The No-Cry Sleep Solution*, by Elizabeth Pantley and William Sears (see "Suggested Supplemental Reading," page 414).

Starting Solid Foods

Probably no area of infant development attracts as much confusion and range of opinion as the starting of solid foods. Your family, friends, and child-care advisors probably all have different ideas on when and how to begin giving solid foods to your baby.

Solid foods are best introduced when a baby becomes developmentally ready for them and is able to benefit from the nutrition they offer. Although this does not happen until a baby is six months of age or older, many mothers feel pressured to begin solids earlier. Some think of feeding solids as a sort of status symbol, something to brag about. Some doctors suggest that when babies are very large, they need solids sooner than six months. This is certainly not the case. Very big babies are large mostly because their mothers have abundant milk supplies. These babies are growing very well on mother's milk.

The American Academy of Pediatrics, as well as many other health organizations, now recommends that breastfed babies not be fed solid foods until they are at least six months old. Rest assured: Your milk provides all the nutrients your baby needs for at least the first six months of life.

There are many good reasons to delay solids until this time. Offering solids prematurely means replacing breast milk, which is nutritionally perfect, with foods that are nutritionally incomplete.

Surprisingly, babies who are started on solid foods before six months of age do not receive additional calories. This is because most of the solids fed to babies are relatively low in calories, and these foods tend to displace higher-calorie breast milk in the diet. Besides, when solids are given, breast-milk production typically lessens. Decreased milk production all too often leads to early weaning.

Babies who are exclusively breastfed for the first six months of life experience slower weight gain but faster growth in length and head size than babies fed solids earlier. After exclusively breastfed babies begin eating other foods, at about six months of age, these children tend to be leaner than the national average. They are less prone to become obese than are their peers who started on solid foods before six months (Wilson, 1998; von Kries, 1999; Kalies, 2005).

Holding off on offering solids may contribute to your baby's health in another way. In the Wilson study, babies who were offered solid foods before six months of age had more colds and other respiratory infections, wheezing, and ear infections than babies who were not given solids until six months. Starting solids early is also associated with food allergies (Fiocchi et al., 2006).

Delaying the introduction of solids is beneficial for mothers as well. Women who exclusively breastfeed for a full six months are more likely to return to their pre-pregnancy weight, as compared with mothers who offer solids prematurely, and have a lower risk of long-term obesity.

Mothers who nurse exclusively are also less likely to resume their periods in the first few months post partum. One advantage of not having periods is the opportunity to rebuild one's iron stores, which are often depleted during pregnancy and birth.

You'll know that your baby is developmentally ready for solid foods when he can sit with support, control his head and neck movements, and tell you he is hungry (by leaning forward with an open mouth) or full (by pulling away and turning his head). He may indicate his readiness for solids by grabbing food off your plate or out of your hand.

At this time he will also begin to lose his tongue-thrust reflex, which causes him to push anything in his mouth forward and out. This means he will be better able to eat from a spoon, move the food to the back of his mouth, and swallow. The baby's digestive system will also be mature enough to handle solids at this time. His kidneys will be able to excrete the waste products of solid foods. His iron stores will lessen, so the iron from solid foods will be beneficial for him.

Holding off on feeding solids is also practical: The closer to six months you introduce them, the more likely it is you'll be able to skip the "baby food" stage and start with table foods. Guidelines for offering solid foods are discussed in Chapter 8.

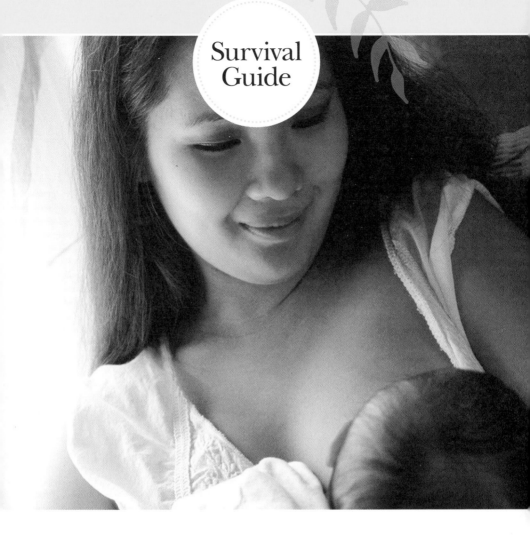

MONTHS TWO
THROUGH SIX

Concerns About Yourself

- Recurrent Plugged Ducts
  and Breasts Infections

- Overabundant Milk

Concerns About the Baby

- Slow Weight Gain

- One-Sided Nursing

- Sudden Refusal to Nurse

313

Concerns about Yourself

Recurrent Plugged Ducts and Breast Infections

Many nursing mothers experience recurrent plugged ducts or breast infections. If you are suffering from either at the moment, carefully review the information in "Survival Guide: The First Two Months," pages 187 to 193. If you have had more than two occurrences, the following suggestions may be helpful in preventing future episodes.

Treatment Measures for Recurrent Plugged Ducts and Breast Infections

1. Be sure that you are nursing the baby frequently, and that at least one breast is emptied well at each feeding.

2. Avoid skipping or delaying feedings. Pick a quiet place to nurse if your baby gets distracted during feedings. Wake the baby at night if your breasts feel too full. If your baby routinely sleeps for long periods at night, consider using an effective breast pump before you go to bed, after the first morning feeding, or both. This way you'll ensure that your breasts are completely drained at least once or twice a day.

3. To encourage complete drainage of the milk ducts, massage your breasts gently while nursing.

4. Change nursing pads whenever they become wet.

5. Get as much rest as possible. Nap whenever you can. Consider sleeping with the baby if you aren't already.

6. Make sure you are getting plenty to drink every day.

7. Check that your bra and other clothing are not too restrictive.

8. If you're using a Medela, Ameda, Lansinoh, Avent, Hygeia, or Nurture III breast pump, try Pumpin' Pal Super Shields. These elliptical shields are inserted into pump flanges to gently milk

the breast instead of pulling on just the nipple and areola. Some mothers have found that the shields help prevent plugged ducts. See Appendix A, page 360, for more information.

9. Consider taking nutritional supplements. Many lactation consultants believe that vitamin C supplements may prevent recurrences of breast infections. Some suggest that taking supplemental lecithin may prevent plugged milk ducts; start with one 1,200-milligram capsule three or four times a day, and reduce the dosage after a few weeks without another episode. (Note that these dosages of lecithin are relatively low; higher doses of lecithin can lead to depression for those who have a history of it.) If you are anemic, take a daily iron supplement.

10. If your periods have resumed, try limiting your salt intake for several days before your period is due. A high salt intake may increase susceptibility to breast infections, and some women seem to be prone to breast infections premenstrually. This may have to do with the fact that they retain water just before their periods.

11. Try to reduce the amount of saturated fats in your diet. Some lactation professionals believe that avoiding saturated fats may prevent plugged milk ducts.

12. If a plugged duct or breast infection does not go away within three days, consult your physician.

13. If your doctor prescribes antibiotics, take the entire course. A 10- or 14-day prescription may be needed; a 5- or 7-day course may be insufficient for complete treatment. If an infection recurs in the same part of the breast shortly after antibiotic therapy has ended, the antibiotic may be ineffective. Some antibiotics do not penetrate breast tissue as well as others. Discuss this possibility with your doctor (see page 190).

14. Recurrent mastitis can also be a sign of methicillin-resistant *Staphylococcus aureus,* or MRSA (see page 191). Ask your doctor whether this might be the case.

Overabundant Milk

Some mothers continue to be bothered by an oversupply of milk after two months post partum. You are not necessarily producing too much milk, however, if you leak or become engorged during the baby's long sleep stretches. Only if you are still feeling uncomfortably engorged most of the time should you consider taking steps to decrease your milk supply.

Treatment Measures for an Overabundance of Milk

1. Continue drinking plenty of fluids. Decreasing fluids does not decrease milk production.

2. Nurse your baby at just one breast per feeding. Let him suck as long as he likes on one side. If you become uncomfortable, express a small amount of milk from the other breast. Switch breasts with each feeding.

3. Should you be caught in a routine of expressing milk while nursing full-time, gradually decrease the amount of milk you take until you are no longer expressing any.

Concerns about the Baby

Slow Weight Gain

A two- to three-month-old baby is considered a slow gainer when he is putting on less than 1 ounce a day. A slow-gaining three- to six-month-old is gaining less than ½ ounce per day.

A baby who is discovered to be gaining weight slowly, not gaining at all, or losing weight may be nursing too infrequently—that is, fewer than seven times in a 24-hour period. Between three and four months of age, most babies find their fingers or become avid pacifier users. Some babies stop letting their mothers know when they are hungry and instead suck away at fingers or a pacifier, decreasing the number of nursings to fewer than seven a day. The baby who sleeps eight or more hours at a stretch each night may fail to get enough milk if he doesn't nurse at least seven times during his waking hours. A baby may also slow his weight gain after losing some interest in nursing because juices or solid foods have been introduced prematurely, especially if they have replaced nursings.

Slow weight gain may occur, too, when a working mother fails to express her milk often enough while she is away from the baby, causing an overall decrease in her milk supply. Estrogen-containing birth control pills, even the low-dose kind, often decrease milk production. Occasionally, a baby who has never had normal weight gain suddenly becomes a worry to his physician and parents. This happens because health professionals do not always identify a newborn who gains less than 1 ounce a day during the early weeks as being underfed. Eventually such a baby may become obviously underweight. This is unfortunate, since a low milk intake can be much more easily remedied if the problem is recognized early on. A milk supply that has been low for two, three, or even four months can be very difficult to improve.

Treatment Measures for Slow Weight Gain

1. Devote at least two or three days to nursing the baby and doing little else. Put the pacifier aside, and offer the breast each time you notice the baby beginning to suck a finger. You may find yourself nursing every hour or so, although increasing feedings to eight or more per 24 hours is usually sufficient to quickly increase milk production. If your baby is sleeping through the night, try to include at least one late-evening feeding. You might also consider waking the baby for a feeding after he has slept for five or six hours.

2. While the baby is nursing, listen for swallowing. As soon as you notice the swallowing taper off, switch breasts. Continue switching back and forth for as long as the baby is willing to continue, ideally at least 10 minutes. If the baby is easily distracted, nurse in a quiet, darkened room.

3. Should your baby refuse to nurse as often as every two hours or resist switching back and forth, you might consider expressing or pumping milk after each nursing to stimulate an increase in milk production. A double electric pump may be most convenient.

After two or three days of this regime, both the baby's nursing pattern and your milk supply should begin to improve.

4. If your baby has been losing weight or has never gained weight adequately, consider giving him supplemental formula while you work on increasing your milk supply. For instructions on estimating the amount of milk you are producing and the amount of milk your baby needs, see "Underfeeding," page 218.

5. Consider taking fenugreek capsules, blessed thistle capsules, More Milk Plus tincture, Go-Lacta, or perhaps even a milk-stimulating pharmaceutical medication to help increase your milk production (see pages 72 and 112).

6. If you are working away from the baby, try to spend two or more consecutive days at home following the recommendations just given. If you can't stay home from work, express milk as often as possible.

7. After two or three days of stepped-up nursing, you should notice that your breasts feel fuller and that the baby swallows over a longer period during feedings. Continue nursing frequently, at least eight times a day. Have the baby's weight checked after a week of frequent nursing, and again a week after that. If the baby still isn't gaining well, supplementation with an ounce or two of formula after some of the feedings may be necessary.

Adding solids to a baby's diet is *not* a good way to deal with slow weight gain. Most solid foods are less calorie-dense than breast milk, and low-calorie foods can displace some of the milk in a baby's diet. So feeding solids tends to slow rather than speed a baby's weight gain.

One-Sided Nursing

Occasionally a baby develops a preference for one breast over the other. Perhaps the favored breast produces more milk or lets it down more rapidly. Sometimes there is no apparent reason—the baby simply prefers one side. Twins usually choose opposite sides.

Sometimes a mother unknowingly nurses the baby more at one breast than the other, increasing milk production on the favored side. Some mothers prefer nursing on one side only; in certain cultures one-sided nursing is common.

One breast can fully support a baby's nutritional needs. But if a single baby nurses substantially more at one breast than at the other, the less used breast may become noticeably smaller. After weaning, the breasts will equal out in size.

Treatment Measures for One-Sided Nursing

1. Offer the baby her least favorite side first. After she has nursed on both sides, encourage her to nurse on the first side again.

2. Should the baby totally refuse one side, try changing positions. Use the football hold, or nurse while lying on your side. The baby may be more willing when she is sleepy or actually asleep, or when you nurse in a darkened room.

3. Increase the milk supply in the less-used breast by manually expressing or pumping milk after each nursing for a few days.

4. If all else fails, simply accept your baby's preference to be a one-sided nurser.

Sudden Refusal to Nurse

Occasionally a baby under six months old suddenly refuses to nurse. A "nursing strike" usually lasts for a few days but sometimes for as long as two weeks. It rarely means the baby is ready to wean; weaning seldom occurs this suddenly. See "Nursing Strike," page 344, for the reasons behind this problem and suggestions for coping with it.

Some babies who suffer from painful reflux may refuse to nurse. Often, though, they will take their mother's milk by bottle. See "Colic and Reflux," page 207.

If your baby suddenly refuses one breast but is happy to nurse at the other, see "One-Sided Nursing," above.

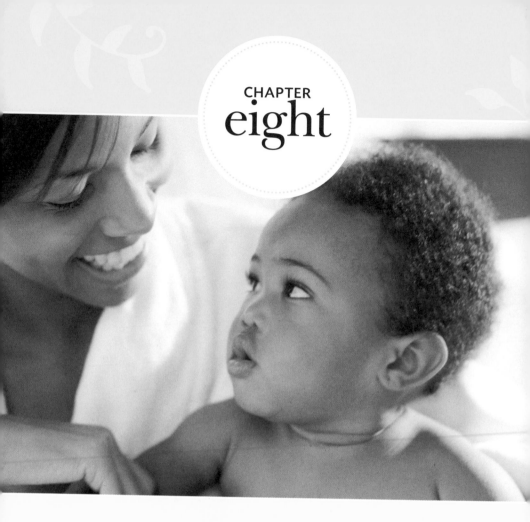

CHAPTER
eight

NURSING THE OLDER BABY

- Caring for Yourself
- Nursing Your Six- to Twelve-Month-Old
- Coping with Night Waking

- Coping with Teething
- The Transition to Table Food
- Considering Weaning

As BREASTFEEDING PROGRESSES TO SIX MONTHS and beyond, the nursing relationship continues to change. Although the baby is busy exploring the world around him and has probably shortened most of his nursings, breast milk continues to be his primary source of nutrients until he is well established on table foods. Breastfeeding also continues to provide protective antibodies against illness.

For you, nursing provides the opportunity to sit down for a few minutes and just enjoy your baby. Nursing may also become your main tool to help your baby fall off to sleep at naptime and bedtime.

Caring for Yourself

You may sometimes feel tired and run-down during your baby's second half-year. Becoming more active and getting overtired seem to be especially common among mothers around six months post partum. Certainly, eating poorly and losing too much weight can contribute to a loss of energy. Taking it a bit easier, getting some extra rest, and paying attention to your diet can do a lot to improve your overall well-being. Taking brewer's yeast or a vitamin B-complex supplement may also be helpful.

Resuming Your Periods

If your periods haven't resumed yet, they may well do so during your baby's second half-year. Although some women see the resumption of their monthly cycles as early as six weeks after birth, most women's periods resume as their babies begin eating regular meals at the table. Other women, especially those who nurse frequently, don't start menstruating until 12 to 24 months post partum. Your initial periods may be lighter, heavier, or less regular than normal.

In most cases, fertility returns before menstruation. If you don't want to become pregnant again soon, you should be using some form of birth control even if your periods haven't resumed.

Both nursing mothers and their babies may feel out of sorts around the time of menstruation. Some mothers report that their babies fuss for a couple of days, or even refuse to nurse for a short time, when periods resume. Other women experience sore nipples for a few days between ovulation and the start of menstruation.

Often, a nursing mother experiences a dip in the milk supply a few days before her period starts. Although this dip tends to be greatest during the first few cycles, some women have low milk production just before their periods for as long as they continue nursing. Calcium and magnesium supplements may help; try taking 1,000 milligrams of calcium and 500 milligrams of magnesium each day from midcycle until your period starts. If your periods are very regular, you can also try taking fenugreek capsules or other herbal preparations in the days before you expect your period to start (see "Underfeeding and Weight Loss," page 107).

Nursing Your Six- to Twelve-Month-Old

The typical baby of this age is venturing out on his own and seemingly becoming more independent, but he often scampers back to the safety and reassurance of his mother's arms. By eight to ten months, in fact, he probably cannot bear to have his mother out of his sight for even a minute. This is known as separation anxiety. Until the baby learns to trust that his mother will return, out of sight means gone forever.

During the first four months, both babies and their mothers tend to be captivated by nursing; they give it all their attention. After the first four months, babies are easily distracted; if anything catches their interest, they may pull off the breast momentarily. As your baby passes six months and develops more motor skills, he may still be somewhat distractible, and he will probably become more active during nursings.

This is a normal stage of development and a healthy part of the nursing relationship. Your baby may play with his foot and smile at you as he nurses. He may adopt some really annoying behaviors—pinching the breast, pulling or twiddling the nipple, or doing acrobatics while nursing. You can put an end to these antics by holding your baby's hand or giving him something else to hold—a beaded necklace, for instance, or a soft blanket.

When your baby is between six and twelve months of age, you should be nursing about seven times a day, on average, and offering him solids only after nursing. Some people might tell you that four or five feedings a day are sufficient, but this number is normal only for formula-fed babies, who take more at a feeding and tend to eat more solids than breastfed babies of the same age. You may also hear that you should expect your baby to go longer between daytime feedings. In fact, as your baby begins to sleep longer stretches at night, he may need to nurse more frequently during the day—as often as every two hours—to get as much breast milk as he needs.

Crawling and cruising babies can be so busy that they may not "ask" to nurse as often as they should. If your baby goes longer than three hours during the day without expressing a desire to nurse, take him to a quiet, dark room and offer your breast, or put on a brightly colored scarf or beaded necklace before picking him up. Some mothers reserve a special toy just for nursing sessions.

At around seven to nine months of age, many babies go through a stage in which they seem to lose interest in nursing. The parents may be told that their babies are "self-weaning." In truth, babies rarely wean themselves without cause before one year of age, and most babies will happily nurse for two to four years without initiating weaning. In most cases of "self-weaning" in seven- to nine-month-old babies, what actually happens is a nursing strike (see page 344). Usually, the baby's normal distractibility results in infrequent nursing, which in turn causes a low milk supply. If the mother takes measures to rebuild her supply, the baby will happily return to nursing. Even if the milk supply is abundant, it's best to assume that when a baby under 12 months loses interest in nursing, he does so because of a problem that can be corrected. Teething pain, a sore throat, a stuffy nose, and an ear infection are all possible reasons that an older baby might temporarily refuse to nurse.

Many women notice that it takes longer for their milk to let down in the second six months of nursing. This may be a sign of a dwindling milk supply. Delayed let-down may contribute to a baby's loss of interest in the breast, especially at nine to ten months of age.

Many parents and physicians worry when weight gain in a healthy breastfed baby dramatically slows in the second six months after birth. Keep in mind that most U.S. babies are totally weaned to formula and solids by six months of age, and that formula-fed babies tend to gain more weight between six and twelve months than breastfed babies. The charts still used in most doctors' offices reflect this unnatural growth pattern. Normal weight gain for a breastfed baby between six and twelve months is 1 to 4 ounces per week. Babies with small parents fall in the lower end of this range.

The World Health Organization's new growth charts are based on a multinational study of children who were exclusively breastfed for six months. These charts show that breastfed babies are slightly leaner and taller in later months than the old charts would lead you to expect. See the new charts in Appendix C, page 371.

Coping with Night Waking

Although some older babies and toddlers sleep well at night, most wake frequently, night after night. Your baby may in fact be waking more at night and napping less during the day than she did in the first few months. You may have thought that when your baby reached six months of age or older and started taking solid food that her nighttime wakings would diminish. You probably even know someone whose baby "sleeps through the night." But such a baby is atypical. When health professionals talk about sleeping through the night, they are referring to a six-hour stretch. Although some babies sleep a six-hour stretch, waking one to three times a night is entirely normal for babies as old as two years. Many babies who slept long stretches in the early months wake more frequently later.

You may think something is wrong if your baby doesn't sleep through the night. Well-meaning family members may say that night waking is not normal. Pediatricians may point out that a baby this age does not "need" to nurse at night. You may wonder if your baby wakes because of teething, illness, digestive problems, wet diapers, chilling or over-heating, superior intelligence, upcoming developmental milestones, or separation anxiety. Although any of these might perhaps contribute to night waking, the basic cause may simply be your baby's need for a cuddle and a snack or drink. Six- to twelve-month-olds may actually wake at night out of thirst or hunger.

As you may suspect, breastfed babies are less likely than formula-fed babies to sleep through the night. Chances are your friend's sleeping baby is already fully weaned or was never nursed at all. One study found that whereas weaned babies slept a median of nine to ten hours at a stretch at every age after four months, nursing babies slept in bouts of four to seven hours to the end of the second year (Elias et al., 1986).

Not only do breastfed babies sleep in shorter bouts than do bottle-fed babies, nursing babies also sleep less overall. In the Elias study, weaned babies slept a median of 13 to 14 hours per day throughout the first two years, but nursing babies gradually lessened their total hours of sleep from a median of 14 to a median of 11 hours.

Why do bottle-fed babies sleep in longer stretches than breastfed babies? Marsha Walker (1993), a lactation consultant, points out that babies formula-fed from birth have poor "vagal nerve tone"; that is, their autonomic nervous systems are measurably disordered. This makes them sleepier and less alert than breastfed newborns. Poor vagal tone in a newborn, by the way, is related to inferior motor and mental develop-ment for at least two years after birth.

Babies who are weaned after several months of breastfeeding may start sleeping through the night for other reasons. They certainly have waking episodes, as everyone does, but these babies fall back into deep sleep without any intervention from parents. Most have probably learned to go back to sleep alone—through the use of a thumb, pacifier, or bottle, through their parents' ignoring them, or perhaps with a sophisticated method such as scheduled awakenings, whereby a parent rouses a child in time to prevent spontaneous awakenings, until both spontaneous and scheduled awakenings are gradually eliminated. In most of these cases, the parents' desire for separation has overcome the baby's natural urge to be close to other human beings.

No one knows for sure why weaned children sleep more overall than those who are still nursing. It seems that babies often nurse during light sleep; they release the nipple when they fall into deep sleep. This may be why a child who was obviously tired will, instead of falling asleep after a long nursing, come off the breast seeming completely refreshed. If nursing in a light-sleep state were counted as sleep, the average total hours of sleep might not vary at all between nursing and weaned children.

A baby's night wakings can be handled in a variety of ways. Some mothers find that sleeping with their babies disrupts their own sleep less, while others prefer to get up, nurse, and return the baby to a crib. If a baby wakes very frequently, it's best to figure out why. Teething, an ear infection, separation anxiety, stomach problems, an allergy, a chill from kicking off the covers, or a low milk supply are all possible causes.

For advice on getting a baby to sleep longer at night, see "Survival Guide: Months Six through Twelve," page 337.

Coping with Teething

By six months of age, most babies begin teething. This can affect their nursing patterns. Some babies are less interested in nursing when their gums are tender, and others want to nurse more often, especially in the night. To soothe your baby's aching gums, give him things to bite on during the day, such as a cold, damp washcloth or a teething ring. You might freeze and slightly thaw the wet washcloth or teething ring before offering it to him. If he fusses during nursing sessions, you can rub his gums with a cold washcloth or apply Baby Orajel just before nursing. If your baby is very uncomfortable, acetaminophen drops (Infants' Tylenol) or ibuprofen drops (Infants' Motrin, Infants' Advil) may help. Check with your baby's doctor before using ibuprofen, an anti-inflammatory, and ask for the correct dosage.

Some mothers swear by amber necklaces to help their babies with teething pain. When worn against the skin, amber is believed to be a natural pain reliever and anti-inflammatory. While there are no studies on the effectiveness of amber, these necklaces have been used by European mothers for quite some time and are now popular in the United States. The necklaces are not recommended to be worn at night, so some parents wrap them around the baby's ankle at night and cover with a sock.

Many mothers worry that the eruption of teeth means that nursing must come to an end. But babies and toddlers with teeth can and usually do nurse without causing pain to their mothers' nipples. While the baby is sucking, the tongue protects you by covering the lower teeth. In other words, so long as a baby is swallowing milk, she cannot bite. If your baby does bite you, you can take measures to make sure it doesn't happen again (see "Biting," page 338).

Some mothers find that their nipples get sore during teething even though their babies aren't actually biting. When babies are cutting teeth, they may adjust their latch on the breast to put pressure on sore areas of their gums. This can make your nipples sore. To avoid the problem, ease the baby's pain before nursing with one or more of the remedies I've just described. If you feel tenderness while nursing, adjust the baby's position at the breast (see "Nipple Soreness from New Teeth," page 338).

The Transition to Table Food

Around the age of six months, your baby will begin to show readiness for solid foods. You'll know he is ready when he can sit up with some support, when he reaches for food at the table, when he explores his world by grabbing objects and placing them in his mouth, and when he generally acts interested in eating what the rest of the family eats.

By six months of age a baby begins to require more nutrients than his body stores and his intake of breast milk can provide. He needs more protein and, especially, more iron and zinc. Even in a healthy, full-term baby, iron stores sometimes fail to last beyond the first months, and when this happens, a baby becomes at risk for developing iron-deficiency anemia. Babies born prematurely may need additional iron even earlier than six months. Iron-deficiency anemia is common in infants between nine and twelve months of age who do not receive iron-rich foods. If the anemia continues unabated for long, it can cause long-lasting harm to mental, motor, and behavioral functioning. Zinc-rich foods are also important, for growth and development as well as for proper immune functioning.

Babies born earlier than 36 weeks' gestation may not be ready for self-feeding at six months, but they may well need extra iron at this age. Some health professionals recommend spoon-feeding prematurely born babies pureed high-iron foods, such as meat, beginning at the age of six months. Others recommend giving liquid iron supplements until these babies are ready for self-feeding.

Throughout the twentieth century, the first foods usually recommended for babies were commercial infant cereals, followed by pureed fruits and vegetables. Most parents started feeding their babies cereal at four to six months of age. Made from refined grain, infant cereal lacks some of the nutrients of whole grain, and the iron and zinc added to the cereal are poorly absorbed by the baby's body. Because cereal is very filling and digested slowly, it tends to replace breast milk and other solids in the baby's diet, especially if the cereal is fed by spoon. When breast milk is replaced with cereal, the baby's protein intake declines.

Recently, nutritionists have developed new guidelines for starting the breastfed baby on solid food. They now recommend introducing foods rich in protein, iron, and zinc as well as fruits and vegetables at around six months of age, and whole-grain cereals and breads, rather than infant cereal, a little later.

Breast milk will continue to be your baby's most important food until he is eating three daily meals of table food, at around nine months of age. Until then, you should always nurse your baby shortly before offering him any solid foods.

Your baby's first solids need not be pureed. Pureed foods require spoon-feeding, which sometimes leads to food battles. Besides, babies always fed pureed rather than more textured foods don't learn to chew at the appropriate stage of development and may have more trouble learning later. And babies *can* chew, with their gums. Store-bought pureed baby foods are an entirely unnecessary expense.

Just as a baby learns to walk by trying, he can learn to feed himself as part of his natural development. To help him, you need only place him in a high chair or on your lap at the family table, with a sheet or mat on the floor to make cleanup easier, and offer him appropriate foods from the family meal. Let him grab handfuls of food, transfer them to his mouth, and chew them. If your baby takes charge of what he eats and how much he eats, he will be able to feed himself regular meals by the time he is a year old.

The British midwife and breastfeeding counselor Gill Rapley is the creator of a wonderful video about what she calls baby-led weaning. You can have a brief look at the video by following the link at www.nursing motherscompanion.com/resources. To purchase the complete video or the book *Baby-Led Weaning: Helping Your Baby to Love Good Food*, by Gill Rapley and Tracey Murkett, see Appendix A, page 359. Rapley also has an informative website, www.rapleyweaning.com.

Your baby will be a clumsy eater at first. A six-month-old is not able to purposely open his fist to place food in his mouth, so you'll need to offer large chunks or sticks of fruits and cooked vegetables that your baby can grasp while still having a portion available to chew on. The baby may seem to spit much of the food out at first; this is because he is not yet good at moving food to the back of his mouth to swallow it. A baby at this stage may also gag when eating. This is not choking but a normal part of learning to eat.

Note that certain foods do pose a choking hazard; these include raw vegetables, nuts, whole grapes, raisins, and dried fruits. But the baby who is being spoon-fed is actually at greater risk for choking than the self-fed baby, because the former has less control of the process of moving food to the back of his mouth and swallowing. Nevertheless, you should never leave your baby alone while he is eating.

Offering a wide variety of fruits and vegetables will allow your baby to pick what is interesting and tasty to him. These foods are useful more for the experience of self-feeding than for the nutrients they provide. Most babies enjoy the taste and texture of fruits such as apples, bananas, apricots, peaches, nectarines, pears, avocados, mangoes, plums, and melons. (Because citrus fruits are very acidic and can cause rashes and upset stomachs, some experts suggest waiting until a baby is 10 to 12 months old before offering them.) Cooked vegetables such as sweet potatoes, potatoes, carrots, squash, asparagus, broccoli, cauliflower, snap beans, and beets are also good choices for babies just starting to learn to feed themselves. (Large quantities of green and orange vegetables can give a baby's skin a yellow tinge, but this is completely harmless.)

Babies do best with little salt, if any. If you are offering cooked vegetables for the family, salt them after taking out the baby's portion, because young babies are unable to handle large amounts of sodium.

As soon as a baby is managing small amounts of fruits and vegetables, you should offer meats or other foods high in protein, iron, and zinc. Meats such as beef, pork, and poultry, especially dark poultry flesh, are especially good sources of these nutrients. Although chicken and fish (carefully boned) are fairly easy for a baby to manage, red meats may need to be slow-cooked and shredded or ground or minced. Avoid lunch meats, hot dogs, cured sausage, and ham, which are high in salt and sodium nitrate and are not the best sources of protein.

Good non-meat sources of protein and iron include scrambled eggs, semi-hard cheeses like cheddar and Monterey Jack, nut butters (such as almond), tofu and tempeh, and tahini. Peanut butter provides protein, iron, and zinc as well as fat, but be sure to choose a brand without added fat or sugar and preferably without salt. Beans, whole wheat, and oats are also rich sources of zinc.

If any of the baby's close blood relatives, however, are allergic to egg whites, cow's milk products, nuts, soy, wheat, or fish or shellfish, you will want to postpone offering these foods to your baby. Families with food allergies should introduce wheat after seven months of age, soy after eight months of age, cow's milk products after one year, egg whites after two years, and peanuts, tree nuts, and fish and shellfish after three years.

If your baby's blood relatives have no food allergies, you shouldn't worry about your baby's developing them. The American Academy of Pediatrics recently advised that feeding commonly allergenic foods need not be postponed unless specific foods have produced allergic symptoms in a family member.

Offering new foods a few days apart can help you identify any allergy your baby may have. Signs of allergy include diarrhea, gassiness, and redness around the anus; vomiting and increased spitting up; and rashes (especially on the face), wheezing, and a runny nose.

Should you prefer that your child have a vegetarian diet, you can feed him accordingly. If cheese and eggs are not included, tofu, tempeh, and cooked legumes, when combined with whole-grain cereals, can provide protein as well as iron and zinc. Winter squash, sweet potatoes, broccoli, and dark leafy vegetables such as spinach and Swiss chard are especially good sources of iron, and iron absorption is increased a great deal when foods containing vitamin C are eaten at the same time. Do take the time to learn all you can about vegetarianism and the nutritional needs of infants and toddlers. You might want to consult with a nutritionist, especially if you are considering a vegan diet for your baby. Young children on such diets are at substantial risk for B-vitamin deficiencies and, because of a lack of protein, general growth deficiencies. The federal Special Supplemental Nutrition Program for Women, Infants, and Children (WIC) or your local public health department can probably refer you to a nutritionist who can offer further guidance.

Once your baby is eating protein foods as well as fruits and vegetables, you can also offer whole-grain breads and cereals. These offer B vitamins, iron, zinc, and all the other nutrients of the grain in its original form. Refined grains—white rice, white breads, regular pasta, and dry cereals not made from whole grains—are less healthful. Whole-grain cereals of rice, corn, and barley are good first choices, as are corn tortillas and whole-wheat pasta (I've found tastier brands of whole-wheat pasta in natural-foods stores). Whole buckwheat flour contains more protein than any other grain flour and makes delicious and nutritious pancakes. Last but not least, most babies enjoy rice cakes, some of which are made with whole-grain rice.

When shopping for breads and cereals, check the ingredients. The first ingredient should be whole wheat or another whole grain. Do not accept products made with partially hydrogenated oils (or trans fats). Try to find breads and cereals that have little or no added sugar.

As your baby progresses with his self-feeding skills, you will gradually begin to see from his diaper that he is taking in more solid foods. His stools will begin looking and smelling more like adult bowel movements.

At some point after your baby's first six months, you may want to offer him a cup to learn drinking skills. Most babies are ready to begin learning how to drink from a cup by the time they are six or seven months old. You can begin with water. A cup is also useful for feeding semi-liquid foods like yogurt. Many parents offer fruit juice, but juice offers no nutritional advantage over fruit, and it often lessens a baby's appetite for milk and solid foods. "Juice abuse" is a common mistake in infant feeding that can lead to diarrhea, dental decay, and possibly childhood obesity.

If you give your baby juice, limit it to 3 ounces a day, and offer it only alongside a meal or snack. Don't let your baby carry around juice in a bottle, cup, or box. Be careful with citrus, tomato, and pineapple juices, which can cause reactions in babies. Avoid "fruit drinks"; they contain mostly water and sugar or corn syrup. Juices bottled especially for infants are expensive and unnecessary. If you buy juice in a metal can, transfer it to another container after the can is opened.

Once your baby begins drinking from a cup, be prepared for her to turn the cup over to see what happens—all part of the learning process. You can try a sippy cup, one with either a spout or a straw, which comes with a tight-fitting lid and therefore won't spill.

At around seven to nine months of age, your baby will be able to use his thumb and fingers to pick up both large and smaller pieces of food. He'll be able to eat brown rice, diced meat, or small pieces of pasta, fruits, and vegetables with his fingers.

Once the baby is doing well with different food groups, you can offer him more complex family foods, such as pasta, casserole dishes, and sandwiches. But try to minimize the salt in your cooking until the baby is at least a year old.

The baby will begin to use cutlery, if you let him, sometime between 10 and 11 months of age. At this point he'll be able to spoon-feed himself yogurt and cooked cereals. By the time he reaches his first birthday, your baby will probably be proficient with a spoon and fork.

When your baby is eating table foods fairly well, you can give him regular meals and snacks. Offer three or four small servings of whole-grain cereal or bread per day and at least four daily servings of fruits and vegetables, at 1 to 2 tablespoons per serving. The baby also needs at least two daily servings of high-protein foods. A serving of meat, poultry, fish, or eggs is about 1 tablespoon, or ½ ounce. The baby can have an egg three or four times a week. Should allergies be a concern, cook the egg until solid and offer only the yolk. Other high-protein servings for a baby of this age might be 1 ounce of semi-hard cheese, ¼ cup of cottage cheese, or ½ cup of cooked shell beans or lentils. Pass up commercially prepared "infant dinners"; mostly vegetables and water with only a small amount of meat, these are a poor source of protein.

While your baby may not always get precisely the suggested amounts of grains, fruits, vegetables, and high-protein foods every day, averaging close to these amounts over a week will ensure he is well nourished. But if by eight to ten months your baby will still take solids only sporadically at best, it may be time to give him a little extra encouragement. In this case, try nursing after meals, not before. If he is desperate for the breast, try to keep the nursing short, and then encourage him to return his attention to other foods. Always include him in family meals, but offer food at other times of the day if he refuses it at mealtimes. Never assume that because he spits something out in disgust one day he won't take it a week later.

One of the last transitions is postponing breastfeeding until after the meal; this encourages the baby to take more solids. I recommend making this transition at 10 to 12 months.

After the baby is established on table foods, the final transition is serving cow's milk along with the meal. Ideally, this should be accomplished when the baby is around 12 months of age (a baby much younger than that can't digest cow's milk well). Use whole milk; low-fat milk does not provide the fat that the older baby or toddler needs. If the rest of the family drinks low-fat milk, you might feed the baby whole evaporated milk, diluted one to one with water. Because evaporated milk is treated with high heat, it is more digestible than whole milk, and it is no more expensive. If your baby is allergic to milk and is not yet one year old, use soy formula or hypoallergenic formula instead. If your baby does not like any milk but yours, offer plenty of cheese and yogurt, and try tofu—it is also very high in calcium.

After your baby's first year, you can feed him regular soy milk in place of cow's milk or formula, provided that the soy milk is whole, not low-fat or nonfat, because fat is important for brain development in children under two years of age. The soy milk you choose should also be fortified with vitamins A and D and calcium. Try to offer plenty of calcium-rich or calcium-fortified foods as well, because soy milk contains phytates, which can reduce the absorption of calcium and other minerals.

You may be wondering if we have just weaned your baby. In a sense, yes. Weaning is the *process* of expanding a baby's diet to include other foods. For another year or two or more, however, nursing may continue to be important and convenient for early morning feedings, snacks, naps, bedtime, and general soothing and comforting.

Considering Weaning

For any of various reasons, you may be considering giving up nursing altogether. If you truly resent breastfeeding, if you need to give it up because of a serious illness, or if you are planning to get pregnant soon, you can wean completely and easily at this stage.

Perhaps the reasons you want to stop nursing are less compelling. Maybe months ago you set a time limit for breastfeeding and now you feel you must carry through with your plan, or maybe you think your baby is simply too old to nurse. You may have heard a myth—that older babies all bite or that weaning a toddler is just too difficult.

Or you may hope that ending breastfeeding will solve various problems like the shape of your body, fatigue, marital troubles, or sibling rivalry. Rarely does total weaning solve problems like these. Many women who end the breastfeeding relationship early come to regret later that they have given up this precious time for no benefit.

It is normal to feel ambivalent about nursing. Sometimes you may wish you could be free of this intense relationship, and other times you may adore putting your baby to your breast and watching him fall off to sleep there. Such ambivalence is a natural part of an intimate relationship. Simply recognizing this may help put your mind at ease.

Perhaps the problem is friends and relatives. If they have started asking when you plan to wean the baby, you may feel embarrassed and pressured to give up nursing. Our society seems to rush babies and toddlers toward independence. Keep in mind that nursing is still providing your baby with protective antibodies; even at 12 months, a baby has only 60 percent of an adult's ability to fight off infection. If a friend's baby weaned early and easily, remember that some babies need the comfort of the breast much longer than others. Babies who are allowed to wean themselves do so when they feel that their source of security will always be there when they need it.

Knowing all this, you may still have trouble dealing with the disapproval of friends and family members. You may be able to cope with criticism from others by ignoring the comments, confronting the people who make them, or keeping your nursing a secret from them.

Since your nursing older baby will soon be a talking nursing older baby, you might consider what word you'll feel comfortable hearing your baby use in public for breastfeeding. Words like *booby* might be fine at home, but they could cause you embarrassment elsewhere. You might choose a term such as *nursie* or *numnums* or use a word that your baby makes up.

You won't, of course, be able to hide your nursing relationship from your partner, whose comments may be the hardest to deal with. If he is bothered by your breastfeeding, you can try telling him about its benefits to your baby's health and to your family's finances. If your baby is waking at night, you might invite your partner to take over night duty.

You can find support for your continued nursing by seeking out mother-to-mother support groups such as La Leche League. See Appendix A, page 358, to learn how to find a local group.

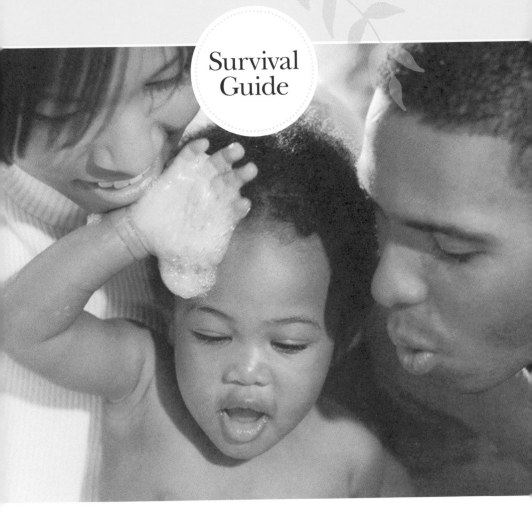

MONTHS SIX
THROUGH TWELVE

Concerns about Yourself

- Nipple Soreness from
  New Teeth

Concerns about the Baby

- Biting
- Night Walking
- Nursing Strike
- Weaning the Older Baby

Concerns about Yourself

Nipple Soreness from New Teeth

Your nipples can become temporarily sore when the baby's new top teeth erupt. New teeth must be very thin and sharp to make their way through the tough gums, and this can cause you some discomfort until they thicken up after a few weeks.

Coping Measures for Dealing with New Teeth

1. Because the baby's mouth tends to drag down the breast tissue, it may help to lift her upward by using a pillow and lifting your breast upward.

2. Experiment with other nursing positions to see which positions are more comfortable.

3. If the baby is letting her chin rest on her chest, try to get her head tilted back a little more.

4. Offer your breast with the nipple pointing downward and wait for a wide-open mouth before latching.

5. After nursings, rinse your nipples with cool water and apply a thin coating of modified lanolin ointment.

Concerns about the Baby

Biting

While not all babies bite, some do. In fact, some mothers actually decide against breastfeeding out of fear of being bitten, or may end breastfeeding prematurely when their babies begin to get teeth. Being bitten can be painful, and it can also make a mother tense for fear it will happen again. Some mothers may wonder if this is the baby wanting to be weaned, which is not the case. Most of the time, biting is a temporary problem, and babies can be taught not to bite. The behavior may continue for a few days, but it usually ends as suddenly as it began.

If your baby has bitten you, there are a few things you should know. Most importantly, babies don't do this intentionally, and they certainly don't understand that they are causing you pain. Second, babies cannot bite when they are actively sucking and drinking milk, as their tongues cover their lower teeth. But with that being said, they can certainly stop sucking, pull their tongue back, and bite down. Your baby is most likely to bite at the end of a feeding or when she is just snacking; she may have a playful look on her face and may push the nipple to the front of her mouth just before she takes a chomp. So if you are bitten by your baby, do not nurse her again until you are sure she is hungry.

If you are bitten, there are a few ways to react. Biting hurts, and there is no reason not to let your baby know by responding with an unpleasant natural noise, like "No!" or "Ouch!" This doesn't work with all babies, however; some get so frightened that they go on a nursing strike. Others enjoy the reaction and want to continue the "game."

This is likely the first disciplining you will do as a mother. The goal is to teach your baby that biting is unacceptable behavior. I think that the most effective thing to do after being bitten is to simply end the nursing session so that the baby learns that biting is not allowed while nursing. If the baby bites down and does not let go, put your finger in between his gums to release the suction.

Many mothers are told to respond to biting by flicking their baby's cheek or pulling him in toward the breast so that he cannot take a breath and will let go. I am not a fan of either of these tactics, as both seem variations on hurting the baby back in some way. Babies are learning to trust in their first year, and I don't think it is an emotionally healthy response for the person that they love and depend on most in the world to hurt them in any way.

A baby most commonly bites before her teeth come in, often just before the top two teeth break through. Your baby may bite your breast because she is biting everything and anything in an attempt to relieve the ache in her gums. Mothers may be given the go-ahead by their baby's doctor to give acetaminophen drops (Infants' Tylenol) or ibuprofen drops (Infants' Motrin, Infants' Advil) for teething pain. Some mothers use these medications an hour or so before nursing, but this may still not prevent biting. For more suggestions to help ease your baby's teething pain, see "Coping with Teething," page 326.

Occasionally a baby's bite can cause a wound on the nipple. In the case of a painful wound, it may be necessary to temporarily express milk by using hand expression or pumping. Nipple wounds (like all human bites) can easily become infected. If a bite wound is not healing after a couple of days, it may contain bacteria, so you should seek help from your doctor and be treated with an antibiotic. Wounded nipples that are not healing may also lead to mastitis. Mastitis comes with fever and flu-like symptoms and can lessen milk production on that breast, which in some cases can become permanent.

Coping Measures for Biting

1. Avoid letting the baby snack at the breast during this period of biting. If the baby has nursed well within the past hour or so, delay the next feeding.

2. Shortly before your baby is due for a feeding, offer her a cold, damp washcloth or a chilled water-filled teething ring.

3. While you're nursing, watch for a change in your baby's nursing pattern. As soon as she stops taking long, even sucks and begins short, choppy ones, end the feeding—with your finger if necessary. If you notice a playful look on her face, end the feeding. Instead of paying attention to the TV, talking on the phone, or engaging in other activities, pay attention to your baby and stay vigilant during nursings so that you can tell when the baby is starting to lose interest and you can end the feeding.

4. If you resume nursing and the baby tries to bite again, she is obviously not hungry anymore. End the feeding.

Night Waking

Whether or not you've identified a reason for frequent night waking, you may be spending a considerable amount of energy trying to end it. Manipulating daytime naps, feeding solids late in the evening, giving pain relievers or cold remedies when the baby isn't sick or in pain, trying to keep the baby from falling asleep at the breast, consulting health-care providers, and trying different tactics in the middle of the night rarely work.

This is not to say that you shouldn't have your baby examined if you suspect a physical discomfort. She could be hurting from an ear infection (especially if she has had a runny nose in the past couple of weeks) or from teeth working their way in. Some babies who are distracted during many of their daytime nursings may wake often at night out of hunger.

If your baby seems to be waking from teething pain, you can try giving her acetaminophen drops (Infants' Tylenol) or ibuprofen drops (Infants' Motrin, Infants' Advil). Of the two, ibuprofen seems more effective for teething pain. If the medication wears off before it's time to give another dose, you can "piggyback" the two pain relievers—that is, give the other in the meantime. But call your doctor's office for advice first.

Offering pacifiers, bottles, or other comfort objects in the night is not likely to get you a full night's sleep. Most parents who try these things must get up at night to find them when their babies wake up crying. Besides, unless a bottle is filled with water, a baby risks developing tooth decay when she falls asleep at night drinking from one.

There are simple ways you can help your baby sleep for longer periods at night. First, leave the baby alone if she doesn't need you immediately. Babies may make a lot of noises as they sleep, and not all of them signal a need to be fed. Listen before responding, and learn to distinguish which sounds are feeding requests and which are not. Soothing music can help a baby relax and drift off to sleep, and to fall back to sleep when she wakes in the night. White noise (sounds of different frequencies combined

Childhood dental health becomes an important concern once a baby's teeth erupt. Clean the new teeth once or twice a day with a tiny amount of fluoride toothpaste and a soft cloth or very soft toothbrush. Although research indicates that breast milk has a protective effect against dental caries, some of that protection seems to be lost once a baby begins eating solids, and the presence of other carbohydrates along with breast milk in the diet can lead to caries. The American Academy of Pediatric Dentists recommends having a child's teeth first checked for decay at about the age of 12 months.

together) is another tool that might lull the baby to sleep. You can buy a white-noise machine or a white-noise CD.

One way some parents succeed at making a baby sleep through the night is by letting her "cry it out" for a few nights or more. Several books tout this technique, perhaps the best known among them being Richard Ferber's *Solve Your Child's Sleep Problems* (a revised edition was published in 2006). The idea is to refuse to pick up your baby when she wakes during the night, and to let her cry herself back to sleep, until she finally learns that her crying is fruitless and stops crying in the night. Many parents report that this method has worked for them.

To other parents, though, the cry-it-out method seems too drastic, and some mental-health experts warn against it. No studies have shown that it is safe, these experts point out, and it certainly seems inconsistent with infants' emotional needs.

> White-noise CDs made for babies have advantages over white-noise machines. Not only are the machines more expensive, they also have a small range of sounds, and they play the same sounds over and over. The small speaker on a white-noise machine can't reproduce the full spectrum of sound on a white-noise CD. And the machine may not be loud enough to block outside noises. See Appendix A (page 366) for information on ordering white-noise CDs made for babies.

If you decide to try the cry-it-out method, or "controlled crying," choose a three- to four-day period in advance. When your baby wakes crying, go to her every 5 minutes. Lay her down, say "It's night-night time," and leave. Most babies cry for up to an hour or more the first night, and for a shorter time the next two or three nights. If this technique solves your night-waking problem, you can still continue nursing during the day.

A kinder way of training babies to sleep through the night is advocated by Elizabeth Pantley, a mother of four and the co-author of *The No-Cry Sleep Solution*. The no-cry method involves long naps early in the day, before-bed routines, and early bedtimes. Nighttime wakings are handled this way: As soon as the baby cries, you nurse her back to sleep. Over time, you gradually shorten the baby's time at the breast, with the aim of ending the nursing as soon as she stops actively sucking, before she is fully asleep (you must stay awake yourself, of course, to manage this). When the baby can fall back to sleep without extended sucking, you comfort her when she wakes just by patting her on the back and repeating a soothing word. Eventually, the baby should be able to go back to sleep on her own with just a word. If the baby shares your bed, you may want to help her stay asleep by holding her hand against your breast. Pantley's book includes sleep charts for tracking the baby's progress.

After developing her method with her own children, Pantley tested it on 200 other mother-baby pairs. More than half of the mothers had their babies sleeping through the night within three weeks, according to Pantley, and 92 percent succeeded within two months.

If Pantley's and Ferber's methods fail to work for you, you might consider the way nursing mothers all over the world have made night waking less disruptive: Sleep with your baby. Despite what people say, your baby won't be smothered by the covers, by you, or by your mate. The baby won't keep you awake; babies with easy access to the breast rarely cry at night. After a few nights you'll adjust to the new sleeping companion, and her presence will not disrupt your sleep as much as would waking to her cries, getting out of bed, tending to her, and coming back to bed again. Neither you nor your baby will need to waken completely to nurse, and Dad won't need to waken at all.

If taking a baby into the parents' bed puts a damper on sexual activity, couples who have adopted this approach seldom complain about a lack of sex. Parents do mention how much they enjoy watching their baby sleep, cuddling her warm little body, and waking up with her in the morning.

Families have come up with many inventive ways to make the "family bed" more comfortable, safe, and convenient. You might buy a larger mattress, build a platform for mattresses placed side by side, or simply put your mattress on the floor. Get a waterproof mattress pad so your mattress stays dry; so *you* stay dry, double-diaper the baby or use disposables at bedtime. This will eliminate most nighttime diaper changes;

when you or your mate must get up, a low-wattage night-light will make things easier.

If you have doubts about sleeping with your baby, you might still try it for a couple of weeks before dismissing the idea. You can find more detailed advice on bed sharing in Dr. James McKenna's *Sleeping with Your Baby: A Parent's Guide to Cosleeping* (see "Suggested Supplemental Reading," page 414).

If you're still feeling worn out after you've found some way to get more sleep at night, you might examine your diet. Some lactating women may be vulnerable to fatigue because of vitamin B deficiencies. Although in such a case the baby will generally grow well and get the nutrients she needs from her mother's milk, her mother may suffer from low energy levels. Be sure you are eating plenty of whole grains, which are rich in B vitamins.

You might also consider supplementing your diet with brewer's yeast, a potent source of B vitamins that is considered more effective and faster acting than B-complex supplements. Available in health-food stores, brewer's yeast can be taken as a tablet or as a powder to be mixed with juice or milk. Starting with the daily dose recommended on the label, you can slowly increase the amount to two to four times the daily recommendation (increasing the amount too quickly could cause diarrhea in you and your baby).

Nursing Strike

Although nursing strikes can occur at any time, they usually happen in the second half of the baby's first year. A nursing strike is distinguished from weaning by its suddenness. Some babies wean themselves between eight and twelve months of age, but they usually do so gradually.

Reasons for nursing strikes vary greatly. They may include teething, a cold, an ear infection, a painful herpes sore in the mouth, or a change in the taste of the milk. They sometimes happen after a prolonged separation between a baby and his mother, or after a baby has bitten his mother and been frightened by her response. Sometimes, when a baby has become used to a bottle and its rapid flow of milk, his refusal to nurse is a response to his mother's dwindling milk supply. Some authorities believe a nursing strike may precede mastery of a major motor skill, such as crawling, standing, or walking.

Although some mothers decide to turn a nursing strike into final weaning, in most cases the baby can be coaxed to resume nursing. Strikes typically last a few days, but they may go on for as long as two weeks.

Treatment Measures for Nursing Strikes

1. Try a change in position, or nurse in a quiet, darkened room.

2. So long as the baby refuses to nurse, pump or manually express your milk frequently throughout the day. Offer the milk in a cup rather than a bottle.

3. Try to determine the cause for the nursing strike. Consider having the baby examined to rule out an ear infection or other physical problem. Check your milk supply, especially if the baby has been nursing infrequently or has become increasingly dependent on a bottle: Do your breasts feel empty most of the time? Is the milk slow to let down? Is the baby swallowing less?

4. Maintain frequent and close skin-to-skin contact with the baby without nursing. Offer the breast whenever the baby is sleepy.

Weaning the Older Baby

Weaning the older baby need not be hard, especially if she is crawling and busily exploring or has lost interest in some of her nursings. Ideally, weaning at any age should occur gradually, over several weeks at least. A good place to begin is with the nursing that the baby seems least interested in, most likely one during the day. Key to your success is providing an appealing substitute for the breast. This means offering not only something else to eat or drink, but also yourself. Nursing provides a mother's love and attention as well as food. You'll need to do a lot of cuddling and rocking and activities like reading a book or playing on the floor together.

You must choose whether to wean to a cup or a bottle. Although the older baby is developmentally ready for a cup, if she has trouble swallowing from one, the bottle may be best. However, giving the baby a bottle can lead to other difficulties. If she is not carefully monitored, she can become overdependent on the bottle, lose interest in solid foods, and end up with tooth decay. And if you wean the baby to a bottle, you will probably need to wean her *from* it later on.

Unless the baby is well established on table foods and eating three meals a day, give formula before offering solid foods.

Although weaning may progress quickly for some babies, concluding in a month or two, other babies take longer, especially those who are especially fond of nursing or are reluctant to give up certain feedings. The first nursing in the morning and those before naptime and bedtime are often most loved by the older baby. It may take longer to eliminate these completely. For helpful advice, read *The Nursing Mother's Guide to Weaning* (see "Suggested Supplemental Reading," page 414).

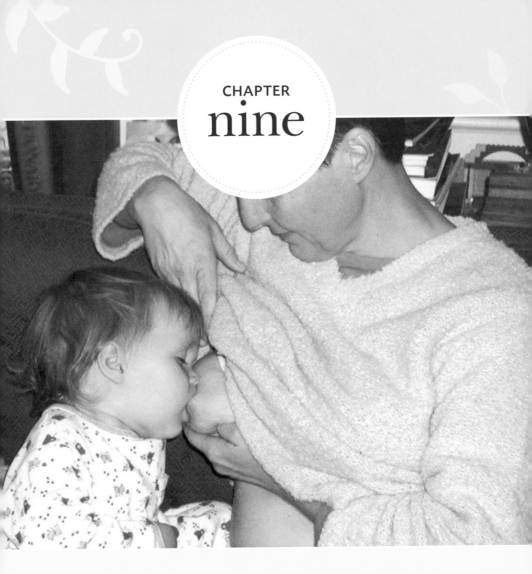

NURSING THE TODDLER

- Nursing during Pregnancy
- Tandem Nursing
- Your Toddler's Diet
- Weaning Your Toddler

THE TODDLER IS TRYING TO ACCOMPLISH the major task of establishing himself as an individual. Although he is no longer a baby, he is still very dependent. One minute he is exploring and getting into everything, and the next he is turning to his mother for comfort and reassurance.

Many toddlers tend to nurse briefly. Some nurse just a few times a day, but many want the breast often. Or a toddler may nurse just a few times one day, and many times the next.

Even if a toddler nurses infrequently, nursing is important to him. The antibodies in breast milk are still present and protective. The toddler wants the breast for quick snacks, help in falling off to sleep, and intermittent comfort and emotional refueling. Sometimes nursing is one of the toddler's few connections to a busy mother. You may discover that nursing into toddlerhood is not only a convenient way of mothering, it is also one of the few times during the day that your child holds still long enough for cuddling and affection.

Some nursing toddlers still wake at night for feedings. See "Night Waking" (page 340) for suggestions and coping strategies. If you are sleeping with your baby, you might find additional help from the suggestions of Dr. Jay Gordon at www.drjaygordon.com/attachment/sleeppattern.html.

The young toddler may be quite insistent when he wants to nurse, regardless of the time or place. As he gets a bit older, he will become more willing to wait a little while.

Although children in many parts of the world are breastfed until they are two, three, or four years of age, nursing a walking, talking toddler is considered somewhat deviant in parts of Western society. Many toddlers are dependent on a bottle, pacifier, thumb, or blanket, and this is quite accepted, but a mother who is nursing a toddler may have to deal with veiled or point-blank suggestions that her child is too old for it. The concerns about nursing beyond infancy often reflect the fear that a child

NURSING THE TODDLER

will become spoiled or overdependent. In fact, when a toddler's need for security is met, he becomes more self-assured and independent.

Mothers who are nursing toddlers usually enjoy socializing with others who are doing the same. La Leche League not only voices support for women who breastfeed beyond the first year but also offers meetings for those who are nursing one-, two-, three-, or even four-year-olds (see Appendix A, page 358, for more information on La Leche). Norma Jane Bumgarner's book *Mothering Your Nursing Toddler* is an excellent resource for those nursing beyond infancy (see "Suggested Supplemental Reading," page 414).

Nursing during Pregnancy

Although many people frown on breastfeeding during pregnancy, there is no reason you cannot continue nursing your child, if you're comfortable doing so, when you find out another is on the way. Fears that nursing will harm a fetus have no basis, even for mothers who are too queasy to eat much. Despite some doctors' warnings, no studies have shown that nursing during pregnancy leads to miscarriage or poor growth. When to stop nursing should be left up to you—but it's best to be sure your child is regularly eating solid foods and drinking from a cup before you give up nursing completely.

Even with frequent nursing, pregnancy often causes a decrease in milk supply, particularly at mid-pregnancy. The milk becomes quite salty as the supply diminishes, and at about the start of the third trimester colostrum replaces milk in preparation for the newborn. If your baby is not yet a year old when you notice your milk supply declining, you may need to supplement your milk with formula. After the first year, though, you can substitute whole dairy milk, served in a cup (see "Your Toddler's Diet," page 351).

It is thought that about half of nursing babies and toddlers wean during their mothers' pregnancies, some on their own and the rest with encouragement from their mothers. The other half do not seem to mind the changes in the milk and show no signs of wanting to give up nursing. This can be problematic, because many women who nurse while pregnant experience tender breasts and sore nipples. Caused by the hormonal changes of pregnancy, this soreness usually goes away as the pregnancy progresses, but in the meantime the pain may be so great that you feel you can't go on breastfeeding. In this case, see "Weaning Your Toddler," page 352.

Some mothers feel agitated while nursing during pregnancy. This is apparently a physiological response.

Many nursing women also feel especially tired after becoming pregnant again. This is a normal response to pregnancy. Plenty of rest helps combat fatigue, especially in the first trimester. Nursing your baby or toddler may actually help you deal with fatigue, since breastfeeding is a relaxing way to mother a baby who is tired, hurt, or demanding of your time.

Some pregnant mothers may notice uterine contractions while nursing. No studies have shown that such contractions lead to premature labor, but if you have had a previous premature labor, you should discuss this possibility with your doctor.

Tandem Nursing

Mothers who have nursed throughout all or most of their pregnancies may find themselves nursing an older baby or toddler along with the new baby. This may be overwhelming for some, particularly if the older child is nursing frequently. But many have found it to be a generally positive experience.

Because the breasts receive more stimulation with two babies than with only one, the milk is usually plentiful. As a rule, the younger baby should be nursed first, but the supply is likely to be so abundant that the timing of feedings may not be essential. In fact, mothers nursing two often end up with an oversupply of milk.

It's hard to know how your nursing toddler will react to the baby's arrival. Some toddlers want to nurse more often after than during pregnancy, and others cut back or wean entirely. Some siblings sweetly bond while nursing together, but often toddlers become possessive of their mothers' breasts. Nursing or not, older children may struggle with having to share Mom with a new baby. You may need to set limits if your toddler acts out because of jealousy.

Should you decide to wean the older sibling while nursing the new baby, ideally you should do so gradually. It may be tricky to keep the older child's mind off nursing while breastfeeding the baby in front of him. Reducing the number and length of nursings and providing distractions can be helpful in gradual weaning. See "Weaning Your Toddler," page 352.

Bumgarner's *Mothering Your Nursing Toddler* includes a detailed section on tandem nursing. A book wholly devoted to this topic is Hilary Flower's *Adventures in Tandem Nursing: Breastfeeding during Pregnancy and Beyond* (see "Suggested Supplemental Reading," page 414).

Your Toddler's Diet

Toddlers are notoriously sporadic eaters. Their appetites decrease during this time—first because their growth slows greatly from that of the first year, and second because they are often too busy to eat. The toddler grows more in length than in weight. Weight gain typically slows to no more than a pound every two months. (In Appendix C, page 371, you'll find the World Health Organization's new growth charts, which show the normal weight of breastfed babies and children all over the world.)

The toddler's feeding skills vary considerably. Sometimes she may feed herself, and other times she may want to be fed. Parents who worry about how little their child eats may be tempted to persuade, trick, or even force her to eat more. This turns meals into battles and may be the start of long-term eating problems. As Ellyn Satter (2000) says, "You are responsible for *what* your child is offered to eat, *where* and *when* it is presented. She is responsible for *how much* of it she eats."

The suggested minimum servings of foods for the toddler are similar to those for the older baby. A handy rule of thumb is this: Give 1 tablespoon per year of age or one-quarter of the adult serving, whichever is easiest to figure for the particular food. You would therefore offer your toddler 2 tablespoons of peas or one-quarter of an apple. The suggested daily minimum servings for each food group are as follows:

- Fruits and vegetables: 4 servings
- Grains (bread, cereal, noodles, rice): 4 servings
- High-protein foods: 2 servings
- Whole milk: 2 to 3 cups

Offering a meal or nutritious snack every three to four hours is a good approach with a toddler. Don't always offer milk just because she likes it; if she drinks more than three cups a day, it may replace other nutritious foods in her diet. Expect that your toddler may enjoy a certain food one day and refuse it the next. Make sure she comes to the table for meals and is offered whatever foods the family is eating. Do not play into her food whims by running out to the kitchen to fix something else for her when she refuses to eat.

Weaning Your Toddler

Ideally, complete weaning occurs when both the child and the mother are ready for it. Many times, though, a mother begins to think about bringing breastfeeding to a close while her toddler is still happily nursing. She may feel that full weaning will make things easier—that it will put an end to night waking, make the baby more independent, or improve her own energy level. Some mothers have a self-imposed deadline for ending breastfeeding and begin to feel pressured once it draws near. Others simply become fearful that their children will nurse forever if allowed. Most often, a mother considers full weaning when other people suggest that the baby should no longer need to nurse. Criticism from friends, family, or health-care workers may be straightforward or subtle, but it often motivates a mother to end the nursing relationship.

All mothers have mixed feelings about nursing at times. Keep in mind that ending breastfeeding will not help your child sleep through the night, improve your relationship with your partner, make you less tired or less bored, or make your child less dependent on you. Toddlers, especially, often demand to nurse more when their mothers become busier and when they receive little mothering except at the breast. At those times that young children need more attention, ironically, mothers often most feel that they need some kind of a break. Stopping breastfeeding during one of these times could be terribly upsetting for a child and for the rest of the family as well. Should the arbitrary date you had in mind for full weaning arrive, there is no need to follow through if you and your child are still enjoying nursing.

Knowing all this, you may still have trouble dealing with the disapproval of friends and family members. Families in particular can wield tremendous influence over a nursing relationship. You may be able to deal with criticism from others by either ignoring it or confronting it. Or you may choose to withdraw from those who are critical and find new friends who believe in nursing older babies; a mother-to-mother support group, such as the Nursing Mothers Counsel or La Leche League (see Appendix A, pages 357 and 358), is one place to do this. Finally, you might simply keep your nursing secret from those who don't approve. This may be easy if you're nursing only at night and in the early morning.

When a baby is still nursing often and enthusiastically at the end of his first year, he will probably want to continue nursing throughout the second year and beyond. Some experts say that a child rarely initiates weaning before the age of four. For this reason friends may tell you to wean by your baby's first birthday if you have definite feelings against nursing a three-year-old. You may fear that if you wait, you will have a major struggle convincing your child to stop nursing in the months to follow. That toddlers seldom initiate weaning, however, doesn't mean that they always fight it. Should you find yourself still happily nursing at your baby's first birthday, be assured that there will probably be several opportune times to wean and numerous techniques to accomplish weaning after a year of age and before the age of four.

You might rightly stop breastfeeding if you have definite feelings against nursing a toddler or nursing while pregnant. Full weaning—or just limiting the number of daily feedings—may also be best if you are starting to resent nursing. The decision to give up breastfeeding should be made carefully, not in reaction to a bad day or a temporary problem.

Timing is important once you've decided to wean. Keep in mind that weaning is a process rather than an event. Weaning initiated by the mother should ideally occur gradually and empathetically over several weeks, at least. And there are better times than others to initiate the process. If the child is particularly clingy and needy, if he has recently had a stressful experience such as moving or starting childcare, or if you are actively trying to get him to sleep through the night, now is not the time to wean.

In general, mother-led weaning involves substituting for nursing something that the child enjoys as much. In this way weaning does not become a series of deprivations or rejections. If the pace of weaning is too rapid, most children will react with obvious unhappiness or increased dependency on a pacifier, a thumb, or a bottle. Occasionally, full weaning must be postponed for a few weeks because the child is simply unable to cope without nursing.

Unfortunately, no one technique works for every mother and toddler. The best recommendations involve finding substitutions and distractions that may satisfy the child while at the same time ensuring that his needs for food, love, and attention are met. No plan is likely to succeed, however, unless a mother is sure of her own desire to wean. Her attitude is most important to her success.

Before you begin, pay close attention to the child's nursing routine, and yours. Keeping a record for a few days, like the one below, may give you some valuable insights for developing an effective plan.

TIME	PLACE	INTEREST LEVEL	REASON FOR NURSING
1:15 P.M.	living room	moderate	attention (I was talking on the phone)
5:30 P.M.	kitchen	moderate	hunger
8:00 P.M.	living room	high	sleepiness

Take note of when and where you nurse, the child's level of interest in nursing, and what you think prompted his demand for the breast. From the toddler's point of view, nursing may be just the thing whenever he is bored, frustrated, or tired, or he wants your attention or comfort—as well as when he is hungry.

From your observations, you should be able to identify which nursings are least crucial to your toddler and get some clues as to what type of substitutions will most likely satisfy him. Some nursings may be easily replaced with a nutritious snack or something to drink. Substitutions for toddlers may include any number of activities—playing with a special toy, reading a book, taking a walk, or visiting with another toddler. Warm-weather months may be an easier time to encourage weaning, as most toddlers enjoy exploring out of doors.

Although you may be able to substitute certain predictable daily nursings with other activities, if your toddler nurses sporadically all day, you may sometimes need to coax him to postpone nursings. Delaying daytime nursings works well for some toddlers as long as some distraction is provided. This can be an effective way to further weaning.

Some of your nursings are probably associated with routines the two of you have established, and with recurrent situations in which your toddler wants to nurse to get your attention. Identify these instances so you can change the pattern. If you nurse in bed early in the morning, get up instead. Get dressed, and offer your child a breakfast of table food. If you have a favorite place to relax and nurse, stay away from it. If your toddler demands to nurse every time you talk on the phone, keep conversations short. If you sit in front of the television and nurse, do something else or he will want to continue with the usual pattern. Think creatively of ways your child can learn new routines.

You can also take advantage of your child's ability to understand language. Talk to him about nursing—especially if you are trying to postpone feedings. He may accept your wish to "save up the milk till naptime and night-night." Older toddlers may be able to agree to future weaning upon an upcoming birthday or other milestone, such as the start of preschool.

The bedtime nursing may continue as the child's favorite. Some mothers find this is a special time for themselves as well and continue with it for weeks or months after other feedings have been abandoned. If you want to wean your toddler completely, your partner or another family member may be able to help the child establish a non-nursing bedtime routine.

More suggestions for easing weaning can be found under "Weaning the Older Baby," page 345, and in *The Nursing Mother's Guide to Weaning* (see "Suggested Supplemental Reading," page 414).

Once nursings become infrequent, your breasts may look smaller and feel less firm. Still, you may be able to express milk for several months after nursing has stopped. Your breasts will probably regain their former size and shape within six months of weaning.

Whether you initiate weaning or whether it is a mutual undertaking, you are bound to feel a little sad as the final days of nursing arrive, marking the end of the precious time you and your child spent together nursing. I hope you will also feel proud of yourself, for the wonderful start in life that you have given your child.

NURSING THE TODDLER

Appendices

APPENDIX A
Resources for Nursing Mothers

BREASTFEEDING SUPPORT AND EDUCATION

Nursing Mothers Counsel

San Francisco Bay Area Chapter:
P.O. Box 5024, San Mateo, CA 94402
650-327-6455
www.nursingmothers.org

Santa Cruz Chapter:
P.O. Box 66634, Scotts Valley, CA 95067
831-688-3954
www.nursingmothers.org

Counselors are available to take calls seven days a week from 9:00 A.M. to 9:00 P.M. PT.
Free breastfeeding classes and home visits are available to mothers who live in the area.
The San Francisco Bay Area Chapter rents and sells breast pumps, and also has grant
pumps available at reduced rates for those in need.

**Boston Association for Childbirth Education
and Nursing Mothers' Council**

P.O. Box 29, Newtonville, MA 02460
617-244-5102
www.bace-nmc.org

Local mothers can call or visit the website to find breastfeeding counselors in the area.

Nursing Mothers Counsel of Oregon

Portland: 503-282-3338
SW Washington: 360-750-0656
www.nursingmotherscounsel.org

Call seven days a week for free breastfeeding support. Free breastfeeding classes are also offered.

Nursing Mothers Advisory Council

P.O. Box 91, Abington, PA 19001
www.nursingmoms.net

NMAC serves mothers in certain areas of Bucks, Montgomery, and Philadelphia counties.

La Leche League International

957 N. Plum Grove Road, Schaumburg, IL 60173
800-525-3243
www.llli.org

Call between 9:00 a.m. and 5:00 p.m. CT for breastfeeding help or a referral to a local La Leche League group or La Leche League leader.

LACTATION PROFESSIONAL REFERRAL SERVICES

International Lactation Consultant Association

2501 Aerial Center Parkway, Suite 103, Morrisville, NC 27560
888-452-2478
www.ilca.org

Call weekdays between 9:00 a.m. and 5:00 p.m. ET or, on the ILCA website, click on "Find a Lactation Consultant."

Breastfeeding National Network (Medela, Inc.)

800-TELL-YOU
www.medela.com

Call at any hour for a referral to a local lactation professional.

HELPFUL WEBSITES

www.babycenter.com

Thousands of original, medically reviewed articles on preconception, pregnancy, babies, and toddlers, plus live chats with experts, bulletin boards, and newsletters.

www.kellymom.com

A popular site with information for breastfeeding mothers.

www.breastfeedingonline.com

Information for nursing mothers.

www.normalfed.com

Information for breastfeeding mothers and their helpers from Diane Wiessinger, a certified lactation consultant.

www.bfar.org
Information for women who are breastfeeding after breast and nipple surgeries.

www.lowmilksupply.org
Information for mothers experiencing low milk supply.

www.fourfriends.com/abrw
Information for women who are or will be nursing adopted babies.

www.pumpingmoms.blogspot.com
Discussion site for breast-pump users, from occasional to full-time. Topics include lactation problems and boosting the milk supply.

www.theleakyboob.com and www.facebook.com/TheLeakyBoob
A popular site for information, support, and discussions for nursing mothers.

DVDS FOR PURCHASE

"Breastfeeding: A Guide to Getting Started"

"Making Enough Milk: The Key to Successful Breastfeeding... Planning for Day One"
These 30-minute videos by Dr. Jane Morton cover getting the baby latched on, avoiding soreness, managing engorgement, hand expressing, and using a breast pump. Each costs $65 plus shipping.

"A Premie Needs His Mother: First Steps to Breastfeeding Your Premature Baby"
This video for mothers of premature babies covers hand expression, breast pumping, transitioning the baby from tube feeding to breastfeeding, and more. It costs $125 plus shipping.

Breastmilk Solutions
3655 Valencia Road, Aptos, CA 95003
831-219-5021
www.breastmilksolutions.com

"I Can Feed Myself! A Baby-Led Approach to Introducing Solid Foods"
This video by Gill Rapley, a British midwife, teaches parents how to help their baby make an easy transition to eating solid foods. You can see a short preview at the website. The video sells for $79.95 plus shipping, but readers of this book get a 20 percent discount (use the code DS20 at checkout).

Platypus Media
725 8th Street SEWashington, DC 20003
877-752-8977
www.platypusmedia.com

SPECIAL SUPPLEMENTAL NUTRITION PROGRAM FOR WOMEN, INFANTS, AND CHILDREN (WIC)
WIC is a federally funded program that provides nutritional information, counseling, and food to low- and moderate-income pregnant and nursing mothers and their young children. Some WIC programs also offer breast pumps to nursing mothers. Eligibility for

WIC services is determined by family income. To locate a WIC office near your home, contact your county or city health department or visit www.fns.usda.gov/wic.

NURSING BRAS AND BUSTIERS

Although nursing bras are available at maternity shops and department stores, the selection of styles and sizes may be too limited for you. The companies listed here sell online and by mail or phone order.

Bravado! Designs

41 Hollinger Road, Toronto, ON M4B 3G4 Canada
800-590-7802
www.bravadodesigns.com

Bravado makes several comfortable and popular nursing bras that are available in many maternity and baby stores in both Canada and the United States as well as at the company's website. Some styles come in extra-large sizes.

Simple Wishes

888-324-9474
www.simplewishes.com

Simple Wishes makes a "bustier" that allows for hands-free pumping. The flanges fit securely into small openings at the nipples, making it possible to move about freely while pumping. The bustier can be adjusted to fit a changing body, it covers more of the trunk than a bra, and it exposes little skin. It sells for $40. Simple Wishes also offers the B3 All-in-One Bra, which can be used as both a regular nursing bra and a pumping bra, for $60. Call or visit the website to locate a retailer near you, or order online. Readers of this book receive a 20 percent discount when ordering online (use the code NMC2014 during checkout).

SPECIAL PUMPING FLANGES

Pumpin' Pal

877-466-8283
www.pumpinpal.com

The angled, elliptical Pumpin' Pal Super Shields can be inserted into various other pump flanges for more comfortable pumping. Used along with the hands-free strap, the flanges allow a mother to sit back while pumping. The shields can also be used in place of the removable flanges of some pumps, like Medela and Lansinoh pumps. The shields come in three sizes, determined by the mother's cup and nipple sizes. One pair costs $15; the set of all three sizes costs

$30, and the strap for hands-free pumping costs $15. Visit the website or call to place an order, speak with a helpful salesperson, or find a local retailer.

ELECTRIC BREAST PUMP RENTAL

Medela, Inc.
1101 Corporate Drive, McHenry, IL 60050
800-435-8316
800-TELL-YOU
www.medela.com
Medela's Breastfeeding National Network can refer you to a local station where you can rent the full-sized Symphony pump or the more portable Lactina.

Ameda, Inc.
485 Half Day Road, Suite 320, Buffalo Grove, IL 60089
866-992-6332
www.ameda.com
Call or check the website to locate an Ameda station, where you can rent the full-sized Platinum pump, the lightweight Lact-E pump, or the more portable Elite pump.

Hygeia Medical Group II
1375 S. Acacia Avenue, Fullerton, CA 92831
888-786-7466
www.hygeiainc.com
Call to find a local station for Hygeia rental pumps.

BREAST SHELLS

Breast shells are used to correct inverted nipples during pregnancy or to protect injured nipples from friction against clothing. Many women find the flexible SoftShells for Inverted Nipples ($16 per pair) effective and comfortable in treating inverted nipples. The SoftShells for Sore Nipples ($19 per pair) and the TheraShells ($19 per pair) are vented to keep nipples protected. Order from online retailers or by telephone from Medela.

Medela, Inc. (for contact information see above)

SILICONE NURSING PADS

An alternative to conventional cloth or disposable pads, LilyPadz ($23 per pair) don't absorb milk but instead apply a gentle pressure on the nipple to keep milk from leaking. The pads adhere gently to the skin, so they can be worn without a bra. Call or visit the website to order a pair or to locate a retailer near you.

Simply Lily
P.O. Box 5801, Cary, NC 27512
800-640-5459
www.lilypadz.com

NURSING SUPPLEMENTATION DEVICES

A nursing supplementation device provides supplementary milk or formula while a baby is breastfeeding. Such a device is most commonly used when a baby is adopted or a mother wishes to resume lactating after a period of not nursing. A supplementer may also help when a mother wishes to both build up and supplement a low milk supply, or when a baby has a weak or ineffective suck.

A supplementer consists of a pouch to hold breast milk or formula and a thin, flexible tube that is placed on the breast, ending at the nipple. The baby must latch on to the nipple and the soft tube at the same time. As the baby sucks, he receives the supplement along with whatever milk his mother is producing. These devices should be used with the guidance of a lactation professional experienced with them, who may also sell nursing supplementers. Medela and Lact-Aid will be happy to refer you to any local source or sell them directly.

Medela, Inc. (for contact information see page 361)

Medela's Supplemental Nursing System is available from the manufacturer and various stores, clinics, and online sources for $67 plus shipping.

Lact-Aid International

P.O. Box 1066, Athens, TN 37371
423-744-9090
www.lact-aid.com

The Lact-Aid Nursing Trainer System is available from the manufacturer and from some lactation professionals for $49 for the standard kit and $63 for the deluxe kit.

MILK EXPRESSION CUP

This is a handy cup for catching milk during hand expression. At a cost of $15, the cup is available through Hygeia or where Hygeia pumps are sold. Check the website to order or call to find a local retailer.

Hygeia Medical Group 11

1375 S. Acacia Avenue, Fullerton, CA 92831
888-786-7466
www.hygeiainc.com

HERBAL REMEDIES FOR LOW MILK SUPPLY

Fenugreek

Fenugreek is available in capsule form in most health-food stores and some drugstores. A bottle of 100 capsules sells for $10 to $12. The typical lactation dose is three capsules three times daily (disregard the dosing recommendations on the label).

More Milk Plus and More Milk Special Blend Capsules and Liquid Extract

More Milk Plus capsules and extract contain fenugreek seed, blessed thistle, nettle leaf, and fennel seed and are designed to increase milk production quickly. More Milk Special Blend capsules and extract, which contain goat's rue as well as the herbs in More Milk Plus, are designed to stimulate the development of breast tissue and increase milk supplies in mothers who have had breast surgery, who have polycystic ovary syndrome (PCOS), who have insufficient glandular tissue, or who are adopting. Capsules let you avoid the licorice-like flavor but are more expensive; extract may be absorbed faster. In either formulation, capsules cost $24 for 60 or $42 for 120. The extracts cost $20 for 2 ounces, $34 for 4 ounces, and $50 for 8 ounces. The usual dose for capsules is one capsule four times daily. The dose for the extracts depends on the woman's weight. Motherlove products are available in some health-food stores, baby supply stores, and lactation practices. You can contact Motherlove to find a local distributor or order direct from Motherlove by phone or through the website.

Motherlove Herbal Company

3101 Kintzley Court, Suite S
P.O. Box 101, LaPorte, CO 80535
888-209-8321
www.motherlove.com

Go-Lacta

Go-Lacta is an herbal remedy containing the dried leaves of the Malunggay tree. One study showed that mothers who delivered premature infants and were using a pump to bring in full milk production produced 200 percent more milk than mothers who did not use it in the early days after giving birth. The powdered leaves are also high in vitamin A, vitamin C, calcium, potassium, iron, and protein. The typical dose is one to three capsules two to three times a day. One bottle of 60 capsules costs $20; if you order from Go-Lacta's website, you can get free shipping when buying two or more bottles.

Sugarpod Naturals

22115 NW Imbrie Drive, Suite 268, Hillsboro, OR 97124
503-468-4278
www.golacta.com

DOMPERIDONE

Usually sold for treating disorders of the gastrointestinal tract, this drug has also been found to stimulate milk production, more safely so than Reglan. Side effects in the mother (headache, abdominal cramps, dry mouth) are uncommon with domperidone, and very little of the medication reaches the baby. With a prescription, domperidone can be made in the United States at special compounding pharmacies, but you can get it without a prescription and for a much lower cost from InHouse Pharmacy in Vanuatu. InHouse carries three different brands of 10-milligram domperidone tablets, each with different package sizes and different prices. The least expensive is Vomistop, at about $65 for a minimum order of 500 tablets. Domperon is available for about $45 for a minimum order of 200 tablets, and Motilium is about $35 for a minimum order of 100 tablets. Shipping to the United States is free and takes 10 to 14 days.

InHouse Pharmacy

800-868-9064

Fax: 866-571-0332

www.inhousepharmacy.vu

NURSING PILLOWS

The wearable My Brest Friend Nursing Pillows, each with a cushioned back support, make positioning the baby easier and sitting to nurse more comfortable. The pillow for a single baby in a variety of prints costs about $42; the deluxe model offers a baby-plush soft fabric and costs about $51. The model for twins costs about $78. Call or check the website to order or to find a dealer near you.

Zenoff Products

25 Tamalpias Avenue, Suite C, San Anselmo, CA 94960

415-785-3890

www.mybrestfriend.com

NURSING STOOLS

Nursing stools help maintain a comfortable position for breastfeeding by lifting the lap and alleviating stress on the back, shoulders, and neck. These adjustable stools are available from the manufacturer and various stores, clinics, and online sources for $34.

Zenoff Products

25 Tamalpias Avenue, Suite C, San Anselmo, CA 94960

415-785-3890

www.mybrestfriend.com

NIPPLE CREAMS

Lansinoh HPA Lanolin

Lansinoh HPA Minis

Lansinoh's modified lanolin costs $10 for a 1.4-ounce tube. HPA "Minis" come in a three-pack of 0.25 ounce each for about $15. The cream is carried by many drugstores and discount stores; call or visit the website to find a local source.

Lansinoh Laboratories

333 N. Fairfax Street, Suite 400, Alexandria, VA 22314

800-292-4794

www.lansinoh.com

Motherlove Nipple Cream

Motherlove nipple cream contains organically grown healing herbs, marshmallow root, calendula, olive oil, shea butter, and beeswax. A 1-ounce jar costs $10. Visit Motherlove's website to order or locate a local distributor.

Motherlove Herbal Company
3101 Kintzley Court, Suite S
P.O. Box 101, LaPorte, CO 80535
888-209-8321
www.motherlove.com

Derma Sciences Medihoney Gel
Medical-grade Manuka honey is well known for its healing and antibacterial properties.
A ½-ounce tube can be ordered from Amazon or other online stores for about $12.

ELECTRONIC BABY SCALES

Highly accurate electronic scales are available from local rental stations and direct from
Medela for about $72 per month.

Medela, Inc. (for contact information see page 361)

SPECIALNEEDS® FEEDER

Formerly called the Haberman Feeder, this device is designed for babies with cleft palates or
other oral problems that make it difficult to maintain suction. A special valve and adjustable
silicone nipple make it easy for a baby to withdraw milk through this feeder, which is available
through Medela and online sources for about $33 for the 80-milliliter bottle.

Medela, Inc. (for contact information see page 361)

BREAST MILK STORAGE BAGS

Many mothers use bottle liners for milk storage, but these bags are sturdier. You can
pump your milk directly into them instead of using bottles. The bags zip closed—no
twists or ties are needed—and can stand upright for storage.

Hygeia Medical Group 11
1375 S. Acacia Avenue , Fullerton, CA 92831
888-786-7466
www.hygeiainc.com
Visit the website to find a Hygeia rental station, which will also carry Hygeia bags. Usable
only with Hygeia pumps, they hold up to 8 ounces of breast milk and cost $10 for a
package of 25 or $25 for a package of 100.

Medela, Inc. (for contact information see page 361)
Medela Pump *&* Save Bags can be used with most Medela pumps except Freestyle. The
bags are available through Medela and online stores for $9 for a package of 20 or $19 for
a package of 50.

PUMP-SANITIZING MICROWAVE BAGS

Medela Quick Clean Micro-Steam Bags allow you to disinfect pump parts in a microwave
in about 3 minutes. Each bag can be used as many as 20 times. The bags are available
from Medela and online stores for $6 for a package of five.

Medela, Inc. (for contact information see page 361)

PUMP WIPES

Medela Quick Clean Breastpump and Accessory Wipes allow for convenient portable cleaning, with no need for soap and water after each pump session. These hygienic wipes are proven safe for cleaning pumps and accessories as well as high chairs, tables, cribs, and countertops. A pack of 24 wipes costs $9 and a pack of 40 wipes costs $15.

Medela, Inc. (for contact information see page 361)

INFANT PROBIOTICS

A study of breastfed infants showed that giving a baby just five drops a day of probiotics decreased colic symptoms by the end of one month. These drops are now being sold by Gerber as Gerber Soothe Colic Drops. A 0.17-ounce bottle (enough for 25 days) costs $30 and can be purchased from Amazon and at some pharmacies.

WHITE-NOISE CDS

Ease colic and fussiness with Baby's First White Noise, a pure white noise CD made especially for baby's sensitive hearing. Designed especially for children from birth to 5 years of age, the soft white noise is formulated to help babies fall asleep. You can order the 74-minute CD for $14 or download the mp3 for $11 at the Pure White Noise website.

Pure White Noise

580 Lakeside Place, Windsor, CO 80550
www.purewhitenoise.com

ATTACHABLE BABY BED

The Arm's Reach Bedside Co-Sleeper is a baby bed that connects to an adult-size bed to allow a mother and her baby to sleep safely and comfortably next to each other. Various models are available, priced from $140 to $350. Each can be converted into a bassinet, a playpen, a changing table, or even a love seat. For beds higher than 24 inches, a leg extension kit is available separately. Visit the Arm's Reach website to find a local retailer.

Arm's Reach Concepts

2081 N. Oxnard Boulevard, PMB #187, Oxnard, CA 93030
800-954-9353
www.armsreach.com

THE HUMAN MILK BANKING ASSOCIATION OF NORTH AMERICA

This nonprofit milk banking association screens its donors and pasteurizes the donated milk for vulnerable newborns and infants whose mothers are unable to provide enough milk.

Women who wish to donate milk must be healthy nonsmokers who take no medications (with some exceptions). Most milk banks require a minimum number of ounces from each donor.

Donors freeze their milk before sending it to the milk bank. The milk banks send a large cooler and pay to have it shipped back to them at no cost to the mothers. There the milk is thawed, pooled with that of other donors, heat-treated to kill any bacteria or viruses, and refrozen (it retains its immunological properties through this processing).

The milk is dispensed only after a cultured sample shows no bacterial growth. Then it is shipped frozen by overnight express to hospitals and individual recipients.

Because of all the work that goes into processing it, donated milk is expensive, and its supply is limited. Parents who want to buy donated milk must have a physician's prescription. Common conditions for which physicians prescribe donated milk include prematurity, allergies, formula intolerance, immunological deficiencies, infectious diseases, and inborn errors of metabolism. Doctors may also prescribe donated milk for short periods to provide superior nutrition for a baby recovering from surgery or to get an adopted baby off to a good start.

As of this writing the Human Milk Banking Association of North America has certified fifteen milk banks in the United States and three in Canada, and many others are in the process of becoming certified. Visit www.hmbana.org to find out if a new milk bank is available in your area.

MILK BANKS IN THE UNITED STATES

CALIFORNIA
Mothers' Milk Bank of California
751 S. Bascom Avenue
San Jose, CA 95128
877-375-6645
www.mothersmilk.org

COLORADO
Mothers' Milk Bank of Colorado
1719 E. 19th Avenue
Denver, CO 80218
303-869-1888
www.milkbankcolorado.org

INDIANA
Indiana Mothers' Milk Bank
4755 Kingsway Drive, Suite 120
Indianapolis, IN 46205
877-829-7470
www.themilkbank.org

IOWA
Mother's Milk Bank of Iowa
University of Iowa Children's Hospital
119 2nd Street
Suite 400
Coralville, IA 52241
877-891-5347
www.uichildrens.org/mothers-milk-bank

MICHIGAN
Bronson Mothers' Milk Bank
601 John Street, Suite N1300
Kalamazoo, MI 49007
269-341-6146
*www.bronsonhealth.com/services/
pregnancy-and-childbirth-at-bronson/
mothers-milk-bank*

MISSOURI
Saint Luke's Heart of America Mothers'
Milk Bank
4401 Wornail Road
Kansas City, MO 64111
816-932-4888
*www.saintlukeshealthsystem.org/servic-
es/saint-luke's-heart-america-mothers'-
milk-bank*

MONTANA
Mothers' Milk Bank of Montana
734 Kensington Avenue
Missoula, MT 59801
406-531-6789
www.mothersmilkbankofmt.org

NEW ENGLAND
Mothers' Milk Bank Northeast
377 Elliot Street
Newton Upper Falls, MA 02464
617-527-6263
www.milkbankne.org

NORTH CAROLINA

WakeMed Mothers' Milk Bank and
Lactation Center
3000 New Bern Avenue
Raleigh, NC 27610
919-350-8599
www.wakemed.org

OHIO

OhioHealth Mothers' Milk Bank
4850 E. Main Street
Columbus, OH 43213
614-566-0630
www.ohiohealth.com/mothersmilkbank

OKLAHOMA

Oklahoma Mother's Milk Bank
901 N. Lincoln Boulevard, Suite 330
Oklahoma City, OK 73104
405-297-5683
www.okmilkbank.org

OREGON

Northwest Mothers Milk Bank
417 SW 117th Avenue, Suite 105
Portland, OR 97225
503-469-0955
www.nwmmb.org

TEXAS

Mothers' Milk Bank at Austin
2911 Medical Arts Street, Suite 12
Austin, TX 78705
877-813-6455
www.milkbank.org

Mothers' Milk Bank of North Texas
600 W. Magnolia Avenue
Fort Worth, TX 76104
866-810-0071
www.texasmilkbank.org

VIRGINIA

King's Daughters Milk Bank at CHKD
400 Gresham Drive, Suite 410
Norfolk, VA 23507
757-668-6455
*www.chkd.org/Our-Doctors/Our-
Pediatricians/Patient-Resources/King-s-
Daughters-Milk-Bank/*

MILK BANKS IN CANADA

ALBERTA

Calgary Mothers' Milk Bank
103-10333 Southport Road SW
Calgary, AB T2W 3X6
403-475-6455
www.calgarymothersmilkbank.ca

BRITISH COLUMBIA

British Columbia Women's
Milk Bank
C & W Lactation Services
1U 50-4450 Oak Street
Vancouver, BC V6H 3N1
604-875-2282
www.bcwomens.ca

ONTARIO

Rogers Hixon Ontario Human Milk Bank
Mount Sinai Hospital
600 University Avenue
Toronto, ON M5G 1X5
416-586-4800
www.milkbankontario.ca

APPENDIX B
Determining Babies' Milk Needs during the First Six Weeks
TEN-PERCENT WEIGHT LOSS

A newborn should lose less than 10 percent of her birth weight before she begins to gain weight. Find your baby's birth weight in the left column of the table. Look at the figure across from your baby's birth weight in the right column. If your baby weighs this amount or less, you'll want to compare her milk needs (see the following sections of this appendix) with your milk production, and take steps to increase her milk intake.

Birth Weight (in pounds-ounces)	10% Less	Birth Weight (in pounds-ounces)	10% Less	Birth Weight (in pounds-ounces)	10% Less
4-8	4-2	7-0	6-5	9-8	8-9
4-9	4-2.5	7-1	6-6	9-9	8-10
4-10	4-3	7-2	6-7	9-10	8-10.5
4-11	4-3.5	7-3	6-7.5	9-11	8-11.5
4-12	4-4	7-4	6-8	9-12	8-12
4-13	4-5	7-5	6-9	9-13	8-13
4-14	4-6	7-6	6-10	9-14	8-14
4-15	4-7	7-7	6-11	9-15	8-15
5-0	4-8	7-8	6-12	10-0	9-0
5-1	4-9	7-9	6-13	10-1	9-1
5-2	4-10	7-10	6-14	10-2	9-2
5-3	4-11	7-11	6-15	10-3	9-3
5-4	4-12	7-12	7-0	10-4	9-4
5-5	4-12.5	7-13	7-0.5	10-5	9-4.5
5-6	4-13	7-14	7-1	10-6	9-5
5-7	4-14	7-15	7-2	10-7	9-6
5-8	4-15	8-0	7-3	10-8	9-7
5-9	5-0	8-1	7-4	10-9	9-8
5-10	5-1	8-2	7-5	10-10	9-9
5-11	5-2	8-3	7-6	10-11	9-10
5-12	5-3	8-4	7-7	10-12	9-11
5-13	5-4	8-5	7-8	10-13	9-12
5-14	5-5	8-6	7-9	10-14	9-13
5-15	5-5.5	8-7	7-9.5	10-15	9-13.5
6-0	5-6	8-8	7-10	11-0	9-14.5
6-1	5-7	8-9	7-11	11-1	9-15
6-2	5-8	8-10	7-12	11-2	10-0
6-3	5-9	8-11	7-13	11-3	10-1
6-4	5-10	8-12	7-14	11-4	10-2
6-5	5-11	8-13	7-15	11-5	10-3
6-6	5-12	8-14	8-0	11-6	10-4
6-7	5-13	8-15	8-1	11-7	10-5
6-8	5-14	9-0	8-2	11-8	10-5.5
6-9	5-14.5	9-1	8-2.5	11-9	10-6.5
6-10	5-15	9-2	8-3	11-10	10-7.5
6-11	6-0	9-3	8-4	11-11	10-8
6-12	6-1	9-4	8-5	11-12	10-9
6-13	6-2	9-5	8-6	11-13	10-10
6-14	6-3	9-6	8-7	11-14	10-11
6-15	6-4	9-7	8-8	11-15	10-12

BABIES' MILK NEEDS DURING THE FIRST FIVE DAYS

Find your baby's age in the left column. At right is the amount of milk he needs at each of eight daily feedings.

Baby's Age, in Hours	Milk Needed per Feeding	
	in Milliliters	in Ounces
24–48	15	½
48–72	20	⅔
72–96	30	1
96–120	45	1½

BABIES' MILK NEEDS FROM FIVE DAYS TO SIX WEEKS OF AGE

Follow these steps to determine how much milk your baby needs.

Step 1. Weigh the baby naked, on an accurate scale, at least one hour after a feeding. Find the baby's weight in kilograms in the chart below. If the baby weighs 7 pounds, 5 ounces, for example, look down the column headed "7" and across the row headed "5." The baby's weight in kilograms is 3.317.

					Pounds						
Ounces	4	5	6	7	8	9	10	11	12	13	14
0	1.814	2.268	2.722	3.175	3.629	4.082	4.536	4.990	5.443	5.897	6.350
1	1.843	2.296	2.750	3.203	3.657	4.111	4.564	5.018	5.471	5.925	6.379
2	1.871	2.325	2.778	3.232	3.685	4.139	4.593	5.046	5.500	5.953	6.407
3	1.899	2.353	2.807	3.260	3.714	4.167	4.621	5.075	5.528	5.982	6.435
4	1.928	2.381	2.835	3.289	3.742	4.196	4.649	5.103	5.557	6.010	6.464
5	1.956	2.410	2.863	3.317	3.770	4.224	4.678	5.131	5.585	6.038	6.492
6	1.984	2.438	2.892	3.345	3.799	4.252	4.706	5.160	5.613	6.067	6.520
7	2.013	2.466	2.920	3.374	3.827	4.281	4.734	5.188	5.642	6.095	6.549
8	2.041	2.495	2.948	3.402	3.856	4.309	4.763	5.216	5.670	6.123	6.577
9	2.070	2.523	2.977	3.430	3.884	4.337	4.791	5.245	5.698	6.152	6.605
10	2.098	2.551	3.005	3.459	3.912	4.366	4.819	5.273	5.727	6.180	6.634
11	2.126	2.580	3.033	3.487	3.941	4.394	4.848	5.301	5.755	6.209	6.662
12	2.155	2.608	3.062	3.515	3.969	4.423	4.876	5.330	5.783	6.237	6.690
13	2.183	2.637	3.090	3.544	3.997	4.451	4.904	5.358	5.812	6.265	6.719
14	2.211	2.665	3.118	3.572	4.026	4.479	4.933	5.386	5.840	6.294	6.747
15	2.240	2.693	3.147	3.600	4.054	4.508	4.961	5.415	5.868	6.322	6.776

Step 2. To determine the approximate amount of milk a baby needs in a 24-hour period, multiply the baby's weight in kilograms by 6, and round the result to the nearest whole number.

Example: 3.317 kilograms × 6 = 19.902 ounces

If the baby weighs 3.317 kilograms, she needs approximately 20 ounces of milk per day.

Step 3. Calculate how much milk the baby needs at each feeding. Divide the amount of milk the baby needs daily by the number of times she nurses in each 24-hour period.

Example: 20 ounces ÷ 8 = 2½ ounces

If the baby needs 20 ounces of milk per day and nurses eight times per day, she needs 2½ ounces of milk at each feeding.

If the baby is taking eight feedings per day, however, you can skip step 2, and instead multiply the baby's current weight in kilograms by 22.5. The result will be the amount of milk the baby needs at each feeding in milliliters.

Example: 3.317 kilograms x 22.5 = 74.6325 milliliters

A baby weighing 3.317 kilograms needs approximately 75 milliliters of milk per feeding. To find this amount in ounces, divide by 30.

Example: 75 milliliters ÷ 30 = 2½ ounces

The baby in our example needs 2½ ounces of milk at each of eight daily feedings.

If the baby is taking nine feedings every 24 hours, you can find how much milk she needs at each feeding by multiplying her weight in kilograms by 20.

Example: 3.317 kilograms x 20 = 66.34 milliliters

The baby weighing 3.317 kilograms and nursing nine times per day needs about 66 milliliters of milk at each feeding.

Example: 66 milliliters ÷ 30 = 2⅕ ounces

Since 30 milliliters equals 1 ounce, the baby needs 2⅕ ounces of milk nine times per day.

APPENDIX C
The World Health Organization Growth Standards

The World Health Organization (WHO) Growth Reference Study was undertaken between 1997 and 2003 to generate new growth curves for assessing the growth and development of infants and young children around the world. Growth data was collected from about 8,500 children from widely different ethnic backgrounds and geographical settings (Brazil, Ghana, India, Norway, Oman, and the United States). The new growth charts provide a single international standard that best represents the normal physiological growth of children from birth to five years of age and establishes the breastfed infant as the model for normal growth. The charts differ from those used by most U.S. health-care providers, which are based mostly on the growth of formula-fed children. In the near future, I hope, the WHO charts will replace the ones currently in use in doctors' offices.

The original WHO weight charts are in kilograms only, but the versions on pages 372 and 373 also show a baby's weight in pounds.

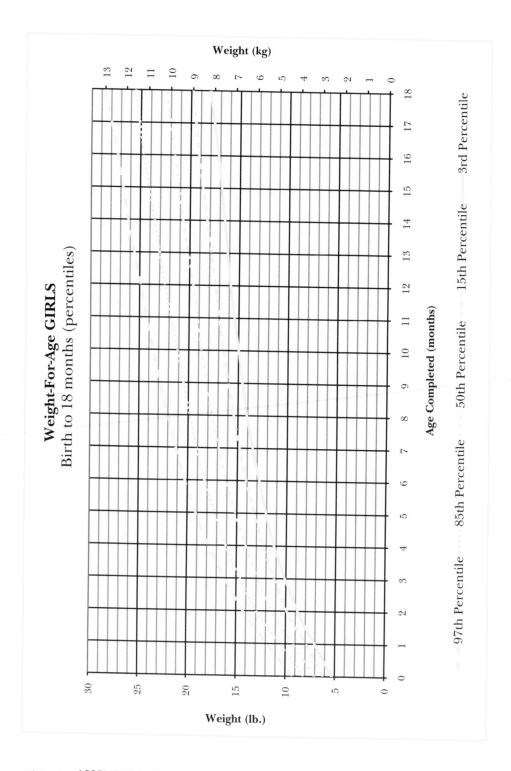

Weight-For-Age GIRLS
Birth to 18 months (percentiles)

Weight (kg)

Weight (lb.)

Age Completed (months)

97th Percentile ···· 85th Percentile ─ ─ 50th Percentile ···· 15th Percentile ─ ─ 3rd Percentile

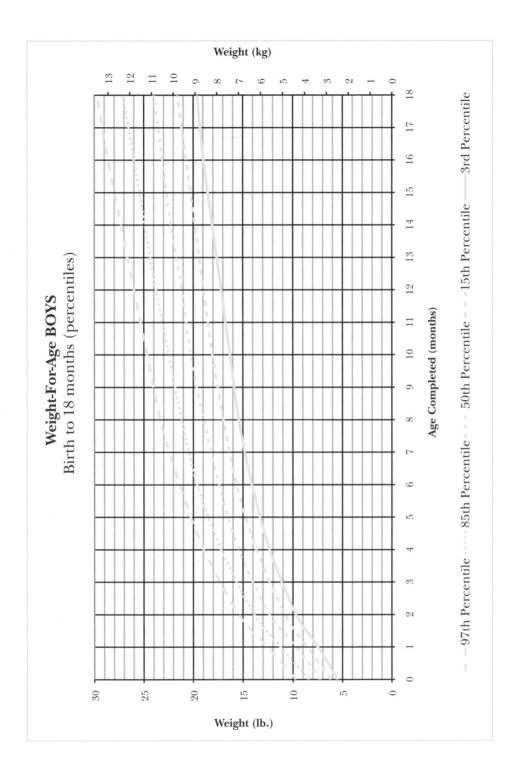

Weight-For-Age BOYS
Birth to 18 months (percentiles)

Weight (kg)

Weight (lb.)

Age Completed (months)

- - 97th Percentile · · · · · 85th Percentile - · - 50th Percentile - - - 15th Percentile —— 3rd Percentile

APPENDIX D
The Safety of Drugs during Breastfeeding

By Philip O. Anderson, Pharm.D., F.A.S.H.P., F.C.S.H.P.

If you are considering taking a drug while nursing, you are likely wondering what effects it may have on your baby and on milk production. Clear guidelines are sometimes hard to come by in this situation. This appendix will explain what you should consider before taking a particular drug, and how, if you take it, you can minimize its effects on your child.

Each brand name that is listed is capitalized; the corresponding generic name is given after it. All generic names that do not appear as headings in the text are followed here by cross-references to the relevant sections. The names of combination products are followed by lists of the ingredients they contain; see the separate entry for each ingredient. Not all brands are listed, so if you can't find the name of a particular product in this list, look under the generic name of its ingredient or ingredients.

THE PASSAGE OF DRUGS INTO MILK

Almost any drug you take will reach your milk in some quantity. Although you would never want to expose your baby to a foreign chemical unnecessarily, the amount of a drug that appears in milk is usually not great enough to harm a nursing child. One group of researchers found that 87 percent of drugs are transmitted in amounts of 10 percent or less of the mother's dose. About half of these are in amounts less than 1 percent of the mother's dose. Only about 3 percent of drugs reach the infant in amounts similar to the mother's dose. If you were taking a medication during pregnancy, the amount your infant is exposed to in breast milk is considerably less than during pregnancy.

Several considerations are important when deciding whether to take a particular drug:

Your baby's age and maturity. Just as your baby becomes better able to move about as he grows older, his ability to detoxify and eliminate foreign chemicals and drugs improves with time. Premature infants have little ability to metabolize drugs; when a preemie needs treatment for a medical condition, drugs are given in much smaller doses than they would be for a full-term newborn or an older infant. The amount of medication in a mother's milk that is safe for a one-month-old might be risky for a premature infant. Likewise, a baby who is several months old has a much greater capability of handling drugs in breast milk than does a one-month-old. And when an infant begins to eat solid food, he consumes less breast milk and, therefore, less of any drug it may contain. Most unwanted drug effects in breastfed infants occur in infants younger than two months old.

The persistence of the drug in the body. Some drugs are eliminated from the body after only a few hours, whereas others remain for a long time and accumulate. Accumulation potential is measured by the "half-life" of the drug; it takes four to five half-lives for a drug to be eliminated from the body. Drugs with long half-lives are more likely to persist in milk than are those with short half-lives.

Drugs with long half-lives are also more likely to accumulate in the baby and affect her. A drug might have a longer half-life in a newborn than in a two-month-old for reasons discussed above.

Your needs. Maybe you have a serious medical condition that threatens your health and your ability to care for your child, and you must take medication for it. Or maybe you're suffering from only a minor discomfort, and can get by without a medication. Whatever your condition, you must evaluate its seriousness and the consequences of not taking a particular drug. Then weigh these consequences against the benefits of breastfeeding, as you see them. You may decide to pump your milk and discard it while you're taking the medication or, if necessary, give up nursing altogether rather than expose your baby to a potentially hazardous drug. Only infrequently does a mother's medication make it necessary for the mother to completely stop nursing, though. Researchers in Canada found that many mothers who were prescribed an antibiotic for an infection failed to take the medication for fear of harming their nursing infants, even after being told that the drug was safe to use during nursing. Such action could easily cause a resurgence of the infection and the need for a more potent antibiotic.

The duration of treatment. If you have a chronic health problem, such as high blood pressure, you may be taking a drug over a long period. But perhaps you need medication for only a few days, as is usual with many antibiotics, or even just once, as with an anesthetic for a dental procedure or a diagnostic agent for an X-ray. If only brief drug therapy is needed, you can usually avoid exposing your infant to harmful amounts of the drug with minimal disruption to your normal pattern of breastfeeding.

The history of the drug. If a drug has been used for many years—especially if it has been given frequently to infants or to nursing mothers—the risks it poses to the breastfed baby are quite predictable. This is not so, however, for drugs that are new on the market, for most herbal remedies, and for drugs that have never been used in children or infants. With no safety record to go on, health-care providers may vary in their assessments of the risks your baby faces from small amounts of the drug in your milk. Drugs given to you as samples by your physician are usually very new and are unlikely to have information about use during breastfeeding. Ask your physician if he can prescribe an older medication that will be just as effective as the free sample of the new drug—the peace of mind is usually worth the cost of paying for the prescription.

You may also get different advice from different physicians—your obstetrician and the baby's pediatrician, for example. Unnecessary alarm and confusion are often caused by statements concerning nursing made by a drug's manufacturer in the *Physicians' Desk Reference* (*PDR*) or package insert. These statements generally are not written to help the nursing mother; instead, they often reflect the manufacturer's desire for protection from legal liability. Unfortunately, many health-care providers use the *PDR* as their primary source of information on the use of drugs during lactation. Many mothers stop nursing after receiving such confusing or inaccurate advice. It is important to consult a health professional with specific expertise in advising nursing mothers about medication use if you have questions about your drug.

Coordinating feedings and dosage. If a drug is quickly eliminated because of a short half-life, you may be able to time the doses in a way that will minimize the amount of drug in your milk at feedings. You might take a dose just after nursing, so the amount of drug in the milk peaks between feedings. If you are on a once-a-day medication, you might take it after the last feeding of the evening. By morning the amount of drug in your milk may be down to an acceptably low level. These strategies work best with older infants who are nursing at infrequent intervals.

Part of the reason you can limit your baby's drug exposure this way is that drugs pass in both directions between your bloodstream and breast milk. As the drug levels in your bloodstream decrease, the drug in your milk will pass back into your bloodstream. When breastfeeding must be withheld because of drug therapy that may harm an infant, expressing and discarding milk ("pumping and dumping") is sometimes advocated in the mistaken belief that the drug will thereby be eliminated from the milk sooner. Because of the reverse passage of drugs from milk to the bloodstream and because only a very small fraction of the drug in your body is in your milk, pumping and dumping has very little effect on the eventual amount of drug your baby gets from your milk. Pumping the breasts can be useful, though, in maintaining your milk supply and decreasing any pain from engorgement when you've temporarily stopped breastfeeding.

Route of Administration. The way that you take a medication partially determines how much of the drug will get into your bloodstream and to your baby. Drugs you're given by injection go directly into your bloodstream and can reach the milk, but some injected drugs cannot be absorbed into the infant's bloodstream from her gastrointestinal tract. Medications you take by mouth usually appear in your bloodstream, except for some that are meant to work locally in the stomach or intestines. Drugs can be absorbed from drops and ointments placed in the eye. Vaginal and rectal products can also be absorbed into the bloodstream. Drugs taken by inhaler generally reach the bloodstream in much smaller amounts than the same drug taken orally.

Since creams and ointments applied to the skin usually do not allow very much drug to enter into your bloodstream, they are generally safe to use while nursing. Be careful, though, not to get a medicated cream on your baby's skin or allow him to get any into his mouth. If you are applying medication to your nipples, wipe them before nursing and reapply the medication after nursing. It is better to use water-washable creams on the breast than greasy petrolatum (Vaseline)-based ointments, because the baby can ingest and absorb some of the petroleum-based oils found in petrolatum.

THE EFFECTS OF DRUGS ON LACTATION

Not only may the drugs you take affect your baby directly, but some may influence your milk production. This can happen in a number of ways, since several hormones work together to control lactation. Some drugs are used deliberately to stimulate or stop milk flow; however, a few medications intended for another purpose can affect lactation. Those that can are identified in this appendix.

SIDE EFFECTS IN THE BABY

Only infrequently must nursing be discontinued completely because of potential drug toxicity. Concern usually arises when the baby is a newborn or preemie or when the mother must take one of the most toxic drugs or a combination of potentially toxic drugs. But even drugs that are usually safe for nursing babies can occasionally cause mild but unpredictable allergic reactions, such as skin rashes. Minor side effects such as fussiness, drowsiness, and diarrhea occur sometimes but usually do not require medical attention. More serious side effects are rare.

COMMON DRUGS AND THEIR SAFETY

If side effects or possible allergies become a problem for your baby while you're taking a drug, do not hesitate to seek help.

In the following list, common drugs are grouped into categories and subcategories according to their uses. Noted are their potential effects on the breastfeeding infant and, where applicable, on lactation itself. Drug names that begin with a lowercase letter are generic names; those that begin with a capital letter are brand names. A more complete listing of brand names is in the "Index to Common Drugs" at the end of this appendix. If you can't find the drug you're looking for here or need more detailed information, you might find it on the U.S. National Library of Medicine's Drugs and Lactation (LactMed) website, at www.toxnet.nlm.nih.gov/cgi-bin/sis/htmlgen?LACTMED. This website has been recommended by the American Academy of Pediatrics as a source of information on medication use during breastfeeding. Although the information on this site is mostly aimed at health professionals, the summaries are easy to understand. You might print out the detailed information for a particular drug so you can discuss it with your health-care provider.

Acne products. Even though the manufacturer cautions against it, *tretinoin* is safe to use during nursing if it is applied only to the face, because very little is absorbed into the bloodstream. Avoid touching the infant's skin with treated areas of your own skin, when you're nursing and when you're not. Other topical products, such as *benzoyl peroxide, clindamycin,* and *erythromycin,* are also safe. *Isotretinoin* taken by mouth or tretinoin by injection should not be used while nursing. Daily long-term use of *tetracycline* for acne is not desirable while nursing.

Anesthetics

General anesthetics. Nitrous oxide is sometimes used for dental procedures and short outpatient procedures; it is rapidly eliminated from the milk. Injectable anesthetics such as *midazolam, propofol,* and *thiopental,* which are used for many short outpatient surgical procedures, have little or no effect on breastfed infants. Gaseous general anesthetics such as *desflurane, enflurane, isoflurane,* and *sevoflurane,* which are used in hospitals for major operations, have not been studied in nursing mothers and their babies. Generally, by the time a mother feels sufficiently recovered from anesthesia to breastfeed, it is safe to resume nursing.

Local anesthetics. These drugs are given by injection for dental or other short procedures. Although many people refer to all of these drugs as "Novocaine" (the trade name for *procaine*), this old drug is rarely used now. Information on the effects of local anesthetics during nursing is available for only three drugs, *ropivacaine, lidocaine,* and *bupivacaine,* all of which are safe to use while nursing. Ask your physician or dentist if one of these can be used. Although other local anesthetics are unlikely to affect a breastfed baby, breastfeeding may be withheld as a precaution for four hours after one of these other drugs is administered.

Antibacterials. Most drugs that are taken for infections reach the milk in only small quantities—quantities that would be too small to treat the same infections in your infant. Occasionally, though, these small drug amounts can disrupt the normal balance of microorganisms in a baby's mouth and intestines. This may result in diarrhea or diaper rash, caused by an overgrowth of yeast or other organisms in the bowel or, less often, thrush, an overgrowth of yeast in the mouth (see "Thrush Nipples" in "Survival Guide: The First Week," page 78, and "Fussiness, Colic, and Reflux" in "Survival Guide: The First Two Months," page 204). The likelihood of diarrhea or thrush occurring depends on the particular drug you are taking, especially if you need more than one course of therapy for a persistent infection. Although these conditions generally are not serious and can be readily treated, it is important to watch for their signs while you are taking an antibacterial drug.

Aminoglycosides. These drugs (***gentamicin, tobramycin, amikacin***) are given primarily in the hospital, by injection. Amounts that appear in milk are very small and pose no danger to the breastfed infant because they are not absorbed.

Antitubercular drugs. Combinations of medications such as ***isoniazid, rifampin,*** and ***pyrazinamide*** are used to treat tuberculosis. Isoniazid is also used alone, to prevent tuberculosis in those exposed to the disease. In general, treating the nursing mother with these drugs is safer than exposing the infant to untreated tuberculosis, although isoniazid and pyrazinamide pose a slight theoretical risk of damage to the baby's liver. Watch the infant for signs of jaundice (yellowing of the skin and eyes) and contact your physician if this occurs.

Cephalosporins. These are similar to penicillins, and the same precautions apply. Occasionally allergies develop to these drugs, so watch for signs of rash. Cephalosporins, especially the more potent ones given by injection, may also cause diarrhea and thrush. ***Cephalexin*** is a cephalosporin commonly prescribed to nursing mothers.

Clindamycin. Clindamycin is best avoided if possible, but a few days of therapy is probably safe, as long as the baby is closely monitored for diarrhea and bloody stools. Clindamycin presents less risk to the infant if it is given vaginally rather than orally or intravenously. *See also* "Acne Products."

Linezolid. Information is limited on this antibiotic for resistant ***Staph.*** infections, but it appears that the dose in milk is much less than the dose given directly to newborn infants.

Macrolides. ***Erythromycin*** is a generally safe drug that is often given directly to infants. The closely related drugs ***azithromycin*** and ***clarithromycin*** appear to be equally safe. *See also* "Acne Products."

Metronidazole and ***tinidazole.*** Breastfeeding should be stopped temporarily during use of these medications but can be resumed 24 hours after the last dose of metronidazole and three days after a dose of tinidazole. For postoperative (including C-section) infections, cephalosporin or clindamycin should be considered as an alternative.

Nitrofurantoin. This drug appears in small amounts in breast milk. These amounts are generally not harmful to infants over one month of age, but the drug should be avoided with younger babies, especially preemies.

Penicillins. These are very safe drugs that are often given directly to infants as treatment for infections. Occasionally allergies develop to penicillins, so the baby should be watched for rashes. If you see signs of rash, diarrhea, or thrush, call your healthcare provider.

Quinolones. *Ciprofloxacin, levofloxacin, moxifloxacin,* and several others have not been well studied in nursing infants because they are usually not given directly to infants or children, although recent experience indicates that they are probably not particularly harmful during nursing.

Sulfonamides (sulfas). *Septra* and *Bactrim* are common drugs that contain *trimethoprim* and the sulfonamide *sulfamethoxazole.* Large doses of sulfas given directly to newborn infants can increase the risk of jaundice (yellowing of the skin and eyes). Other medications are usually preferred if the baby is premature or less than two months of age.

Tetracyclines. These are generally not given to children or pregnant women because they can cause permanent staining of the infant's teeth. The amounts that appear in milk, however, are very small and are partially inactivated by the calcium in milk. In fact, tooth staining caused by a tetracycline in breast milk has never been reported. Tetracyclines can be used safely by the nursing mother for up to two weeks, but they should be used only if no other drug will work. One tetracycline, *minocycline,* can cause the milk to turn black. *See also* "Acne Products."

Vancomycin. Vancomycin and the related drug *daptomycin* are excreted into milk in only small amounts and are not absorbed into the baby's bloodstream. They are acceptable during nursing.

Anticoagulants. Some anticoagulants, such as *heparin, enoxaparin,* and *dalteparin,* are injected; others, such as *warfarin,* are taken orally. Injected anticoagulants can be safely used during lactation because they do not pass well into milk; nor does the infant absorb them from milk. *Warfarin* is likewise acceptable, because only small amounts are found in breast milk. Some newer oral anticoagulants such as dabigatran and rivaroxaban have not yet been studied in nursing mothers and should be avoided because they might be absorbed by the nursing infant.

Ticlopidine and *clopidogrel* act in a different way to decrease blood platelet function. Neither has been studied during nursing, and so both should be avoided.

Anticonvulsants. Anticonvulsants are used to treat epilepsy, mood disorders, and nerve pain. Because these medications are used continuously and are often long acting, they should be taken with caution during breastfeeding. Your baby may show no effects other than subtle behavioral changes, so be vigilant. Infants of mothers taking anticonvulsants tend to have more difficulty nursing and to wean earlier than other babies. You may need to have your infant's blood drawn to determine if the drug is affecting him. Infants of mothers taking other medications along with an anticonvulsant are more likely to have problems with drowsiness, feeding difficulties, and growth. Recent studies on some of these drugs indicate no harmful effects on the infant's development.

Carbamazepine. This drug is known to pass into milk in moderately large amounts. Although most breastfed infants of women taking the drug show no effects from it, three infants have had liver problems. Watch for jaundice (yellowing of the skin and eyes) while using carbamazepine. Also make sure that your infant is nursing and growing well. Breastfeeding with carbamazepine taken alone does not appear to adversely affect infant growth or development.

Clonazepam. Use of clonazepam during nursing can cause drowsiness and sluggishness in breastfed infants. Other drugs are preferred, if possible.

Felbamate. No information is available on use of this medication during breastfeeding. It should be avoided if possible.

Gabapentin. Only small amounts of gabapentin are found in breast milk. Monitor the infant for drowsiness, adequate weight gain, and developmental milestones.

Lamotrigine. Numerous infants have been safely breastfed during maternal therapy, but infants have measurable blood levels of the drug. It can cause very severe skin reactions, so use caution until more information is available; if your infant develops a rash, stop breastfeeding immediately and check with your health-care provider. Breastfeeding with lamotrigine taken alone does not appear to adversely affect infant growth or development.

Levetiracetam. Limited information is available on this drug, but only small amounts appear in milk.

Oxcarbazepine. A few infants have been breastfed while their mothers used oxcarbazepine. All of the infants have done well, but use caution until more information is available.

Phenobarbital. This drug has been given directly to infants for many years, usually with no severe adverse effects. You can probably use it safely during breastfeeding, although it may make the baby drowsy and less interested in nursing. The baby's behavior, weight gain, and blood levels should be monitored if there is concern. Women taking phenobarbital sometimes have to stop nursing because of its sedating effects on their infants.

Phenytoin. This drug has been used for many years by breastfeeding women. Very low amounts enter milk, and there have been no reports of drug-induced problems in breastfed infants.

Pregabalin. Limited information indicates that the amounts of this drug in milk are low.

Primidone. This drug is similar to phenobarbital; the same precautions apply.

Tiagabine. Information on tiagabine is very limited. Use this medication with caution, and observe your infant carefully for drowsiness and feeding difficulties, especially in the newborn period.

Topiramate. A few infants have been breastfed while their mothers used this drug, and no adverse effects have been reported. Most of the infants had no detectable topiramate in the bloodstream. One infant had diarrhea from topiramate in breast milk. Use caution until more information is available.

Valproic acid and *divalproex.* Both of these drugs are converted to valproate in the body. Only very small amounts of valproate enter milk, and many nursing mothers have used it safely. Rarely, the drug may cause liver damage or interference with blood platelets. The infant should be watched for unusual bruising and signs of jaundice (yellowing of the skin and eyes). Breastfeeding with valproate taken alone does not appear to adversely affect infant growth or development.

Vigabatrin. Limited information indicates that the amounts of this drug in milk are low.

Zonisamide. Information on the safety of this drug during breastfeeding comes from only a few mother-infant pairs. Rather large amounts are found in breast milk, and some breastfed infants have detectable zonisamide in their blood. No adverse effects have been reported, but use zonisamide with caution until more information is available, especially in newborns.

Antifungals

Clotrimazole (dissolved from a troche) and **miconazole** have been safely used in the mouths of infants with thrush, often successfully after **nystatin** has failed, and these antifungals are also safe to use for a mother's vaginal infections. Numerous related drugs, such as *butoconazole, econazole, oxiconazole,* and *terconazole,* are also available for vaginal use. Since little is known about their absorption into the bloodstream of a nursing infant, it is preferable to use clotrimazole or miconazole when a vaginal antifungal is needed.

Fluconazole. Fluconazole is a potent, low-risk antifungal that is taken orally. A single dose for vaginal infections is safe while nursing. Fluconazole can also be used simultaneously in the mother and infant to treat breast infections and thrush when other drugs have failed. At least two weeks of therapy is required in this situation.

Ketoconazole. You should not take ketoconazole orally or apply the cream to your nipples because it can be absorbed into the baby's bloodstream and may be toxic. Application of the cream elsewhere on your body is not harmful to the baby.

Polyenes. Since *amphotericin B* and *nystatin* aren't absorbed into the baby's bloodstream, you can safely use them in your infant's mouth or on your nipples to treat thrush. You can also safely take them orally.

Antinauseants. Most drugs used for nausea and vomiting are phenothiazine derivatives (see "Psychotherapeutic Agents"), such as *prochlorperazine* and *promethazine,* taken in low doses. Another commonly used drug is *trimethobenzamide.* These drugs may cause transient drowsiness or, rarely, abnormal movements in infants, but are safe to use for a short time. Newer antinauseants such as *dolasetron, ondansetron,* and *granisetron* are used for more severe nausea due to cancer chemotherapy or general anesthesia. Although these drugs have not been studied in breastfeeding women, they are not absorbed well into the baby's bloodstream if they do get into the mother's milk, so the risk they pose to the baby seems minimal.

Antiparasitics. Insecticides are used to treat scabies, a skin condition caused by mites, and pediculosis, or infestation with lice. An old medication, *lindane,* is a very fat-soluble insecticide that can persist in milk for a long time. Although no harm has been reported in breastfed infants due to lindane, it does persist in the infant's body, so this drug is best avoided. Safer alternatives include *pyrethrins (A-200,* for example) or *permethrin (Nix)* for lice, and a higher potency permethrin *(Elimite)* for scabies.

Mebendazole. Mebendazole is used for various worm (parasite) infestations. Since it is poorly absorbed from the intestinal tract, it is unlikely to cause adverse effects in breastfed infants. Contrary to one old report, it does not inhibit lactation.

Antivirals

Acyclovir. This antiviral drug, used to treat newborns, is well tolerated by the nursing infant.

Amantadine and **rimantadine.** These antiviral agents for influenza may decrease lactation and cause side effects in the breastfed baby. They should therefore be avoided while nursing.

Famciclovir. Famciclovir and its derivative, *penciclovir,* which is available as a topical cream, have not been studied in infants or during nursing. It is best to avoid famciclovir, but application of penciclovir away from the breast is acceptable.

Oseltamivir. This antiviral drug for influenza enters milk in very low levels and is acceptable to use during breastfeeding. The similar drug *zanamivir* has not been studied, but since it is inhaled and little drug reaches the mother's bloodstream, its use is also acceptable.

Valacyclovir. Valacyclovir breaks down in the mother's body to acyclovir, so it also is safe to use during nursing.

Arthritis, Pain, and Migraine Medications

Acetaminophen. This drug is often used in infants and is safe to use during breastfeeding.

Antirheumatic drugs. Several drugs are used for severe rheumatoid arthritis. *Hydroxychloroquine* has been fairly well studied and is acceptable during breastfeeding. Low weekly doses of *methotrexate* appear to be acceptable during breastfeeding as well, although some believe it should be avoided (*see also* "Immunosuppressants and Immunomodulators"). *Penicillamine* has been used safely in the mothers of three breastfed infants. Newer biotechnology drugs, such as *etanercept, infliximab,* and *adalimumab,* are excreted in only tiny amounts into breast milk and are probably not absorbed by the infant. Of these drugs, however, information on safety during breastfeeding is available only for infliximab and adalimumab. *Leflunomide* has not been studied in nursing infants and is currently considered incompatible with breastfeeding.

Aspirin. When large doses are taken daily, as for arthritis, problems can sometimes occur. Generally, it is best to avoid aspirin; ibuprofen is a better choice. If you take an occasional aspirin, do not breastfeed for at least one hour after the dose.

Ergotamine. This is a component of several products, such as *Cafergot,* used in the treatment of migraine headaches. Some ergot alkaloids cause vomiting in breastfed infants whose mothers have taken the drugs. Although ergotamine itself has not been studied, avoiding it while breastfeeding is a good idea.

Narcotics. Drowsiness due to narcotics in milk occurs more commonly in infants than formerly thought—about 20 percent of breastfed babies whose mothers have taken narcotics are affected. The degree of drowsiness varies with the dosage, and babies under one month old are particularly susceptible. Limiting the dosage to one tablet (such as 30 milligrams of *codeine,* 5 milligrams of *hydrocodone* or *oxycodone,* or 65 milligrams of *propoxyphene*) every four hours for four days is advisable; acetaminophen (Tylenol) or ibuprofen (Motrin, Advil) can be taken in addition. Larger amounts of narcotics have caused sedation and decreased breathing in some infants as well as interfered with nursing. Single injections of narcotics during nursing usually cause no problems, but intravenous narcotics given during labor can sometimes interfere with the establishment of lactation. *Meperidine* is the worst in this regard; *morphine* causes fewer problems and *fentanyl* the least. Epidural administration causes fewer nursing problems. Only a small amount of *tramadol* appears in milk, and infants are not adversely affected by this amount, so tramadol can be used during breastfeeding. *Methadone,* when used for maintenance in narcotic addicts during pregnancy, appears not to adversely affect breastfed infants. The methadone in breast milk minimizes the methadone-withdrawal symptoms of newborn infants. Beginning methadone after delivery while breastfeeding is not safe for the baby.

Nonsteroidal anti-inflammatory drugs (**NSAIDs**). *Ibuprofen, diclofenac,* and *flurbiprofen* appear in only minute amounts in milk; they seem safe to use while nursing an infant of any age. If your infant is over one month old, you can also use *fenoprofen, ketoprofen, ketorolac, naproxen, tolmetin, celecoxib, indomethacin,* and long-acting drugs such as *diflunisal, meloxicam, piroxicam,* and *sulindac.* The more toxic drug *mefenamic acid* should be avoided during breastfeeding. Until more information becomes available, ibuprofen is the best choice among the NSAIDs.

"*Triptans.*" Very little *sumatriptan* appears in milk, even when it is given by injection, and the small amount that reaches the infant is poorly absorbed. *Eletriptan* has also been found to pass poorly into breast milk. Similar drugs for migraine (*almotriptan, frovatriptan, naratriptan, rizatriptan, zolmitriptan*) have not been studied, so sumatriptan and eletriptan are preferred.

Bisphosphonates. These drugs are used to treat and prevent osteoporosis and to decrease bone loss during cancer chemotherapy. Drugs in this class include *alendronate, etidronate, pamidronate, risedronate, tiludronate,* and *zoledronic acid.* The only information available on these drugs concerns pamidronate, which was found to be excreted into breast milk in only very small amounts, but safety information in breastfeeding is not available.

CancerChemotherapy. Because the older drugs in this class are among the most toxic used in medicine, very few women have breastfed while taking them. Little is known about the passage of these drugs into milk, but even small amounts, should they reach the baby, could cause harm. Because these drugs are used for only very severe conditions, it is usually more important for the mother to take the drug than it is for her to nurse her baby. Generally, therefore, breastfeeding should be avoided, although occasionally short-acting chemotherapy drugs that are given intermittently may allow a woman to resume nursing after stopping temporarily. Also included in this group are some drugs used to treat severe arthritis and certain skin diseases, and others used after organ transplantation. Some of these latter drugs are less toxic than the drugs for cancer and might sometimes be acceptable to use in nursing mothers. Some of the newer targeted biotechnology drugs, such as monoclonal antibodies, might be safer during breastfeeding than the older drugs.

Cough, Cold, Allergy, and Asthma Medications. The various drugs used for these respiratory conditions are often taken together in combination products, which should generally be avoided during breastfeeding. Usually only one or two symptoms are really troublesome, and a single-ingredient product can treat them effectively. For example, hay fever and other allergies can be treated with an antihistamine alone, and a cough can be treated with a cough syrup that has only one or two active ingredients. Oral sustained-release products should be avoided. Common sore throat lozenges (such as *Sucrets, Chloraseptic,* and *Halls*) are safe to use. Drugs taken as nasal sprays or by inhaler reach the milk in lesser quantities than those taken orally and pose little risk of harm to the nursing infant.

Antihistamines. Antihistamines are used in many products for allergy, colds, coughs, and inducing sleep, although their use for colds is not justified. These drugs can reach the infant through breast milk in amounts large enough to cause drowsiness or fussiness. High doses of antihistamines, particularly when in combination with a decongestant, may decrease milk flow. Use no more than necessary to control symptoms; often a single dose at bedtime is sufficient. If you are planning to use an oral product, choose one with 2 milligrams or less of *chlorpheniramine* or *brompheniramine* per dose, 25 milligrams or less of *diphenhydramine* per dose, or 5 milligrams or less of *cetirizine* per dose, and avoid sustained-release products. *Loratadine, desloratadine,* and *fexofenadine* are well tolerated by infants and are preferable to the older, sedating antihistamines. *Cetirizine* and its derivative, *levocetirizine,* which can cause drowsiness and may affect lactation, are not good choices while nursing.

Most nonprescription medications for motion sickness, such as **dimenhydrinate** and **meclizine,** are also antihistamines. One or two doses of these medications should have no effect on the infant other than temporary drowsiness. They are preferred over **scopolamine** in the patch form, which is more likely to suppress lactation.

Asthma inhalers and **nasal inhalers.** These may contain a bronchodilator (such as *albuterol, salmeterol,* or *ipratropium*) or a corticosteroid (such as *beclomethasone, fluticasone, flunisolide,* or *triamcinolone*). All of these reach the mother's bloodstream in very low levels, and levels in milk are even lower. Try to avoid swallowing excess medication after using an inhaler, because swallowed medication may enter the blood from the intestinal tract and reach the milk. Rinse your mouth and throat, and spit out the excess medication.

Cough medicines. The two most common drugs are *guaiafenesin* and *dextromethorphan,* both of which are acceptable to use during breastfeeding.

Decongestants. Nasal sprays (*Afrin*) are preferable to oral drugs, especially if your baby is a newborn. A saltwater spray (such as *Ocean*) or rinse is safe to use during nursing. Oral decongestants can cause agitation or fussiness in an infant. Most important, they can decrease the milk supply and might eventually cause the milk to dry up. If you are planning to use an oral product, choose one with 30 milligrams or less of *pseudoephedrine* or *phenylephrine* per dose. Avoid sustained-release and combination products.

Theophylline. *Aminophylline* and other theophylline products have been well studied in breast milk. Occasionally they can cause jitteriness or fussiness in infants, usually newborns. In general, though, they are acceptable to use.

Diuretics. Large doses of diuretics, especially the most potent ones and those that are long acting, can decrease milk production. Their passage into milk has not been well studied, but the amounts that reach infants are likely to be small. These small amounts might in rare instances cause rashes or other allergic reactions.

Chlorthalidone. This very long-acting diuretic should not be used during breastfeeding because it suppresses lactation. It might also accumulate in the infant's body.

Furosemide. This potent drug has been used to suppress lactation. It should be used only with caution during breastfeeding, in small doses.

Hydrochlorothiazide. Given once daily in doses of 25 milligrams or less, this drug appears safe. Larger doses given several times daily have been used to suppress lactation.

Other thiazides. Long-acting thiazides should be avoided during breastfeeding.

Spironolactone. This drug appears in insignificant amounts in milk.

Ergot Alkaloids

Bromocriptine has been used after birth to suppress lactation, but it is no longer approved for this use because it can be severely toxic to mothers. In mothers with increased prolactin levels, an appropriate dose of bromocriptine might still allow breastfeeding.

Cabergoline. This potent, long-acting drug can stop lactation after a single dose. You shouldn't use it if you intend to nurse your baby.

Ergonovine and *methylergonovine.* These drugs are often given to mothers right after delivery to diminish uterine bleeding. Methylergonovine is preferred, because ergonovine can suppress lactation. With the usual doses and the normal length of treatment, these drugs cause no problems in the breastfed newborn. Large amounts, however, might cause nausea, vomiting, and diarrhea in the baby. These effects may occasionally occur when the drugs are used beyond the immediate postpartum period.

See also "Ergotamine," page 382.

Gastrointestinal Drugs. Many of the drugs in this class act in the stomach and intestine and are not absorbed into the bloodstream; they cannot, therefore, appear in milk. Other gastrointestinal drugs are absorbed and can affect the infant through breast milk. If a choice exists, choose a drug that is not absorbed.

Antacids. These drugs are poorly absorbed and are safe to use during breastfeeding.

Antidiarrheals. Loperamide and *diphenoxylate* have not been well studied, but one or two small daily doses should pose little risk to the nursing infant. *Bismuth subsalicylate* is best avoided because of the large amount of absorbable salicylate it contains. Salicylate in large amounts can be toxic to the baby.

Domperidone. This drug is used to stimulate intestinal movement. Like metoclopramide, it has been used to increase milk production. It appears to be less likely to cause serious side effects in the mother than metoclopramide. However, domperidone is not licensed for use in the United States, so drug acquisition and quality can be problematic.

Histamine H-2 antagonists. During breastfeeding, *famotidine* and *nizatidine* are the preferred drugs in this class, especially if the baby is young, because they reach the mother's milk in the lowest amounts. *Ranitidine* is less desirable in this respect, but probably safe, and *cimetidine* is the least desirable of this group and should be avoided. If your baby is older and is no longer nursing at night, you can take a single daily dose of any of these drugs at bedtime just after the baby's last feeding.

Laxatives. Many of the more potent laxatives are absorbed into the bloodstream and have caused increased frequency of stools in breastfed infants. *Cascara* and *senna* can affect the breastfed infant if taken in high doses, but they are safe to use occasionally in small amounts.

Bulk-forming laxatives such as bran and other fibers such as *psyllium* (*Metamucil*) and *calcium polycarbophil* (*FiberCon*) are not absorbed into the bloodstream and are therefore safe to use. Likewise, stool-softening agents such as *docusate* are not absorbable. *Bisacodyl* is a stronger laxative that is also not absorbed into the bloodstream. Saline cathartics such as *Phospho-Soda* and *milk of magnesia* are poorly absorbed and do not affect the composition of milk. *Glycerin* suppositories are also safe to use.

Mesalamine derivatives. Diarrhea and bloody stools have occurred on rare occasions in infants of mothers using *mesalamine, olsalazine,* or *sulfasalazine.* These drugs may be used during nursing, but the baby should be observed for side effects.

Metoclopramide. This medication is used mainly to stimulate intestinal movement. It has also been used to increase the milk supply in women who are producing insufficient quantities of milk, such as mothers of premature or sick infants, and in adoptive mothers. Metoclopramide does not appear to harm the infant if it is used for two weeks or less. Because this drug may cause or worsen depression, it should not be used by women with a history of depression, and it should not be used for long periods of time or repeatedly because of the risk of causing depression or movement disorders.

Proton pump inhibitors. *Omeprazole* and *pantoprazole* are the only drugs of this type that have been studied during nursing, and information is limited. But levels in milk appear to be very low, and no harm has occurred in breastfed infants. Omeprazole is also used in infants. *Esomeprazole* is a form of omeprazole and should be similarly safe. Other drugs in this class (*lansoprazole* and *rabeprazole*) have not been studied during breastfeeding, so for now omeprazole is preferred.

Sucralfate. This drug acts locally in the mother's intestinal tract and poses no harm to the breastfed infant.

Heart and Blood-Pressure Drugs. These drugs are not often used in women of breastfeeding age, and information about them is therefore limited. Very little is known, in particular, about newer agents.

ACE inhibitors. *Benazepril, captopril, enalapril,* and *quinapril* are safe to use while nursing. No other drugs in this class have been studied during breastfeeding.

Amiodarone. This drug has caused low thyroid levels and delayed growth in a breastfed infant. However, a few other infants have been breastfed without harm. Using this medication while nursing requires close monitoring of the infant, including tests of thyroid function.

Angiotensin-II blockers. There is no information on the use of drugs in this class (such as *losartan, irbesartan,* and *valsartan*) during nursing or in infants. It is best to avoid them until more is known.

Beta blockers. The oldest drug in the group, *propranolol,* is also the best studied and safest. *Metoprolol* and *labetalol* are safe to use, too, because these drugs reach the milk in insignificant amounts. The long-acting beta blockers, such as *acebutolol, atenolol, nadolol, sotalol,* and *timolol,* reach the milk in higher quantities and are also more likely to accumulate in the infant's bloodstream. These should be avoided while breastfeeding a newborn.

Calcium channel blockers. Information on *diltiazem, nitrendipine,* and *verapamil* is limited, but amounts in milk do not appear to be large enough to affect nursing infants. *Nifedipine* has been well studied and is safe to use; it is sometimes used to treat painful nipple vasospasm (Raynaud's syndrome) that occurs occasionally during nursing.

Clonidine. Clonidine and the related drug *guanfacine* may either increase or decrease milk production. Clonidine reaches the milk in high levels, and breastfed infants have blood concentrations of the drug approaching those of their mothers. Other blood-pressure drugs are preferable, but if these drugs can't be avoided, they should be used with caution during breastfeeding.

Digoxin. This drug is excreted into milk in only small amounts. It can be used safely during lactation.

Hydralazine. Amounts of this drug excreted into milk are small. Hydralazine can be used safely during lactation.

Methyldopa. Amounts of this drug excreted into milk are small, and methyldopa has been used safely during nursing for many years.

Procainamide. Amounts that reach the milk are small. This drug appears safe to use while nursing.

Reserpine. Because this drug can cause nasal stuffiness in infants, it should be avoided during lactation.

Herbals and Nutraceuticals. There is a mistaken tendency to think that because herbal drugs are "natural" they are never toxic. This is not true. Each herbal product must be evaluated individually on its own merits and risks. Unfortunately, almost none of these products have been studied during lactation, and very few have been studied in infants. Because these drugs are poorly regulated in the United States, the quality and amounts of ingredients and even the ingredients themselves can vary widely from batch to batch and from one manufacturer to another. Additionally, because plant products may contain dozens of chemicals that can cause allergies, they may be more likely than conventional medications to cause problems like asthma and skin rashes in your infant or lead to plant allergies later in his life. For all these reasons, it is somewhat of a gamble to use herbal products during nursing. Information on some of the most commonly used herbals and nutraceuticals is listed below.

Blessed thistle. This herb is sometimes used to stimulate lactation, but there are no scientific studies that confirm its effectiveness. In fact, there have been no studies at all of the herb's effects during lactation. Blessed thistle appears to be fairly safe, but allergies have been reported.

Chamomile. Various preparations have been used to treat mastitis and cracked, bleeding nipples and to increase lactation. No scientific data support these uses, but chamomile is generally safe during breastfeeding. Allergic skin reactions occur occasionally.

Chasteberry. Some weak evidence shows that chasteberry might be useful for breast pain (mastalgia). It is well tolerated, but it might inhibit lactation.

Echinacea. There have been no studies of this herb during lactation. Although it is often used to prevent colds, scientific studies have shown it to be of little benefit. Some of its chemical components have been found in breast milk.

Elderberry. Elderberry is most often used for influenza and immune stimulation. There is no information on the appearance of elderberry in breast milk or on the safety of elderberry in nursing mothers or infants.

Evening primrose oil. This oil contains various fatty acids and vitamin E. Some weak evidence shows that it might be useful for cyclic breast pain (mastalgia). It is well tolerated and safe to take while breastfeeding.

Fennel. Fennel is included in some proprietary mixtures that are promoted to increase the milk supply. Only a minimal amount of data supports its effectiveness.

Fenugreek. Most commonly used as a spice, fenugreek seeds are often used to stimulate lactation and increase milk supply. Although there have been no high-quality scientific studies to substantiate this use, fenugreek is considered a safe food substance in small amounts; it is used as a flavoring in artificial maple syrup. It can lower blood sugar, so diabetic women should not use it without consulting a physician. Allergic reactions have also been reported.

Fish oil. Fish oil, which is a source of omega-3-fatty acids such as DHA and EPA, appears to have some benefit in mothers with severe postpartum depression. Although not harmful to breastfed infants, evidence for beneficial effects in the infants is weak.

Ginkgo biloba. There have been no studies on the use of ginkgo during lactation. Side effects are generally mild, but allergic skin reactions have occurred, and these could occur in the nursing infant as well as in the mother. People who take ginkgo sometimes experience headaches and gastrointestinal problems.

Ma huang. Also called *ephedra,* this common herbal ingredient in diet products contains an amphetamine-like stimulant that can suppress lactation and may affect a nursing infant. These diet products, many of which contain other stimulants as well, should definitely be avoided during lactation. *See also* "Weight-Loss Products."

Moringa. The leaves of this tree, called Malunggay in the Philippines, have been used to increase milk supply. Two small but flawed studies indicate that it might have some activity as a galactogogue in mothers of preterm infants.

Peppermint. This plant contains menthol and supposedly increases milk supply, but no scientifically valid information supports this use.

Raspberry. The leaf supposedly increases milk supply; however, no scientifically valid clinical trials support this use.

Sage. Sage has been used to decrease lactation and to aid with weaning or an overabundant milk supply; however, no scientific studies substantiate this use or the safety of sage in nursing mothers or infants.

Saint John's wort. Colic, drowsiness, and lethargy have occurred in breastfed infants whose mothers were taking St. John's wort, and compounds from the plant are found in the bloodstream of breastfed infants. In fair-skinned persons, the drug may cause allergic skin reactions with light exposure. The drug is not very effective for depression, and the wisdom of self-medication for a serious condition such as depression is doubtful anyway. St. John's wort should be avoided during lactation.

Valerian. Valerian is most commonly used to treat anxiety and sleep disturbances, and occasionally for self-treatment of postpartum blues or depression. No data exist on the safety and efficacy of valerian in nursing mothers or infants, but some of its components are potentially toxic. It is probably best avoided during nursing.

Hormones. Several classes of drugs fall into the category of hormones, and each class must be considered separately. Because hormones are potent agents that might affect a baby's development, it is of paramount importance to consider both the dosage and the duration of therapy.

Antidiabetes drugs. Acarbose is not absorbed from the mother's intestinal tract, so its use is safe during breastfeeding. *Insulin* therapy for diabetes mellitus restores low or missing insulin to normal levels. Diabetic mothers using insulin can nurse their infants, but they may need to reduce their insulin doses to below their prepregnancy doses. Since insulin is inactivated in the baby's stomach, none that enters the milk will be absorbed into the infant's bloodstream. Mothers with type 1 diabetes who use insulin may have a more difficult time initiating lactation, but once breastfeeding is established, they can nurse for as long as those without diabetes. *Metformin* has been studied well during breastfeeding with no adverse effects reported in breastfed infants. It is a good choice for nursing mothers. A small amount of information on the sulfonylureas *glyburide, tolbutamide,* and *chlorpropamide* indicates that they can be used during breastfeeding. Other oral sulfonylureas, *thiazolidinediones (pioglitazone, rosiglitazone), exanitide, pramlintide,* and *sitagliptin,* have not been studied during breastfeeding.

Antithyroid agents. Breastfeeding during treatment with *propylthiouracil* is safe. Doses of *methimazole* up to 20 milligrams daily are also safe; larger doses have not been studied and may adversely affect the infant. Monitoring of the infant's blood for adequate thyroid function may be necessary.

Bone marrow stimulants. *Epoetin alfa* is an injection that stimulates the production of red blood cells. Although small amounts enter breast milk, the drug is not absorbed from the infant's intestinal tract and so has no adverse effects on the infant. *Filgrastim* and *sargramostim* are similar to epoetin alfa but stimulate production of white rather than red blood cells. These drugs are also not absorbed from breast milk. All of these drugs are acceptable to use during breastfeeding.

Clomiphene. This synthetic hormone-like drug affects the activity of estrogen in the body and stimulates ovulation. There is no information on the drug during nursing; however, it is known to suppress lactation. Because it could have serious adverse consequences on the sexual maturation of your infant, and because it could remain in your body and milk for weeks after you take it, you should discontinue nursing if you take it.

Contraceptives. Hormonal contraception is the second choice after barrier methods for birth control during breastfeeding. Hormonal contraceptives can be divided into two categories: combination and progestin-only. The combination products contain estrogen, decrease lactation, and speed the end of nursing, although long-term effects on growth and development have not been found. Included among the combination contraceptives are the vaginal ring (*NuvaRing*), the contraceptive patch (*Ortho Evra*), and one injectable product (*Lunelle*). Because hormonal contraceptives might interfere with the establishment of lactation or affect the newborn, it is usually best to wait four to six weeks after birth before starting on any hormonal contraceptive. It is best not to use a combination contraceptive during breastfeeding unless you intend to stop nursing soon.

The short duration of exposure to morning-after contraceptives, such as **levonorgestrel (Plan B)**, should not adversely affect the nursing infant and should have only a minimal, temporary effect on lactation.

If you plan to use hormonal contraception, a progestin-only oral product such as **norethindrone (Micronor** or **Nor-Q.D.)** or **norethynodrel (Ovrette)**, or a progestin given by injection (**Depo-Provera),** is preferable. Some intrauterine devices (**IUDs**) release small amounts of progesterone or progestin (for example, **Progestasert** and **Mirena)** and are considered as safe as other progestin-only contraceptives. Nonhormonal intrauterine devices, including copper-containing devices (Copper-T), can be used during lactation without concern of adverse effects on the infant or lactation. Progestin-only contraceptive injections or implants are sometimes given within a few days after birth, but there is limited information on how this use affects breastfeeding and the breastfed infant.

Corticosteroids. Drugs in this category include *cortisone, methylprednisolone, prednisone,* and *triamcinolone.* Low doses and short courses of therapy (up to two weeks) appear to pose no harm to the nursing infant. Of concern are long courses of treatment (several weeks to months) with moderate to large doses. Although only a small fraction of each dose appears in breast milk, no one knows what these amounts might do to the developing infant. *Dexamethasone* and *betamethasone* are long-acting agents that have not been studied during nursing. It is best to avoid these two drugs.

Estrogens. Estrogens have been used after birth to suppress lactation, but they are no longer used this way because they are sometimes toxic to the mother. Estrogen products such as *Premarin* and *Estrace,* taken orally or vaginally, can probably interfere with nursing.

Progesterone. This natural hormone is sometimes given in suppositories for premenstrual syndrome. Progesterone is also found in one type of intrauterine contraceptive device, or IUD (*Progestasert*). Amounts of progesterone that appear in breast milk are small, and they are not absorbed by the infant.

Thyroid. Thyroid products have one major, valid use—to replace the thyroid hormone that is lacking in the bloodstream. When a woman takes proper doses, her thyroid levels become approximately normal. Thyroid replacement, therefore, poses no risks to the breastfed infant. Large daily doses of thyroid hormone (more than about 100 micrograms daily of *levothyroxine*) might affect the infant.

Immunosuppressants and Immunomodulators

Azathioprine. Numerous mothers have safely breastfed their infants while taking azathioprine following organ transplantation.

Cyclosporine. Some mothers have breastfed while taking this medication without harm to the baby, but the nursing infant should be carefully monitored, possibly with blood testing.

Glatiramer. Limited information exists on the use of this drug during breastfeeding. Because it is unlikely to be absorbed by the infant from breast milk, harmful effects are unlikely in the infant.

Interferons. Several interferon drugs are available. These drugs are made up of large molecules that are unlikely to pass into milk and affect an infant, as was found to be the case in studies of three breastfeeding women who were taking *interferon alfa.* Also, these drugs are active only when given by injection, so any interferon that would enter breast milk would have little or no effect on the infant. Some information on breastfeeding and *interferon beta* found no harm to breastfed infants, and most experts feel that this drug can be used during breastfeeding.

Methotrexate should not be used during breastfeeding in the doses required for cancer chemotherapy, but this drug might be acceptable in the low doses used for arthritis. *See also* "Arthritis, Pain, and Migraine Medications."

Tacrolimus. Experience with tacrolimus during nursing has found no harm to breastfed infants, and amounts in milk appear small. The infant should be carefully monitored, possibly with blood testing. Tacrolimus can be used on the skin during breastfeeding as long as it is not applied to the breast or other areas where the infant would come into direct contact with it.

Everolimus and **sirolimus.** These drugs have not been studied during breastfeeding and should be avoided if possible.

Iodine and Iodide. Use of *povidone iodine,* especially as a douche, but even on the skin, can result in high iodine blood levels in the mother. Iodine becomes concentrated in milk and subsequently in the infant's thyroid gland, possibly causing abnormal thyroid function; iodide rashes have also occurred in breastfed infants. Iodides should not be used during lactation. *See also* "Radio-Opaque Agents."

Lipid-Lowering Drugs. None of the cholesterol-lowering drugs have been studied during nursing. Because cholesterol is essential for the proper development of the infant's brain and nervous system, drugs that can enter the milk should not be taken during nursing. The most potent and commonly used drugs are called "statins" and include *atorvastatin, fluvastatin, lovastatin, pitavastatin, pravastatin, rosuvastatin,* and *simvastatin.* Other drugs that can enter the milk are called "fibrates" and include *fenofibrate* and *gemfibrozil.* All of these drugs should be avoided during nursing. *Ezetimibe* has not been studied during breastfeeding and should also be avoided. *Cholestyramine, colestipol,* and *colesevelam* are resins that work only in the mother's intestinal tract and can be used during nursing. It is unclear whether high-dose *niacin* can affect the nursing infant.

Muscle Relaxants. Most of these drugs have not been studied during nursing. Muscle relaxants taken by mouth, such as *carisoprodol, chlorzoxazone, diazepam,* and *methocarbamol,* are sedatives and can be expected to cause drowsiness in breastfed infants. *Cyclobenzaprine* probably doesn't reach high levels in milk, but it has not been studied during nursing. In general, it is best to avoid these drugs while breastfeeding, if possible. Taking ibuprofen (Motrin, Advil) or acetaminophen (Tylenol) along with mild to moderate exercise will usually ease muscle spasms and pain as well as muscle relaxants could.

Nonmedical Drugs. Since drugs used for nontherapeutic purposes are not essential to the well-being of the mother, and their effects on a breastfed infant are often unknown, their use is generally discouraged. Additionally, even small amounts can cause positive drug tests in your infant's urine, which with some drugs could lead to legal problems.

Alcohol. Alcohol readily passes into the milk. Large amounts of alcoholic beverages consumed over a short time can make a baby drunk and can inhibit the let-down reflex. Even small amounts of alcohol taken right before nursing can cause disruption in nursing behavior and the mother-infant interaction. Right after you drink an alcoholic beverage, your infant may suck more but consume up to 25 percent less milk (the baby may make up for this later in the day if you take no more alcohol). Heavy daily drinking can lead to hormonal imbalances in a breastfed infant, and even small to moderate amounts of alcohol taken daily or nearly every day while nursing appear to cause delayed muscular development and coordination in infants, although the severity of this problem depends on the amount of alcohol used. An occasional alcoholic beverage does not pose a serious danger to the infant, but it is prudent to wait at least two hours *per drink* before nursing.

Amphetamines. *Amphetamine* and *methamphetamine* ("crystal," "crystal meth") have not been formally studied during nursing. However, they are potent stimulants. Breastfeeding mothers who take these drugs might have fussy infants who cry a lot, cannot be comforted easily, and do not sleep well. Amphetamines probably also inhibit the mother's milk production. These drugs should not be used during nursing; if they are, the mother should temporarily stop nursing for 24 to 48 hours after taking them recreationally. Lower doses of amphetamine or *methylphenidate* prescribed to treat medical conditions appear not to affect breastfed infants.

Caffeine. Low to moderate intake of beverages containing caffeine is unlikely to cause problems in the infant, since the amount of caffeine that reaches the milk is usually small. But very high caffeine intake (more than ten cups of coffee or cola per day, for example) can make the baby jittery and agitated.

Cocaine. Cocaine is extremely toxic to infants because they metabolize it very slowly. Great agitation and continuous crying are often noted in breastfed infants of cocaine users, and cocaine applied to the nipples to treat soreness can cause convulsions in the infant. Cocaine should be avoided during nursing. If a mother does take it, she should stop breastfeeding for at least 24 hours afterward.

Hallucinogens. Information is lacking on the effects of these drugs during breast-feeding; however, levels in milk should be low by the time the mother has stopped feeling the effects of the drug.

Marijuana. There are few reports of the effects of marijuana in breastfed babies. After a single use, marijuana levels in milk are apparently low, but the active component of the drug can build up in the body with daily or near-daily use. Marijuana levels are probably high in the milk of chronic users. Note, too, that an infant in the same room with a smoker will breathe in significant quantities of marijuana. Breast-fed infants whose mothers use marijuana heavily have sometimes shown delayed muscular development and coordination. Marijuana and its metabolites are detect-able in the urine of breastfed infants whose mothers use marijuana.

Narcotics. Large doses can cause narcotic effects and addiction in breastfed infants. Narcotic addicts should not breastfeed; however, mothers on methadone mainte-nance can usually breastfeed their infants safely. *See also* "Arthritis, Pain, and Mi-graine Medications."

Phencyclidine (*PCP*). Large amounts of this drug have been measured in the breast milk of users. PCP must be entirely avoided during breastfeeding.

Tobacco. Nicotine from smoking tobacco appears in breast milk. Other toxic sub-stances in smoke reach the milk as well. Smoking interferes with lactation, which causes smokers to start supplementing and stop nursing sooner than nonsmokers. Infants of smokers are more likely than other babies to have colic symptoms and respiratory infections. Additionally, although breastfeeding reduces the risk of sud-den infant death syndrome (SIDS), smoking negates this advantage. If you can't stop smoking while you are nursing, you should (1) decrease your smoking as much as possible, (2) avoid nursing just after smoking, (3) avoid smoking in the same room with your baby, and (4) cover your regular clothing while you smoke and remove the covering before holding your infant. Although amounts of nicotine in breast milk during the use of a nicotine patch appear to be about the same as those in the milk of smokers, using a nicotine patch or nicotine chewing gum during breastfeeding is preferable to smoking.

Psychotherapeutic Agents. For many of these drugs, little is known about excretion into milk or effects on breastfed infants. Undertake nursing with caution if you are using one of these medications. Combinations of two or more of these drugs are more likely to be detrimental to the infant than a single drug.

Major tranquilizers. These drugs include the *phenothiazines,* such as *chlorpromazine, thioridazine, trifluoperazine, perphenazine,* and *fluphenazine;* the closely related *thioxanthenes,* such as *thiothixene;* the *butyrophenones,* such as *haloperidol;* and the newer "atypical" drugs such as *clozapine, olanzapine, paliperidone, quetiapine, risperidone,* and *ziprasidone.* Small amounts of these drugs appear in breast milk, and occasionally they have caused drowsiness in breastfed infants. Long-term effects on the infant are not well known. One study found no altered development in infants exposed to one of these drugs through breast milk; however, use of two or more of the drugs together could adversely affect the infant's development. Nursing is not recommended during *clozapine* therapy, which could cause harmful side effects in the infant.

Antidepressants. Postpartum depression occurs in about one of eight women. Untreated depression can have serious and long-lasting effects on infant growth and development, so treatment is essential. None of the medications used in treating depression are known to decrease milk production.

The small amounts of tricyclic antidepressants (such as **amitriptyline, imipramine, nortriptyline,** and **desipramine**) found in milk do not seem to affect the growth and development of the breastfed infant. Drowsiness can result with some of the more sedating drugs, such as **doxepin,** which should be avoided. Nortriptyline appears to be the safest and best studied of all the tricyclic antidepressants. It is found in only small amounts in milk, and little or none reaches the infant's bloodstream. If possible, take tricyclic antidepressants in the evening, after the final nursing session of the day, to minimize the dose that the breastfed infant receives.

If you took one of the following drugs during pregnancy, it is best to continue on the same medication during breastfeeding.

Fluoxetine appears in milk in higher amounts than most other antidepressants; it is very long acting; and side effects in the infant (colic, fussiness, and drowsiness) have been reported during its use, although infants older than one month can probably tolerate it better than younger babies. If fluoxetine is being continued from pregnancy or is needed for another reason, the benefits of using this medication while breastfeeding usually outweigh the risks to the infant, but watch the infant carefully for side effects. **Citalopram** is also found in relatively large amounts in milk, and it may cause drowsiness in the infant, especially when the baby is a newborn. **Escitalopram** is a form of citalopram that is taken in a lower dose; it might be preferred over citalopram. Other drugs in the class (**fluvoxamine, paroxetine,** and **sertraline**) are found in lower amounts in milk and are shorter acting than fluoxetine. Sertraline and paroxetine are the best studied and do not seem to affect nursing infants in the short or long run. They are good choices when an antidepressant is needed during nursing, with sertraline recommended most frequently.

Bupropion has been studied in a small number of mother-infant pairs and appears not to adversely affect nursing infants. Limited data indicate that **duloxetine, mirtazapine,** and **trazodone** are probably also acceptable to take during breastfeeding, but watch for excessive drowsiness if you are nursing a newborn.

Nefazodone has also not been well studied, but it has caused drowsiness and poor feeding in one newborn infant, so it is best avoided if you are nursing a newborn.

Venlafaxine is found in relatively high amounts in milk and in the nursing infant's bloodstream. Experience with it during breastfeeding is limited, but side effects in infants have not been seen. If possible, avoid venlafaxine if you are nursing a newborn. **Desvenlafaxine** produces lower levels in milk than venlafaxine, and may be preferable.

Amoxapine, maprotiline, and **vilazodone** have been less well studied, so no judgment can be made on their safety.

The monoamine oxidase inhibitors, **phenelzine** and **tranylcypromine,** are very potent drugs and should not be used while breastfeeding.

Lithium. This drug reaches breast milk in rather high levels. Lithium can accumulate in the infant's bloodstream and cause side effects in a premature or newborn infant who becomes dehydrated due to diarrhea or a viral illness. A healthy infant can be breastfed during lithium therapy, but only with careful monitoring—including, in some cases, blood tests for lithium. If your infant becomes ill for any reason during lithium therapy, discontinue breastfeeding and contact your health-care provider.

Radiologic Diagnostic Agents. A number of compounds are used in the X-ray diagnosis of various conditions. These compounds fall into three categories: MRI contrast agents, radio-opaque contrast agents, and radioactive agents. The radiologist administering these tests usually has guidelines on breastfeeding with the specific agents. X-rays themselves, of teeth, bones, or the chest, pose no hazard to the breastfed infant.

MRI contrast agents. These agents, *gadodiamide, gadopentetate, gadoteridol,* and *gadoversetamide,* contain *gadolinium* rather than iodine and are relatively safe and rapidly eliminated. There is no need to stop nursing for any length of time after receiving one of these agents.

Radio-opaque agents. These are generally compounds that contain iodine, but the iodine is tightly bound to the compound and does not enter breast milk. None of these agents require cessation or withholding of breastfeeding.

Radioactive agents. Breastfeeding must be stopped for a time after many of these agents are administered. The period of time varies depending on the agent and the dose given; a few of these agents persist in breast milk for so long that complete weaning of the baby is necessary. After exposure to some of these agents your body could give off radiation, particularly at close range. This means that not only would you have to stop breastfeeding temporarily, but you might not be able to hold your baby for some time, since doing so would expose her to radioactivity. Be sure to tell the radiologist that you are breastfeeding before you receive any of these agents.

For nursing mothers with overactive thyroid glands, the most commonly prescribed of these agents are **iodine-123** (for diagnosis) and **iodine-131** (for treatment). Although iodine-123 is eliminated in two to three days, it leaves the long-lasting byproduct **iodine-124.** Experts disagree about the safety of iodine-123, but it seems prudent to wean the baby completely after using it. Discontinuation of nursing is definitely required after iodine-131. A future baby can be safely breastfed after receiving these agents. **Technetium 99m pertechnetate** is a suitable alternative for diagnostic use.

Sedatives and Sleep Medications. Several types of drugs are included in this category. Although all of them can make an infant drowsy, some are more likely to do so than others. The drugs also differ in how long they persist in the body, which affects their tendency to accumulate in the infant.

Barbiturates. Drugs in this class include *amobarbital, butalbital, pentobarbital, phenobarbital, secobarbital,* and others. All of them, especially phenobarbital, may occasionally cause drowsiness in breastfed infants, but none are particularly hazardous to the baby otherwise, unless she becomes so drowsy that she nurses less.

Benzodiazepines. Of all sedative drugs, these are the most frequently used. They include *alprazolam, chlordiazepoxide, diazepam, flurazepam, lorazepam, oxazepam, triazolam,* and others. Although these drugs are safe in adults, newborn infants do not readily metabolize them; the long-acting drugs in this group accumulate in the infant's body. This may make the baby drowsy and, in some cases, may interfere with the binding of bilirubin in the bloodstream. These problems are accentuated in premature and newborn babies. Preferable benzodiazepines are short acting and reach breast milk in lesser amounts, and are therefore unlikely to cause drowsiness. These include *oxazepam, lorazepam,* and *triazolam.*

Two sleeping medications similar to the benzodiazepines are **zaleplon** and **zolpidem**. These are very short acting and appear in milk in very small amounts, so they can be used while nursing.

Eszopiclone has not been studied during breastfeeding and is longer acting than the other sleep medications, so one of the others is preferred.

Buspirone. Extremely little information exists on this drug during lactation. It is best avoided during nursing.

Chloral hydrate. This drug is rarely used. It has caused drowsiness in infants, but it is probably acceptable for occasional use. *Dichloralphenazone,* which is in *Midrin,* releases chloral hydrate in the mother's body and can cause drowsiness in the breastfed infant.

Over-the-counter sleep medications. These usually contain *diphenhydramine;* the general precautions for the sedating antihistamines apply. (*See also* "Cough, Cold, Allergy, and Asthma Medications.")

Vaccines and Skin Tests. No vaccine or skin test (such as the one for tuberculosis, PPD), when given to a mother, is known to pose a hazard to her breastfed infant. Killed vaccines, including *diphtheria, hepatitis A* and *B, injectable influenza, injectable polio,* and *tetanus* vaccines, are inactive in breast milk. Although live vaccines are occasionally transmitted through breast milk, they do not endanger the baby. Live vaccines include *inhaled influenza, measles, mumps, oral polio, rubella, oral typhoid,* and *varicella.* With the exception of the smallpox and yellow fever vaccines, the U.S. Centers for Disease Control and Prevention (CDC) states that no vaccination should be withheld from a woman or delayed because she is breastfeeding.

Weight-Loss Products. Rapid, excessive weight loss during lactation should be avoided, because many fat-soluble environmental contaminants (such as some insecticides) are stored in body fat. When body fat is lost rapidly, contaminants are released into the bloodstream and appear in the fat of breast milk in larger than usual amounts. In addition, some weight-loss agents can affect infants or the milk supply. Many weight-loss products contain vitamins that may also be in multivitamin products prescribed by your physician. If you take both products, your vitamin intake may be excessive.

INDEX TO COMMON DRUGS

Each brand name is listed in capital letters; the corresponding generic name is given after it. All generic names that do not appear as headings in the text are followed here by cross-references to the relevant sections. The names of combination products are followed by lists of the ingredients they contain; see the separate entry for each ingredient. Not all brands are listed, so if you can't find the name of a particular product in this list, look under the generic name of its ingredient or ingredients.

chlorzoxazone. *See* muscle relaxants, 391
cholestyramine. *See* lipid-lowering drugs, 391
cimetidine. *See* histamine H-2 antagonists, 385
Cipro: ciprofloxacin. *See* quinolones, 379
ciprofloxacin. *See* quinolones, 379
cisplatin. *See* cancer chemotherapy, 383
citalopram. *See* antidepressants, 393–394
clarithromycin. *See* macrolides, 378
Clarinex: desloratadine. *See* antihistamines, 383–384
Claritin: loratadine. *See* antihistamines, 383–384
clavulanate. *See* penicillins, 379
clindamycin, 378
Clinoril: sulindac. *See* nonsteroidal anti-inflammatory drugs, 383
Clomid: clomiphene, 389
clomiphene, 389
clonazepam, 380
clonidine, 386
clopidogrel. *See* anticoagulants, 379
clotrimazole. *See* antifungals, 381
cloxacillin. *See* penicillins, 379
Cloxapen: cloxacillin. *See* penicillins, 379
cocaine, 392
codeine. *See* narcotics, 382
Colace: docusate. *See* laxatives, 385
cold medications, 383–384
Colesevelam. *See* lipid-lowering drugs, 391
Colestid: colestipol. *See* lipid-lowering drugs, 391
colestipol. *See* lipid-lowering drugs, 391
Compazine: prochlorperazine. *See* antinauseants, 381
contraceptives, 389
Copaxone: glatiramer. *See* immunosuppressants and immunomodulators, 390
Copper T. *See* contraceptives, 389

Cordarone: amiodarone. *See* heart and blood pressure drugs, 386–387
Corgard: nadolol. *See* beta blockers, 386
corticosteroids, 390
cortisone. *See* corticosteroids, 390
Cosmegen: dactinomycin. *See* cancer chemotherapy, 383
cough medicines, 384
Coumadin: warfarin. *See* anticoagulants, 379
Cozaar: losartan. *See* angiotensin-II blockers, 386
Crestor: rosuvastatin. *See* lipid-lowering drugs, 391
crystal meth: methamphetamine. *See* amphetamines, 391–392
crystal: methamphetamine. *See* amphetamines, 391–392
Cubicin: daptomycin. *See* vancomycin, 379
Cuprimine: penicillamine. *See* antirheumatic drugs, 382
cyclobenzaprine. *See* muscle relaxants, 391
cyclophosphamide. *See* cancer chemotherapy, 383
cyclosporine. *See* immunosuppressants and immunomodulators, 390
Cymbalta: duloxetine. *See* antidepressants, 393–394
cytarabine. *See* cancer chemotherapy, 383
Cytosar: cytarabine. *See* cancer chemotherapy, 383
Cytoxan: cyclophosphamide. *See* cancer chemotherapy, 383

dabigatran. *See* anticoagulants, 379
dacarbazine. *See* cancer chemotherapy, 383
dactinomycin. *See* cancer chemotherapy, 383
Dalmane: flurazepam. *See* benzodiazepines, 395
dalteparin. *See* anticoagulants, 379
daptomycin. *See* vancomycin, 379

Darvon: propoxyphene. *See* narcotics, 382
daunorubicin. *See* cancer chemotherapy, 383
Decadron: dexamethasone. *See* corticosteroids, 390
decongestants, 384
Demerol: meperidine. *See* narcotics, 382
Denavir: penciclovir. *See* antivirals, 381–382
Depakene: valproic acid, 380
Depakote: valproic acid, 380
Depen: penicillamine. *See* antirheumatic drugs, 382
Depo-Provera: medroxyprogesterone acetate. *See* contraceptives, 389
desflurane. *See* general anesthetics, 377
desipramine. *See* antidepressants, 393–394
desloratadine. *See* antihistamines, 383–384
Desquam-X: benzoyl peroxide. *See* acne products, 377
Desvenlafaxine. *See* antidepressants, 393–394
Desyrel: trazodone. *See* antidepressants, 393–394
dexamethasone, *See* corticosteroids, 390
dextromethorphan. *See* cough medicines, 384
DiaBeta: glyburide. *See* antidiabetes drugs, 388–389
Diabinese: chlorpropamide. *See* antidiabetes drugs, 388–389
diazepam. *See* benzodiazepines, 395; muscle relaxants, 391
dichloralphenazone. *See* chloral hydrate, 395
diclofenac. *See* nonsteroidal anti-inflammatory drugs, 383
Diflucan: fluconazole. *See* antifungals, 381
diflunisal. *See* nonsteroidal anti-inflammatory drugs, 383
digoxin, 387
Dilantin: phenytoin. *See* anticonvulsants, 379–381

diltiazem. *See* calcium channel blockers, 386
dimenhydrinate. *See* antihistamines, 383–384
Diovan: valsartan. *See* angiotensin-II blockers, 386
Dipentum: olsalazine. *See* mesalamine derivatives, 386
diphenhydramine. *See* antihistamines, 383–384; over-the-counter sleep medications, 395
diphenoxylate. *See* antidiarrheals, 385
diphtheria vaccine, 395
Diprivan: propofol. *See* anesthetics, 377
diuretics, 384
divalproex. *See* valproic acid, 380
docusate. *See* laxatives, 385
dolasetron. *See* antinauseants, 381
Dolobid: diflunisal. *See* nonsteroidal anti-inflammatory drugs, 383
domperidone. *See* gastrointestinal drugs, 385–386
Dostinex: cabergoline: *See* ergot alkaloids, 385
doxepin. *See* antidepressants, 393–394
doxorubicin. *See* cancer chemotherapy, 383
Dramamine: dimenhydrinate. *See* antihistamines, 383–384
Dulcolax: bisacodyl. *See* nonabsorbable laxatives, 385
duloxetine. *See* antidepressants, 393–394
Dyazide: contains hydrochlorothiazide, 384
Dymelor: acetohexamide. *See* antidiabetes drugs, 388–389
Dynapen: dicloxacillin. *See* penicillins, 379

echinacea. *See* herbals and nutraceuticals, 387–388
econazole. *See* antifungals, 381
Effexor: venlafaxine. *See* antidepressants, 393–394

Elavil: amitriptyline. *See* antidepressants, 393–394
eletriptan. *See* triptans, 383
Elimite: permethrin. *See* antiparasitics, 381
enalapril. *See* ACE inhibitors, 386
Enbrel: etanercept. *See* antirheumatic drugs, 382
enflurane. *See* general anesthetics, 377
enoxaprin. *See* anticoagulants, 379
ephedra. *See* herbals and nutraceuticals, 387–388
Epoetin alfa. *See* bone marrow stimulants, 389
Epogen: epoetin alfa. *See* bone marrow stimulants, 389
eprosartan. *See* angiotensin-II blockers, 386
Ergomar: ergotamine, 382
ergonovine. *See* ergot alkaloids, 385
Ergostat: ergotamine, 382
ergot alkaloids, 385
ergotamine, 382
Ergotrate: ergonovine. *See* ergot alkaloids, 385
erythromycin, 377, 378
escitalopram. *See* antidepressants, 393–394
Esidrix: hydrochlorothiazide, 384
esomeprazole. *See* proton pump inhibitors, 386
Estrace. *See* estrogens, 390
estrogens, 390
eszopiclone. *See* benzodiazepines, 395
etanercept. *See* antirheumatic drugs, 382
Ethrane: enflurane. *See* general anesthetics, 377
etidronate. *See* bisphosphonates, 383
etoposide. *See* cancer chemotherapy, 383
evening primrose oil. *See* herbals and nutraceuticals, 387–388
everolimus. *See* immunosuppressants and immunomodulators, 390
exenatide. *See* antidiabetes drugs, 388–389; hormones, 388–390

ezetimibe. *See* lipid-lowering drugs, 391

famciclovir. *See* antivirals, 381–382
famotidine. *See* histamine H-2 antagonists, 385
Famvir: famciclovir. *See* antivirals, 381–382
felbamate. *See* anticonvulsants, 379–381
Felbatol: felbamate. *See* anticonvulsants, 379–381
Feldene: piroxicam. *See* nonsteroidal anti-inflammatory drugs, 383
Femstat: butoconazole. *See* antifungals, 381
fennel. *See* herbals and nutraceuticals, 387–388
fenofibrate. *See* lipid-lowering drugs, 391
fenoprofen. *See* nonsteroidal anti-inflammatory drugs, 383
fentanyl. *See* narcotics, 382
fenugreek. *See* herbals and nutraceuticals, 387–388
fexofenadine. *See* antihistamines, 383–384
FiberCon. *See* laxatives, 385
filgrastim. *See* bone marrow stimulants, 389
Fiorinal: contains butalbital. *See* barbiturates, 395
Fish oil. *See* herbals and nutraceuticals, 387–388
Flagyl: metronidazole, 378
Flexeril: cyclobenzaprine. *See* muscle relaxants, 391
Floxin: ofloxacin. *See* quinolones, 379
fluconazole. *See* antifungals, 381
Flumadine: rimantadine. *See* antivirals, 381–382
flunisolide. *See* asthma inhalers and nasal inhalers, 384
fluorouracil. *See* cancer chemotherapy, 383
fluoxetine. *See* antidepressants, 393–394
fluphenazine. *See* major tranquilizers, 392–393
flurazepam. *See* benzodiazepines, 395

flurbiprofen. *See* nonsteroidal anti-inflammatory drugs, 383

fluticasone. *See* asthma inhalers and nasal inhalers, 384

fluvastatin. *See* lipid-lowering drugs, 391

fluvoxamine. *See* antidepressants, 393–394

Forane: isoflurane. *See* general anesthetics, 377

Fosamax: alendronate. *See* bisphosphonates, 383

Frova: frovatriptan. *See* triptans, 383

frovatriptan. *See* triptans, 383

Fungizone: amphotericin B. *See* antifungals, 381

Furadantin: nitrofurantoin, 378

furosemide, 384

gabapentin. *See* anticonvulsants, 379–381

Gabitril: tiagabine. *See* anticonvulsants, 379–381

gadodiamide. *See* MRI contrast agents, 394

gadolinium. *See* MRI contrast agents, 394

gadopentetate. *See* MRI contrast agents, 394

gadoteridol. *See* MRI contrast agents, 394

gadoversetamide. *See* MRI contrast agents, 394

Gantanol: sulfamethoxazole. *See* sulfonamides, 379

Garamycin: gentamicin. *See* aminoglycosides, 378

gastrointestinal drugs, 385–386

Gelusil. *See* antacids, 385

gemfibrozil. *See* lipid-lowering drugs, 391

general anesthetics, 377

gentamicin. *See* aminoglycosides, 378

Geodon: ziprasidone. *See* major tranquilizers, 392–393

ginkgo biloba. *See* herbals and nutraceuticals, 387–388

glatiramer. *See* immunosuppressants and immunomodulators, 390

glimepiride. *See* antidiabetes drugs, 388–389

glipizide. *See* antidiabetes drugs, 388–389

Glucophage: metformin. *See* antidiabetes drugs, 388–389

Glucotrol: glipizide. *See* antidiabetes drugs, 388–389

glycerin. *See* laxatives, 385

Glynase: glyburide. *See* antidiabetes drugs, 388–389

Go-Lacta: Moringa. *See* herbals and nutraceuticals, 387–388

granisetron. *See* antinauseants, 381

guaifenesin. *See* cough medicines, 384

guanfacine. *See* clonidine, 386

Gynergen: ergotamine, 382

Halcion: triazolam. *See* benzodiazepines, 395

Haldol: haloperidol. *See* major tranquilizers, 392–393

Halls. *See* cough and cold medicines, 383–384

hallucinogens, 392

haloperidol. *See* major tranquilizers, 392–393

halothane. *See* general anesthetics, 377

heart and blood pressure drugs, 386–387

heparin. *See* anticoagulants, 379

hepatitis A and B vaccines, 395

herbals and nutraceuticals, 387–388

histamine H-2 antagonists, 385

hormones, 388–390

Humira: adalimumab. *See* antirheumatic drugs, 382

hydralazine, 387

hydrochlorothiazide, 384

hydrocodone. *See* narcotics, 382

HydroDiuril: hydrochlorothiazide, 384

hydroxychloroquine. *See* antirheumatic drugs, 382

Hygroton: chlorthalidone, 384

ibuprofen. *See* nonsteroidal anti-inflammatory drugs, 383

imipramine. *See* antidepressants, 393–394

Imitrex: sumatriptan. *See* triptans, 383

immunosuppressants and immunomodulators, 390

Imodium: loperamide. *See* antidiarrheals, 385

Imuran: azathioprine. *See* immunosuppressants and immunomodulators, 390

Inderal: propranolol. *See* beta blockers, 386

Indocin: indomethacin. *See* nonsteroidal anti-inflammatory drugs, 383

indomethacin. *See* nonsteroidal anti-inflammatory drugs, 383

infliximab. *See* antirheumatic drugs, 382

influenza vaccine. *See* vaccines and skin tests, 395

INH: isoniazid, 378

insulin, 388

interferon alfa. *See* immunosuppressants and immunomodulators, 390

interferon beta. *See* immunosuppressants and immunomodulators, 390

Intron A: interferon alfa. *See* immunosuppressants and immunomodulators, 390

Invega: paliperidone. *See* major tranquilizers, 392–393

iodine and iodide, 391

iodine-123. *See* radioactive agents, 394

iodine-131. *See* radioactive agents, 394

ipratropium. *See* asthma inhalers and nasal inhalers, 384

irbesartan. *See* angiotensin-II blockers, 386

isoflurane. *See* general anesthetics, 377

isoniazid, 378

methimazole. *See* antithyroid agents, 389
methocarbamol. *See* muscle relaxants, 391
methotrexate. *See* antirheumatic drugs, 382; immunosuppressants and immunomodulators, 390
methyldopa, 387
methylergonovine. *See* ergot alkaloids, 385
methylphenidate. *See* amphetamines, 391–392
methylprednisolone. *See* corticosteroids, 390
metoclopramide, 386
metoprolol. *See* beta blockers, 386
metronidazole, 378
Mevacor: lovastatin. *See* lipid-lowering drugs, 391
Micardis: telmisartan. *See* angiotensin-II blockers, 386
Micatin: miconazole. *See* antifungals, 381
miconazole. *See* antifungals, 381
Micronase: glyburide. *See* antidiabetes drugs, 388–389
Micronor: norethindrone. *See* contraceptives, 389
midazolam. *See* general anesthetics, 377
Midrin: contains dichloralphenazone. *See* chloral hydrate, 395
milk of magnesia. *See* laxatives, 385
Minocin: minocycline. *See* tetracyclines, 379
Mirena. *See* contraceptives, 389
mirtazapine. *See* antidepressants, 393–394
Mithracin: mithramycin. *See* cancer chemotherapy, 383
mithramycin. *See* cancer chemotherapy, 383
mitomycin. *See* cancer chemotherapy, 383
Monistat: miconazole. *See* antifungals, 381
monoamine oxidase inhibitors, 394

Moringa. *See* herbals and nutraceuticals, 387–388
morphine. *See* narcotics, 382
Motilium: domperidone. *See* gastrointestinal drugs, 385–386
Motrin: ibuprofen. *See* nonsteroidal anti-inflammatory drugs, 383
moxifloxacin. *See* quinolones, 379
MRI contrast agents, 394
mumps vaccine. *See* vaccines and skin tests, 395
muscle relaxants, 391
Mutamycin: mitomycin. *See* cancer chemotherapy, 383
Mycelex: clotrimazole. *See* antifungals, 381
Mycostatin: nystatin. *See* antifungals, 381
Mylanta. *See* antacids, 385
Myleran: busulfan. *See* cancer chemotherapy, 383
Mysoline: primidone. *See* anticonvulsants, 379–381

nadolol. *See* beta blockers, 386
Nalfon: fenoprofen. *See* nonsteroidal anti-inflammatory drugs, 383
Naprosyn: naproxen. *See* nonsteroidal anti-inflammatory drugs, 383
naproxen. *See* nonsteroidal anti-inflammatory drugs, 383
naratriptan. *See* triptans, 383
narcotics, 382, 392
Nardil: phenelzine. *See* antidepressants, 393–394
nasal inhalers. *See* asthma inhalers and nasal inhalers, 384
nasal sprays, 384
Nasalide: flunisolide. *See* asthma inhalers and nasal inhalers, 384
nateglinide. *See* antidiabetes drugs, 388–389
Navane: thiothixene. *See* major tranquilizers, 392–393

Nebcin: tobramycin. *See* aminoglycosides, 378
nefazodone. *See* antidepressants, 393–394
Nembutal: pentobarbital. *See* barbiturates, 395
Netromycin: netilmicin. *See* aminoglycosides, 378
Neupogen: filgrastim. *See* bone marrow stimulants, 389
Neurontin: gabapentin. *See* anticonvulsants, 379–381
Nexium: esomeprazole. *See* proton pump inhibitors, 386
niacin. *See* lipid-lowering drugs, 391
nicotine. *See* tobacco, 392
nifedipine. *See* calcium channel blockers, 386
Nilstat: nystatin. *See* antifungals, 381
nitrendipine. *See* calcium channel blockers, 386
nitrofurantoin, 378
nitrous oxide. *See* general anesthetics, 377
Nix: permethrin. *See* antiparasitics, 381
nizatidine. *See* histamine H-2 antagonists, 385
Nizoral: ketoconazole. *See* antifungals, 381
Noctec: chloral hydrate, 395
nonmedical drugs, 391–392
nonsteroidal anti-inflammatory drugs, 383
Nor-QD: norethindrone. *See* contraceptives, 389
norethindrone. *See* contraceptives, 389
norethynodrel. *See* contraceptives, 389
norfloxacin. *See* quinolones, 379
Normodyne: labetalol. *See* beta blockers, 386
Noroxin: norfloxacin. *See* quinolones, 379
Norpramin: desipramine. *See* antidepressants, 393–394
nortriptyline. *See* antidepressants, 393–394

Pravachol: pravastatin. *See* lipid-lowering drugs, 391
pravastatin. *See* lipid-lowering drugs, 391
prednisone. *See* corticosteroids, 390
pregabalin. *See* anticonvulsants, 379–381
Premarin. *See* estrogens, 390
Prevacid: lansoprazole. *See* proton pump inhibitors, 386
Prilosec: omeprazole. *See* proton pump inhibitors, 386
primidone. *See* anticonvulsants, 379–381
Pristiq: desfenlafaxine. *See* antidepressants, 393–394
procainamide, 387
procaine. *See* local anesthetics, 377
procarbazine. *See* cancer chemotherapy, 383
prochlorperazine. *See* antinauseants, 381
Procrit: epoetin alfa. *See* bone marrow stimulants, 389
Progestasert: contains progesterone, 390
progesterone, 390
Prograf: tacrolimus. *See* immunosuppressants and immunomodulators, 390
Prohance: gadoteridol. *See* MRI contrast agents, 394
Prolixin: fluphenazine. *See* major tranquilizers, 392–393
promethazine. *See* antinauseants, 381
propofol. *See* anesthetics, 377
propoxyphene. *See* narcotics, 382
propranolol. *See* beta blockers, 386
propylthiouracil. *See* antithyroid agents, 389
Protonix: pantoprazole. *See* proton pump inhibitors, 386
proton pump inhibitors, 386
Prozac: fluoxetine. *See* antidepressants, 393–394

pseudoephedrine. *See* decongestants, 384
psychotherapeutic agents, 392–394
PTU: propylthiouracil. *See* antithyroid agents, 389
pyrazinamide. *See* antitubercular drugs, 378
pyrethrins. *See* antiparasitics, 381
Pyridium: phenazopyridine. *See* sulfonamides, 379

Questran: cholestyramine. *See* lipid-lowering drugs, 391
quetiapine. *See* major tranquilizers, 392–393
Quineprox: hydroxychloroquine. *See* antirheumatic drugs, 382
quinolones, 379

rabeprazole, 386
radio-opaque agents, 394
radioactive agents, 394
radiologic diagnostic agents, 394
ranitidine. *See* histamine H-2 antagonists, 385
Rapamune: sirolimus. *See* immunosuppressants and immunomodulators, 390
raspberry. *See* herbals and nutraceuticals, 387–388
Rebif: interferon beta. *See* immunosuppressants and immunomodulators, 390
Reglan: metoclopramide, 386
Rela: carisoprodol. *See* muscle relaxants, 391
Relenza: zanamivir. *See* antivirals, 381–382
Relpax: eletriptan. *See* triptans, 383
Remeron: mirtazapine. *See* antidepressants, 393–394
Remicade: infliximab. *See* antirheumatic drugs, 382
repaglinide. *See* antidiabetes drugs, 388–389
reserpine, 387
Retin-A: tretinoin. *See* acne products, 377
Rheumatrex: methotrexate. *See* antirheumatic drugs, 382

Rifadin: rifampin. *See* antitubercular drugs, 378
rifampin. *See* antitubercular drugs, 378
rimantadine. *See* antivirals, 381–382
risedronate. *See* bisphosphonates, 383
Risperdal: risperidone. *See* major tranquilizers, 392–393
risperidone. *See* major tranquilizers, 392–393
Ritalin: methylphenidate. *See* amphetamines, 391–392
rivaroxaban. *See* anticoagulants, 379
rizatriptan. *See* triptans, 383
Robaxin: methocarbamol. *See* muscle relaxants, 391
Roferon: interferon alfa. *See* immunosuppressants and immunomodulators, 390
Rolaids. *See* antacids, 385
ropivacaine. *See* local anesthetics, 377
rosiglitazone. See antidiabetes drugs, 388–389; hormones, 388–390
rosuvastatin. *See* lipid-lowering drugs, 391
rubella vaccine. *See* vaccines and skin tests, 395

Sabril: vigabatrin. *See* anticonvulsants, 379–381
sage. *See* herbals and nutraceuticals, 387–388
Saint John's wort. *See* herbals and nutraceuticals, 387–388
saline cathartics, 385
salmeterol. *See* asthma inhalers and nasal inhalers, 384
Sandimmune: cyclosporine. *See* immunosuppressants and immunomodulators, 390
sargramostim. *See* bone marrow stimulants, 389
Scopolamine. *See* antihistamines, 383–384
secobarbital. *See* barbiturates, 395
Seconal: secobarbital. *See* barbiturates, 395

References

American Academy of Pediatrics. "Policy Statement: Breastfeeding and the Use of Human Milk." *Pediatrics* 115 (2005): 496–506.

————. "Prevention of Pediatric Overweight and Obesity." *Pediatrics* 112 (2003): 424–30.

————. "Report on the Assessment of Scientific Evidence Relating to Infant-Feeding Practices and Infant Health." *Pediatrics* 74 (1984): 191–97.

Anderson, A. M. "Disruption of Lactogenesis by Retained Placental Fragments." *Journal of Human Lactation* 17 (2001): 142–44.

Arenz, S., et al. "Breast-Feeding and Childhood Obesity: A Systematic Review." *International Journal of Obesity and Related Metabolic Disorders* 28 (2004): 1247–56.

Auerbach, Kathleen G. "Employed Breastfeeding Mothers: Problems They Encounter." *Birth* 11 (1984): 17–20.

Auerbach, Kathleen G., and Laurence Gartner. "Breastfeeding and Human Milk: Their Association with Jaundice in the Neonate." *Clinics in Perinatology* 14 (1987): 89–107.

Auerbach, Kathleen G., and E. Guss. "Maternal Employment and Breastfeeding: A Study of 567 Women's Experiences." *American Journal of Disease in Childhood* 138 (1984): 958–60.

Bachrach, V. R., et al. "Breastfeeding and the Risk of Hospitalization for Respiratory Disease in Infancy: A Meta-Analysis." *Archives of Pediatrics and Adolescent Medicine* 157 (2003): 237–43.

Ballard, Jeanne L., et al. "Ankyloglossia: Assessment, Incidence, and Effect of Frenuloplasty on the Breastfeeding Dyad." *Pediatrics* 110 (2002): 62–68.

Bauer, G., et al. "Breastfeeding and Cognitive Development of Three-Year-Old Children." *Psychology Report* 68 (1991): 1218.

Bener, A., et al. "Longer Breast-Feeding and Protection against Childhood Leukaemia and Lymphomas." *European Journal of Cancer* 37 (2001): 234–38.

Bier, J. A., et al. "Human Milk Improves Cognitive and Motor Development of Premature Infants during Infancy." *Journal of Human Lactation* 18 (2002): 361–67.

Bishara, R. "Volume of Foremilk, Hindmilk, and Total Milk Produced by Mothers of Very Preterm Infants Born at Less Than 28 Weeks of Gestation." *Journal of Human Lactation* 25 (2009): 272–79.

Bishop, N., M. McGraw, and N. Ward. "Aluminum in Infant Formulas." *Lancet* 1 (1989): 490.

Bowen, A. B., and C. R. Braden. "Invasive *Enterbacter sakazakii* Disease in Infants." *Emerging Infectious Diseases Journal* 12 (2006): 1185–89.

Brazelton, T. Berry. *Infants and Mothers: Differences in Development*, rev. ed. New York: Delta/Seymour Lawrence, 1983.

Brent, N., et al. "Sore Nipples in Breast-Feeding Women: A Clinical Trial of Wound Dressings versus Conventional Care." *Archives of Pediatric and Adolescent Medicine* 152 (1998): 1072–82.

Brewster, Dorothy Patricia. *You Can Breastfeed Your Baby . . . Even in Special Situations.* Emmaus, PA: Rodale Press, 1979.

Byers, T., et al. "Lactation and Breast Cancer: Evidence for a Negative Association in Pre-Menopausal Women." *American Journal of Epidemiology* 121 (1985): 664–74.

Bystrova, K., et al. "Skin to Skin Contact May Reduce Negative Consequences of 'the Stress of Being Born': A Study on Temperature in Newborn Infants, Subjected to Different Ward Routines in St. Petersburg." *Acta Pediatrica* 3 (2003): 320–26.

Christensson, K. "Temperature, Metabolic Adaptation, and Crying in Healthy, Full-Term Newborns Cared for Skin-to-Skin or in a Cot." *Acta Paediatrica Scandinavica* 81 (2009): 488–93.

Coles, J. "Qualitative Study of Breastfeeding After Childhood Sexual Assault." *Journal of Human Lactation* 25 (2009): 317–24.

Collaborative Group on Hormonal Factors in Breast Cancer. "Breast Cancer and Breastfeeding: Collaborative Reanalysis of Individual Data from 47 Epidemiological Studies in 30 Countries, Including 50,302 Women with Breast Cancer and 96,973 Women without the Disease." *Lancet* 360 (2002): 187–95.

Colson, S. D., et al. "Optimal Positions for the Release of Primitive Neonatal Reflexes Stimulating Breastfeeding." *Early Human Development* 84 (2008): 441–49.

Cotterman, K. J. "Reverse Pressure Softening: A Simple Tool to Prepare Areola for Easier Latching During Engorgement." *Journal of Human Lactation* 20 (2004): 227–37.

Courtney, K. "Maternal Anesthesia: What Are the Effects on Neonates?" *Nursing for Women's Health* 11 (2007): 499–502.

Cumming, R. G., and R. J. Klineberg. "Breastfeeding and Other Reproductive Factors and the Risk of Hip Fractures in Elderly Women." *International Journal of Epidemiology* 22 (1993): 684–69.

Davis, M. K., D. A. Savitz, and B. I. Graubard. "Infant Feeding and Childhood Cancer." *Lancet* 2 (1988): 365–68.

DeCarvalho, M., M. Hall, and D. Harvey. "Effects of Water Supplementation on Physiological Jaundice in Breast-fed Babies." *Archives of Disease in Childhood* 56 (1981): 568–69.

Dewey, K. G., et al. "Breast-Fed Infants Are Leaner than Formula-Fed Infants at 1 Year of Age: The DARLING Study." *American Journal of Clinical Nutrition* 57 (1993): 140–45.

—————. "Maternal Weight-Loss Patterns during Prolonged Lactation." *American Journal of Clinical Nutrition* 58 (1993): 162–66.

Dowling, D. A., et al. "Cup-Feeding for Preterm Infants: Mechanics and Safety." *Journal of Human Lactation* 18 (2002): 13–20.

Eglash, A., et al. "History, Physical and Laboratory Findings, and Clinical Outcomes of Lactating Women Treated with Antibiotics for Chronic Breast and/or Nipple Pain." *Journal of Human Lactation* 22 (2006): 429–33.

Ehrenkranz, R., and B. Ackerman. "Metoclopramide Effect on Faltering Milk Production by Mothers of Premature Infants." *Pediatrics* 78 (1986): 614–20.

Elias, Marjorie F., et al. "Sleep/Wake Patterns of Breastfed Infants in the First Two Years of Life." *Pediatrics* 77 (1986): 322–29.

Estrella M. C., et al. "A Double-Blind, Randomized Controlled Trial on the Use of Malunggay (*Moringa oleifera*) for Augmentation of the Volume of Beastmilk among

Non-Nursing Mothers of Preterm Infants." *Philippine Journal of Pediatrics* 49 (2000): 3–6.

Ferber, Richard. *Solve Your Child's Sleep Problems: The Complete Practical Guide for Parents.* New York: Simon and Schuster, 1985.

Fiocchi, A., et al. "Food Allergy and the Introduction of Solid Foods to Infants: A Consensus Document." *Annals of Allergy, Asthma, and Immunology* 1 (2006): 10–20.

Friedland, G., and R. Klein. "Transmission of the Human Immunodeficiency Virus." *New England Journal of Medicine* 317 (1987): 1125–35.

Gardiner, D. T., et al. "Breast-Feeding Increases Sleep Duration of New Parents." *Journal of Perinatal and Neonatal Nursing* 21 (2007): 200–206.

Gillman, M. W., et al. "Risk of Overweight among Adolescents Who Were Breastfed as Infants." *Journal of the American Medical Association* 285 (2001): 2461–67.

Gordan, C. M., et al. "Prevalence of Vitamin D Deficiency among Healthy Infants and Toddlers." *Archives of Paediatric Medicine* 162 (2008): 505–12.

Gupta, J. K., and V. C. Nikoderm. "Position for Women during Second Stage of Labor." *Cochrane Library* 3. Oxford: Update Software, 2003.

Gwinn, M. L., et al. "Pregnancy, Breastfeeding, and Oral Contraceptives and the Risk of Epithelial Ovarian Cancer." *Journal of Clinical Epidemiology* 43 (1990): 559–68.

Hahn-Zoric, M., et al. "Antibody Responses to Parenteral and Oral Vaccines Are Impaired by Conventional and Low Protein Formulas as Compared to Breastfeeding." *Acta Paediatrica Scandanavica* 79 (1990): 1137–42.

Hill, P. D., et al. "Comparison of Milk Output Between Mothers of Preterm and Term Infants: The First 6 Weeks After Birth." *Journal of Human Lactation* 21 (2005): 22–30.

————. "Initiation and Frequency of Pumping and Milk Production in Mothers of Non-Nursing Preterm Infants." *Journal of Human Lactation* 17 (2001): 9–13.

Horne, R. S., et al. "Comparison of Evoked Arousability in Breast and Formula Fed Infants." *Archives of Disease in Childhood* 89 (2004): 22–25.

Horwood, L. J., et al. "Breast Milk Feeding and Cognitive Ability at 7–8 Years." *Archives of Disease in Childhood—Fetal and Neonatal Edition* 84 (2001): 23–27.

Huggins, Kathleen, and Sharon Billon. "Twenty Cases of Persistent Sore Nipples: Collaboration Between Lactation Consultant and Dermatologist." *Journal of Human Lactation* 9 (1993): 155–60.

Huggins, Kathleen, et al. "Markers of Lactation Insufficiency: A Study of 34 Mothers." *Current Issues in Clinical Lactation* 1 (2000): 25–35.

Hurst, N. M., et al. "Mothers Performing In-Home Measurement of Milk Intake During Breastfeeding of Their Preterm Infants: Maternal Reactions and Feeding Outcomes." *Journal of Human Lactation* 20 (2004): 178–87.

Jain, L. "Morbidity and Mortality in Late-Preterm Infants: More Than Just Transient Tachypnea!" *Journal of Pediatrics* 151 (2007): 445–46.

Jensen, Rima. "Fenugreek: Overlooked but Not Forgotten." *UCLA Lactation Alumni Association Newsletter* 1 (1992): 2–3.

Jernstrom, H., et al. "Breast-Feeding and the Risk of Breast Cancer in BRCA1 and BRCA2 Mutation Carriers." *Journal of the National Cancer Institute* 96 (2004): 1094–98.

Kalies, H., et al. "The Effect of Breastfeeding on Weight Gain in Infants: Results of a Birth Cohort Study." *European Journal of Medical Research* 10 (2005): 36–42.

Karp, Harvey. "The 'Fourth Trimester': A Framework and Strategy for Understanding and Resolving Colic." *Contemporary Pediatrics* 21 (2004): 94–114.

Kavanaugh, Karen, et al. "Getting Enough: Mothers' Concerns about Breastfeeding a Preterm Infant after Discharge." *Journal of Obstetric, Gynecologic, and Neonatal Nursing* 24 (1995): 23–32.

Keating, J. P., G. J. Schears, and P. R. Dodge. "Oral Water Intoxication in Infants: An American Epidemic." *American Journal of Disease in Childhood* 145 (1991): 985–90.

Kennedy, K. I., et al. "Lactational Amenorrhea Method for Family Planning." *International Journal of Gynaecology and Obstetrics* 54 (1996): 55–57.

Klingelhafer, S. K. "Sexual Abuse and Breastfeeding." *Journal of Human Lactation* 23 (2007): 194–97.

Koetting, C. A., and G. M. Wardlaw. "Wrist, Spine, and Hip Bone Density in Women with Variable Histories of Lactation." *American Journal of Clinical Nutrition* 48 (1988): 1479–81.

Kotaska, A., et al. "Epidural Analgesia Associated with Low-Dose Oxytocin Augmentation Increases Cesarean Births: A Critical Look at the External Validity of Randomized Trials." *American Journal of Obstetrics and Gynecology* 194 (2006): 809–14.

Kramer, M. S., et al. "Breastfeeding and Child Cognitive Development: New Evidence from a Large Randomized Trial." *Archives of General Psychiatry* 65 (2008): 578–84.

Labbok, M. H., and G. E. Hendershot. "Does Breastfeeding Protect against Malocclusion? Analysis of the 1981 Child Health Supplement to the National Health Interview Survey." *American Journal of Preventative Medicine* 3 (1987): 227–32.

Lawrence, Ruth A., and Robert M. Lawrence. *Breastfeeding: A Guide for the Medical Profession.* St. Louis: Mosby, 2010.

————. *A Review of the Medical Benefits and Contraindications to Breastfeeding in the United States.* Arlington, VA: National Center for Education in Maternal and Child Health, 1997.

Layde, P. M., et al. "The Independent Associations of Parity, Age of First Full-Term Pregnancy, and Duration of Breastfeeding with the Risk of Breast Cancer." *Journal of Clinical Epidemiology* 42 (1989): 963–93.

Lee, S. Y., et al. "Effect of Lifetime Lactation on Breast Cancer Risk: A Korean Women's Cohort Study." *International Journal of Cancer* 105 (2003): 390–93.

Lieberman, E., and C. O'Donoghue. "Unintended Effects of Epidural Anesthesia: A Systematic Review." *American Journal of Obstetrics and Gynecology Supplement* 186 (2002): s31–68.

Lindenberg, C. S., et al. "The Effect of Early Post Partum Mother-Infant Contact and Breastfeeding Promotion on the Incidence and Continuation of Breastfeeding." *International Journal of Nursing Studies* 27 (1990): 179–86.

Livingstone, Verity, and L. Judy Stringer. "The Treatment of *Staphyloccus aureus* Infected Sore Nipples: A Randomized Comparative Study." *Journal of Human Lactation* 15, no. 3 (1999): 241–46.

Lopez, J. M., et al. "Bone Turnover and Density in Healthy Women during Breastfeeding and after Weaning." *Osteoporosis International* 6 (1996): 153–59.

Lucas, A., et al. "Breastmilk and Subsequent Intelligence Quotient in Children Born Preterm." *Lancet* 339 (1992): 261–64.

Main, E. K., et al. "Is There a Useful Cesarean Birth Measure? Assessment of the Nulliparous Term Singleton Vertex Cesarean Birth Rate as a Tool for Obstetric Quality Improvement." *American Journal of Obstetrics and Gynecology* 194 (2006): 1644–52.

Marasco, L., et al. "Polycystic Ovary Syndrome: A Connection to Insufficient Milk Supply?" *Journal of Human Lactation* 16 (2000): 143–48.

Mayer, E. J., et al. "Reduced Risk of IDDM among Breastfed Children." *Diabetes* 37 (1988): 1625–32.

McJunkin, J. E., W. G. Bithoney, and M. C. McCormick. "Errors in Formula Concentration in an Outpatient Population." *Journal of Pediatrics* 111 (1987): 848–50.

McTiernan, A., and D. B. Thomas. "Evidence for a Protective Effect of Lactation on Risk of Breast Cancer in Young Women." *American Journal of Epidemiology* 124 (1986): 353–58.

McVea, K. L., et al. "The Role of Breastfeeding in Sudden Infant Death Syndrome." *Journal of Human Lactation* 16 (2000): 13–20.

Meier, Paula. "A Program to Support Breastfeeding in the High-Risk Nursery." *Perinatology/Neonatology* 4 (1980): 43–48.

————. *Professional Guide to Breastfeeding Premature Infants.* Columbus, OH: Abbott Laboratories, 1997.

Meier, Paula, and G. Anderson. "Responses of Small Preterm Infants to Bottle- and Breast-Feeding." *Maternal-Child Nursing* 12 (1987): 97–105.

Meier, Paula, et al. "Nipple Shields for Preterm Infants: Effect on Milk Transfer and Duration of Breastfeeding." *Journal of Human Lactation* 16 (2000): 106–14.

Merchant, J. R., et al. "Respiratory Instability of Term and Near-Term Healthy Newborn Infants in Car Safety Seats." *Pediatrics* 108 (2001): 647–52.

Merrett, T. G., et al. "Infant Feeding and Allergy: Twelve-Month Prospective Study of 500 Babies Born in Allergic Families." *Annals of Allergy* 61 (1988): 13–20.

Mikiel-Kostyra, K., et al. "Effect of Skin to Skin Contact after Delivery on Duration of Breastfeeding: A Prospective Cohort Study." *Acta Paediatrica* 91 (2002): 1301–6.

Minutes of the Panel on Recommendations Relating to PBB and Nursing Mothers. Lansing: Michigan Department of Public Health, 1976.

Mitchell, E. A., et al. "Cot Death Supplement: Results from the First Year of the New Zealand Cot Death Study." *New Zealand Medical Journal* 104 (1991): 71–76.

Morino, C., and Susan M. Winn. "Raynaud's Phenomenon of the Nipples: An Elusive Diagnosis." *Journal of Human Lactation* 23 (2007): 191–93.

Morrow-Tlucak, M., R. H. Haude, and C. B. Ernhart. "Breastfeeding and Cognitive Development in the First Two Years of Life." *Social Science Medicine* 26 (1988): 635–39.

Morse, Janice M., and Margaret J. Harrison. "Social Coercion for Weaning." *Journal of Nurse Midwifery* 32 (1987): 205–10.

Mortensen, E. L., et al. "The Association between Duration of Breastfeeding and Adult Intelligence." *Journal of the American Medical Association* 287 (2002): 2365–71.

Morton, Jane, et al. "Combining Hand Techniques with Electric Pumping Increases Milk Production in Mothers of Preterm Infants." *Journal of Perinatology* 29 (2009): 757–64.

Moscone, S. R., and M. J. Moore. "Breastfeeding during Pregnancy." *Journal of Human Lactation* 9 (1993): 83–88.

Mosko, S., et al. "Infant Arousals during Mother-Infant Bed Sharing: Implications for Infant Sleep and Sudden Infant Death Syndrome Research." *Pediatrics* 100 (1997): 841–49.

Neifert, M. R., and J. M. Seacat. "Contemporary Breastfeeding Management Clinics." *Perinatology* 12 (1995): 319–42.

Newman, J., and T. Pitman. *Dr. Jack Newman's Guide to Breastfeeding.* Toronto: HarperCollins Canada, 2009.

Nommsen-Rivers, L. A., et al. "Newborn Wet and Soiled Diaper Counts and Timing of On-set of Lactation as Indicators of Breastfeeding Inadequacy." *Journal of Human Lactation* 24 (2008): 27–33.

Oddy, W. H., et al. "Breast Feeding and Respiratory Morbidity in Infancy: A Birth Cohort Study." *Archives of Disease in Childhood* 88 (2003): 224–28.

————. "Association between Breast Feeding and Asthma in 6-Year-Old Children: Find-ings of a Prospective Birth Cohort Study." *British Medical Journal* 319 (1999): 815–19.

Owen, C., et al. "Does Breastfeeding Influence Risk of Type 2 Diabetes in Later Life? A Quantitative Analysis of Published Evidence." *American Journal of Clinical Nutrition* 84 (2006): 1043–54.

————. "Infant Feeding and Blood Cholesterol: A Study in Adolescents and a Systematic Review." *Pediatrics* 110 (2002): 597–608.

Quigley, M. A., et al. "Breastfeeding and Hospitalization for Diarrheal and Respiratory Infection in the United Kingdom: Millennium Cohort Study." *Pediatrics* 119 (2007): e837–42.

Rayburn, W. F., and J. Zhang. "Rising Rates of Labor Induction: Present Concerns and Future Strategies." *Obstetrics and Gynecology* 100 (2002): 164–67.

Reynolds, A. "Breastfeeding and Brain Development." *Pediatric Clinics of North America* 48 (2001): 159–71.

Rickert, V. I., and C. Merle Johnson. "Reducing Nocturnal Awakening and Crying Episodes in Infants and Young Children: A Comparison between Scheduled Awakenings and Systematic Ignoring." *Pediatrics* 81 (1988): 203–12.

Righard, L., and M. O. Alade. "Effect of Delivery Room Routines on the Success of First Breastfeed." *Lancet* 336 (1990): 1105–7.

Rinker, B. D., et al. "The Effect of Breastfeeding upon Breast Aesthetics." *Aesthetic Surgery Journal* 28 (2008): 534–37.

Riordan, Jan, and Francine Nichols. "A Descriptive Study of Lactation Mastitis in Long-term Breastfeeding Women." *Journal of Human Lactation* 6 (1990): 53–58.

Riordan, Jan, and Karen Wambach. *Breastfeeding and Human Lactation.* St. Louis: Mosby, 2009.

Riordan, Jan, et al. "The Effect of Labor Pain Relief Medication on Neonatal Suckling and Breastfeeding Duration." *Journal of Human Lactation* 16 (2000): 7–12.

Roberts, J. E. "The 'Push' for Evidence: Management of the Second Stage." *Journal of Mid-wifery and Women's Health* 47 (2002): 2–15.

Roberts, J. E., et al. "The Effects of Maternal Position on Uterine Contractility and Ef-ficiency." *Birth* 10 (1983): 243–49.

Romano, A., and J. Lothian. "Promoting, Protecting, and Supporting Normal Birth: A Look at the Evidence." *Journal of Obstetric, Gynecologic, and Neonatal Nursing* 37 (2008): 94–105.

Rosenblatt, K. A., D. B. Thomas, and WHO Collaborative Study of Neoplasia and Steroid Contraceptives. "Lactation and the Risk of Epithelial Ovarian Cancer." *International Journal of Epidemiology* 22 (1993): 192–97.

Sanchez-Ramos, L., et al. "Expectant Management versus Labor Induction for Suspected Fetal Macrosomia: A Systematic Review." *Obstetrics and Gynecology* 100 (2002): 997–1002.

Satter, Ellyn. *Child of Mine: Feeding with Love and Good Sense.* Palo Alto, CA: Bull Publishing, 2000.

Savino, F., et al. "*Lactobacillus reuteri* versus Simethicone in the Treatment of Infantile Colic: A Prospective Randomized Study." *Pediatrics* 119 (2007): e124–30.

Schach, B., and M. Haight. "Colic and Food Allergy in the Breastfed Infant: Is It Possible for an Exclusively Breastfed Infant to Suffer from Food Allergy?" *Journal of Human Lactation* 18 (2002): 50–52.

Simpkin, Penny, and M. O'Hara. Non-Pharmacologic Relief of Pain during Labor: Systematic Reviews of Five Methods. *American Journal of Obstetrics and Gynecology Supplement* 186 (2002): s131–59.

Souto, Gláucia C., et al. "The Impact of Breast Reduction Surgery on Breastfeeding Performance." *Journal of Human Lactation* 19 (2003): 43–49.

Tita, A. T., et al. "Timing of Elective Repeat Cesarean Delivery at Term and Neonatal Outcomes." *New England Journal of Medicine* 360 (2009): 111–20.

Tonkin, S., et al., "Apparently Life Threatening Events in Infant Car Safety Seats." *British Medical Journal* 333 (2006): 1205–6.

Torvaldsen, S., et al. "Intrapartum Epidural Analgesia and Breastfeeding: A Prospective Cohort Study." *International Breastfeeding Journal* 1 (2006): 24.

Vennemann, M. M., et al. "Does Breastfeeding Reduce the Risk of Sudden Infant Death Syndrome?" *Pediatrics* 123 (2009): e406–10.

Victora, C. G., et al. "Use of Pacifiers and Breastfeeding Duration." *Lancet* 341 (1993): 404–6.

Von Kries, R., et al. "Breast Feeding and Obesity: Cross-Sectional Study." *British Medical Journal* 319 (1999): 147–50.

Walker, Marsha. "A Fresh Look at the Risks of Artificial Infant Feeding." *Journal of Human Lactation* 9 (1993): 97–107.

Weintraub, R., G. Hams, M. Meerkin, and A. Rosenberg. "High Aluminum Content of Infant Milk Formulas." *Archives of Disease in Childhood* 61 (1986): 914–16.

Wickizer, Thomas M., Lawrence B. Brilliant, Richard Copeland, and Robert Tilden. "Polychlorinated Biphenyl Contamination of Nursing Mothers' Milk in Michigan." *American Journal of Public Health* 71 (1981): 132–37.

Wilson, A. C., et al. "Relation of Infant Diet to Childhood Health: Seven-Year Follow-up of Cohort of Children in Dundee Infant Feeding Study." *British Medical Journal* 316 (1998): 21–25.

Wilson-Clay, B. "Case Report of Methicillin-Resistant *Staphylococcus aureus* (MRSA) Mastitis with Abscess Formation in a Breastfeeding Woman." *Journal of Human Lactation* 24 (2008): 326–29.

Woolridge, M. W., and Chloe Fisher. "Colic, 'Overfeeding,' and Symptoms of Lactose Malabsorption in the Breast-fed Baby: A Possible Artifact of Feed Management?" *Lancet* 2 (1988): 3828.

Suggested
Supplmental Reading

Balaskas, Janet. *Active Birth: The New Approach to Giving Birth Naturally*, rev. ed. Boston: Harvard Common Press, 1992.

Bumgarner, Norma Jane. *Mothering Your Nursing Toddler*. Shaumburg, IL: La Leche League International, 2000.

Flower, Hilary. *Adventures in Tandem Nursing: Breastfeeding during Pregnancy and Beyond*. Shaumburg, IL: La Leche League International, 2003.

Fraiberg, Selma H. *The Magic Years*. New York: Charles Scribner's Sons, 1996.

Gromada, Karen Kerkhoff. *Mothering Multiples*. Shaumburg, IL: La Leche League International, 2007.

Huggins, Kathleen. *The Expectant Parents' Companion: Simplifying What to Do, Buy, or Borrow for an Easy Life with Baby*. Boston: Harvard Common Press, 2006.

Huggins, Kathleen, and Jan Ellen Brown. *The Nursing Mother's Companion Breastfeeding Diary*. Boston: Harvard Common Press, 2010.

Huggins, Kathleen, and Jan Ellen Brown. *25 Things Every Nursing Mother Needs to Know*. Boston: Harvard Common Press, 2009.

Huggins, Kathleen, and Linda Ziedrich. *The Nursing Mother's Guide to Weaning*, rev. ed. Boston: Harvard Common Press, 2007.

Karp, Harvey. *The Happiest Baby on the Block*. New York: Bantam Books, 2003.

Kleiman, Karen R., and Valerie D. Raskin. *This Isn't What I Expected: Overcoming Postpartum Depression*. New York: Bantam Books, 2013.

Kropp, Tori. *The Joy of Pregnancy: The Complete, Candid, and Reassuring Companion for Parents-to-Be*. Boston: Harvard Common Press, 2008.

McKenna, James. *Sleeping with Your Baby: A Parent's Guide to Cosleeping*. Washington, DC: Platypus Media, 2007.

Pantley, Elizabeth, and William Sears. *The No-Cry Sleep Solution*. New York: Contemporary Books, 2002.

Pryor, Gale, and Kathleen Huggins. *Nursing Mother, Working Mother*, rev. ed. Boston: Harvard Common Press, 2007.

Robertson, Laurel, Carol Flinders, and Brian Ruppenthal. *The New Laurel's Kitchen*. Berkeley, CA: Ten Speed Press, 1986.

Sears, William, Martha Sears, Robert Sears, and James Sears. *The Baby Book: Everything You Need to Know about Your Baby from Birth to Age Two*, rev. ed. Boston: Little, Brown, 2013.

Simkin, Penny. *The Birth Partner: A Complete Guide to Childbirth for Dads, Doulas, and All Other Labor Companions*, 3rd ed. Boston: Harvard Common Press, 2007.

Simkin, Penny, Janet Whalley, and Ann Keppler. *Pregnancy, Childbirth, and the Newborn: The Complete Guide*. Minnetonka, MN: Meadowbrook, 2001.

Vartabedian, Bryan. *Colic Solved: The Essential Guide to Infant Reflux and the Care of Your Crying, Difficult-to-Soothe Baby*. New York: Ballantine Books, 2007.

Index

evening primrose oil, 201
exercise
  antidepressant effect of, 199
  D-MER treatment with, 201
  in first two months after birth,
    156, 157, 199
expressing milk
  areola, softening by, 76
  for babies with birth defects,
    149
  for babies with cleft lip and
    palate, 151
  for babies with hydrocephalus
    or spina bifida, 152
  bottles for, 152
  breast lesions, cases of, 131
  colostrum, 71, 84, 85, 100, 101,
    104, 242–243
  discarding after, 376
  engorgement treatment, 62
  equipment for, 227, 345, 362
  feeding, 254–257
  feeding frequency, 104, 243
  during first week, 244
  formula and, 219
  during hospitalization, 177
  iodine, radioactive treatment
    and, 133
  for latch-on problems, 84
  methods of, 225–236
  milk overabundance and, 316
  for near-term babies, 137–138
  nipple wounds, 340
  for non-nursing babies,
    242–246
  after nursing, 71, 118, 220,
    229, 317–318
  before nursing, 105
  one-sided nursing, treating
    with, 319
  overview of, 224–225
  precautions, 202–203
  for premature or sick babies,
    138, 140, 143, 145, 191
  refusal to nurse, treatment
    measures for, 95, 96, 100,
    204, 345
  resources, 85
  before returning to work,
    237–238
  for sick babies, 138
  for slow weight gain, 220, 318
  for sucking problems, 102, 104
  supply, maintaining by, 94, 110
  techniques, 226–227, 244
  weaning off of expressed milk,
    73
  working mothers, 298, 306,
    317

in workplace, 238, 240, 252,
    293–294, 298
eye development, 3, 138
eyedropper, 221
eyedrops and ointments, 376

Fair Labor Standards Act, 294
family, nursing in presence of,
    285
family day care, 291
Family Medical Leave Act
    (FMLA), 289
famotidine (Pepcid), 215
fat
  accumulated, milk production
    role of, 7, 160
  losing excess, 7, 159
  milk as source of, 140
  saturated, reducing, 315
fatigue (mother)
  depression-related, 197
  dietary considerations, 344
  postpartum, 87–88, 148, 157,
    188, 196
  during pregnancy, 350
  weaning and, 335
fatigue (baby), 149
fatty acids, role of, 3
fatty fish, 168
fears about breastfeeding, 8–9
feeding cues, reduced
  in crawling babies, 323
  pacifier, 296, 306
feedings, difficult, with laryngo-
    malacia, 149
feedings, skipping, 314
feeding schedule, 163, 167–168
feeding skills
  of babies, 328, 333
  of toddlers, 351
feeding tube. See tube feeding
feet, tingling or burning, 162
fennel seed, 117, 363
fenugreek
  after breast surgery, 120
  as ingredient, 363
  for hypoplasia, 116–117
  Newman-Goldfarb protocols
    and, 125, 126
  obtaining, 362
  overview of, 72
  before period, 322
  for Polycystic Ovary Syndrome,
    119
  pumping and, 250
  relactation and, 129
  slow weight gain and, 318
  as underfeeding treatment
    measure, 222
Ferber, Richard, 342, 343

fertility, return of, 322
fever
  following epidural, 23–24
  nursing frequency during,
    177–178
fever blisters, 132, 177
fiber, foods containing, 156
fiber guidelines, 160
finger foods, 333
First Years Breastflow Memory
    pump, 270–271
First Years Easy Breastflow Man-
    ual pump, 281
First Years miPump Double Elec-
    tric Breast pump, 271
First Years Quiet Expressions
    Double Breast pump, 271
fish (baby)
  introduction of, 331
  recommendations for, 333
fish (mother)
  eating guidelines, 19
  as omega-3 fatty acid source,
    199
flange (breast pump)
  fit, 239, 243, 247, 250
  need for, 104
  obtaining, 360–361
  placement of nipple in, 233–
    234, 235, 236, 298
  selecting, 263, 264, 265, 275
  shields for, 314–315
  special, 276
flat nipple, 26, 27, 68, 83, 84
flextime schedule, 289–290
Flower, Hilary, 351
fluconazole (Diflucan), 184
fluid intake
  in first two months after birth,
    156, 158, 195
  for headaches, 196
  during illness, 176
  for mastitis, 192
  plugged ducts and prevention,
    188, 300, 314
  two to six months after birth,
    302, 316
  for working mothers, 300
fluoride, 168, 171, 213
folate, 121
folded nipple, 26, 27
food. See baby food; solid foods;
    table food; specific type of food
food allergies
  categories of, 210–214
  dairy products, 211, 334
  development, causes of, 166
  family members with, 330–331
  signs of, 210
  solid food introduction, 311

refined *vs.* whole-grain, 331
  for toddlers, 352
  whole-grain, 160
gripe water, 215
growth and development
  deficiencies, 328
  heart abnormality, 149
  infant formula and breast milk
    compared, 3
  poor, causes of, 216
  of toddlers, 351
  two to six months, 307–308,
    311
  WHO growth standards, 308,
    324, 371–373
guilt feelings, 197
gum gels, 309
gums, 326. *See also* teething

Haberman Feeder, 151, 365
hair loss, postpartum, 156
Hale, Thomas, 112
hallucinogens, 392
hand expression of milk
  after pumping, 245, 246, 261
  as pumping alternative, 36,
    226, 227
  technique of, 225–227
hand-operated pump, 228, 230,
  236, 270, 280–283
hands, washing, 61
hands-free bra, 244, 298
hands-free pumping, 247, 264,
  265, 276, 279, 298, 360–361
hands-on pumping, 244, 250
Happiest Baby on the Block, The
  (Karp), 205
harming baby, fears of, 198
hay fever, 383
headache, 186, 190, 196
heartburn (baby), 208, 209, 219
heart defects, nursing babies
  with, 149–150
heart disease, 8
heart medications, 386–387
heart problems, babies with, 140
heart rate (baby), 23, 63, 139,
  141
hemorrhage, postpartum, 42,
  70, 155
hemorrhoids, 88, 155
hepatitis A, 395
hepatitis B, 114–115, 395
hepatitis B-specific immunoglobulin (HBIG), 114
hepatitis B surface antigen
  (HBsAg), 114–115
hepatitis C, 115
herbals, 387–388

herbs
  for colic, 215
  for depression, 200
  risks associated with, 375
herbs, milk production stimulation with
  adoptive mothers, 128–129
  breast surgery and, 120
  contraindications for, 124
  vs. drugs, 109
  hypoplastic breasts, 119
  Newman-Goldfarb protocol
    role of, 125, 126
  obtaining, 362–363
  overview of, 72, 73, 109
  before period, 322
  pumping and, 250
  relactation and, 129, 130
  testing, 117
  underfeeding treatment with,
    222
herpes, nursing mothers with,
  115, 131–132
herpes sore in mouth, 344
Herpes Type I lesions, 132
hiccuping, 60, 96
high chair, 329
high-protein foods
  for babies, 333
  for mothers, 87, 145, 148
  for toddlers, 352
hindmilk
  for babies with heart defects,
    149–150
  colic treatment and prevention
    with, 214, 229
  one-breast nursing and, 164
  for premature babies, 140, 141
  for sick babies, 140
HIV (human immunodeficiency
  virus), 115, 122, 235
home birth, 30
honey, 84, 100
hopelessness, feelings of, 197
hormonal contraceptives, 305,
  389
hormone replacement therapy,
  127
hormones
  breastfeeding readiness, 123
  drop, headaches caused by,
    196
  drug category, 388–390
  postpartum shift, 65, 157, 196
hospital-grade pump, 231, 232,
  258. *See also* clinical-grade
  pump
hospitalization
  nursing and, 176–177, 287–288

risk, formula *vs.* breast milk
  compared for, 3
hospitals and birthing centers,
  selecting, 29–30
human immunodeficiency virus
  (HIV), 115, 122, 235
Human Milk 4 Human Babies,
  167
Human Milk Banking Association of North America, 167,
  251, 366–367
human T-cell leukemia virus
  type 1 (HTLV-1), 115
hydrocephalus, 151, 152
hydrogel dressings, 75
hydrogenated oils, 332
Hygeia EnDeare pump, 262
Hygeia EnHande One-Hand
  Manual Breast pump, 282
Hygeia EnJoye pump, 234, 247,
  267–268, 275
Hygeia EnJoye Q pump, 275
Hygeia Medical Group II, 361,
  362, 365
Hygeia milk expression cup, 227
Hygeia Two-Handed Manual
  Breast pump, 283
hyperlactation syndrome, 210,
  214
hypertension, severe, 123
hyperthyroidism, 133
hypoallergenic detergents, 79
hypoallergenic formula, 210
hypoplasia/hypoplastic breasts
  appearance and identification
    of, 117
  milk production insufficient
    due to, 107, 111, 223
  overview of, 116–118, 223
  pumping in cases of, 241
hypothyroidism, 132–133

ibuprofen. *See also* Advil; Motrin
  after birth, 65
  after cesarean birth, 52, 156
  for engorged breasts, 70
  for headache, 196
  for mastitis, 192
  as nipple dermatitis ointment
    ingredient, 185
  before nursing, 42, 74, 82
  safety of, 383
  for teething pain, 309, 341
ice cream, 211, 213
ice packs, 155
illness (baby)
  baby care and, 292–293
  night waking due to, 325

premature baby safety issues, 139
for thyroid condition, 133
Meier, Paula, 260
melamine, 4
Melodi Advanced One pump, 263
Melodi Advanced pump, 262–263
Melodi Prime pump, 266, 275
meningitis, bacterial, 4
menopausal Newman-Goldfarb protocol, 127
menopause, nursing after, 127
menstrual periods
    milk production decline at start of, 250, 322
    resuming after birth, 9, 305–306, 312, 321–322
    salt intake, limiting before, 315
mental function
    depression effect on, 197
    postpartum problems with, 157
mental health care for depression, 200
mercury sources, 19
metformin, 119
methyldopa (Aldomet), 124
metoclopramide (Reglan), 112, 215
Micatin, 183
miconazole, 185
Microgestin, 123, 126, 127
microwave oven, 254
midwives, 30
migraine headaches, 196, 382, 383
migraine medications, 382–383
milk. See also cow's milk; donated milk; expressing milk; foremilk; hindmilk; leaking milk
    appearance and characteristics of, 82–83, 252
    bacterial testing of, 166
    blood in, 83, 189, 194
    composition and characteristics of, 167, 170
    content during pregnancy, 349
    defrosting and warming, 252, 254–255, 296, 366
    digestion of, 202, 208
    discarding, 114, 115, 140, 375, 376
    drug content in, 18, 374–376
    handling and feeding, 297
    jaundice treatment with, 91
    leaking (see leaking milk)

nutrients in, 311
overabundant, 195, 229, 247, 316, 350
pasteurizing, 166, 167
quality of, 9, 167
quantity of, 9
solid foods as replacement, 311
spitting up, 60
taste, change in, 344
transporting, 243, 254, 295, 298
vitamin C levels in, 163
milk allergy, 334
milk banks, 166–167, 251, 366–368
milk collection and storage
    for adopted baby, 125, 126
    advances in, 9
    benefits of, 234
    equipment for, 251, 365
    freezing milk, 94, 136, 140, 222, 229, 237–238, 247, 251, 252, 253, 287, 297, 366
    before or during hospitalization, 176, 177, 243, 254
    overview of, 250–253
    for premature or sick baby, 140, 253–254
    refrigerating milk, 177, 229, 245, 251, 252, 253, 255, 287, 295, 297, 298
    refusal to nurse, 105
    using stored milk, 297
    at workplace, 252, 295
milk ducts, plugged
    breast infection, 188
    breast lumps as sign of, 193
    breast pain accompanying, 80
    causes of, 229
    overview of, 187–188
    preventing, 147, 164, 276, 300, 302, 314–315
    treatment measures for, 131, 188–189
milk ducts, severed, 119–120
milk fistula, 194
milk intake (baby)
    adequate, signs of, 55–56, 58, 59, 89, 94, 107, 137, 166, 178, 204, 218–219, 242, 307
    estimating, 55–56, 110, 143–144, 151
    inadequate, risk factors for, 57, 85
    inadequate, signs of, 88–89
    during mother-baby separation, 287–288

requirements, estimating, 107–108, 110, 144, 151, 220, 222, 229, 237, 247–248, 299, 369–371
requirements vs. production, 220, 242, 318, 369–371
milk intake (mother)
    guidelines and requirements, 161
    milk overabundance and, 316
    multiple births, 148
milk intake (toddler), 352
milk production
    of adoptive mothers, 120–121
    of bed-sharing mothers, 172
    capability of, 15
    constant nature of, 163
    decline or insufficient, causes of, 70, 107, 111, 116, 134, 136, 165, 168, 176, 219, 222–223, 228, 236, 240, 241–242, 245, 250, 307, 317
    estimating, 73, 108, 130, 220, 222, 232, 318
    estrogen effect on, 303, 305, 307, 317
    factors affecting, 58
    fat, accumulated role in, 160
    late onset of, 17, 21, 23, 57, 61, 70–73, 232, 241
    loss of, 190
    maintaining, 96, 102, 105, 114, 147, 152, 244, 247
    mature, overview of, 61–62
    monitoring, 118
    for multiple babies, 144
    nursing impact on, 55
    nutritional intake considerations, 160
    overview of, 17–18
    peak period of, 229
    post-menopause, 127
    preparation for, 127
    pumping and bottle feeding, 101
    rebuilding, 129
    requirements for, 71, 73, 129, 145
    signs of, 55, 57
    stimulating (see also drugs, milk production stimulation with; herbs, milk production stimulation with)
        after breast surgery, 120
        for babies in underfeeding risk groups, 58
        expressing milk, 226, 238, 244, 245, 317–318
        hypoplasia, 116–117

milk production
stimulating (*cont.*)
  nursing frequency impact
    on, 165, 206, 221, 306–
    307, 323
  Polycystic Ovary Syn-
    drome (PCOS), 119
  for premature babies, 139
  by pumping, 58, 81, 109,
    129, 145, 203, 219, 221,
    245–246, 249–250, 300,
    317–318, 376
  slow weight gain, treating,
    317
suppressing, 124
tandem nursing and, 350
milk purity, 28–30
milk release, 18, 82, 164, 201. *See
also* let-down
milk sharing, casual, 167
milk supplementation for premature babies, 140–141
milk supply
breast surgery effect on,
  119–120
bringing in, 96
building, 112, 136, 145
decrease in, 216
demand as factor in, 179, 299
ensuring, 52–58, 89
established, 134
in first two months, 165–167
increasing, 89, 103, 124, 125,
  127–128, 220, 242, 300
low, 82, 85, 119, 120, 132, 223,
  359
maintaining, 75, 94, 114, 143,
  152, 177, 289, 300, 376
normal, 299
overabundant, 214
pregnancy effect on, 349
rebuilding, 108
refusal to nurse and, 345
requirements, 247–248
supplementing, 126
Mimijumi bottle nipples, 256
minerals, 160
modesty, heightened in sexual
abuse survivors, 134
Mojab, Cynthia Good, 169, 170
monilia. *See* thrush
Monistat 7, 183
monophasic birth control pills,
  123
Montgomery's tubercles, 14
moodiness, 157
mood swings, 65–66
More Milk Plus, 72, 129, 222,
  250, 318, 363

More Milk Special Blend, 72,
  117, 119, 120, 129, 363
Moro reflex, 205
Morton, Jane, 47–48, 71, 85, 98,
  226, 244, 245, 359
mother-baby exercises, 157
mother-child bonding
beginning of, 39
breastfeeding role in, 6, 11, 39,
  288, 335
home, time at, 289
physical contact, 35, 139
rooming in, 29
mother-child separation
after complicated birth, 21
expressing milk (*see* expressing
  milk, for mother-baby
  separation)
fever treatment as cause of, 24
milk storage for, 234
planning for, 287–288,
  290–293
after premature birth, 24–25
refusal to nurse after, 344
motherhood, adjustment to, 66,
  88, 157, 180
Mothering Your Nursing Toddler
  (Bumgarner), 251, 349
mother-led weaning, 354–356
Motherlove Herbal Company,
  72, 117, 363, 365
Motherlove Nipple Cream, 75,
  76, 364
mothers
breastfeeding benefits to, 6–10
workload, easing for new, 37,
  64, 66, 87, 88, 198, 300
mothers' groups, 157, 158
motility drugs, 215
Motilium. *See* domperidone
motion, baby love of, 206, 209,
  217–218
motion sickness, drugs for, 384
motor development, 3
motor skills, acquiring, 322–323,
  345
Motrin. *See also* ibuprofen
Infants', 309, 327, 339, 341
mouth conformation problems,
  57, 241
MRI, 194
MRSA (methicillin-resistant
  Staphylococcus aureus), 191,
  315
mucus, spitting up, 60
multiple babies, 144–148
multiple sclerosis, 168
multiple-user pump, 235, 267,
  268

mupirocin, 80, 185
Murkett, Tracey, 329
muscle relaxants, 391
muscle tone, excessive, 153
muscle tone, poor
in babies with cerebral palsy,
  153
in babies with Down syn-
  drome, 57, 152
milk pumping for babies with,
  232
in premature babies, 141
muscular growth, 3
music, soothing, 341
My Best Friend Nursing Pillow,
  364
Mycostatin, 182–183, 207
Mylanta, 214
Mylicon, 214

nanny, hiring, 291, 292
napping (baby), 157, 286, 304
napping (mother)
before expressing milk, 245
in first two months, 157, 198
in first week, 87
plugged ducts and breast
  infections, preventing, 314
before sexual intercourse, 304
timing, 198
in two to six months after
  birth, 302
for working mothers, 300
narcotic pain relievers, 65, 137
narcotics, 382–383, 392
nasal inhalers, 384
nasal sprays, 383
National Highway Traffic Safety
  Administration, 34
National Women's Health Information Center, 231
National Women's Law Center,
  231
natural family planning, 306
nausea during nursing, 195
near-clinical-grade pump
vs. clinical-grade pump, 245
overview of, 287
refusal to nurse, use during,
  204
near-term babies
birth complications in, 24
breastfeeding of, 136–138
milk supply for, 145
underfeeding risks in, 57, 242
neck, difficulty turning, 97
neck stretching exercises, 97
needle aspirations, 193
needle biopsies, 194

one-breast nursing
  burping after, 89–90, 106, 209
  and hindmilk, 164
  overabundant milk, 214, 316
  reflux, treating with, 209
one-sided nursing, 96–97,
  318–319
onions, 162, 211
online classes, 289
oral antifungal agents, 184
oral contraceptives
  combination birth control
    pills, 249
  domperidone, taking without,
    125, 126, 128
  health risks associated with,
    127
  milk production stimulation
    with, 125, 126
  pregnancy simulated with,
    123–124
organic solvent exposure, 19
Ortho Evra, 305
Ortho-Novum 1/35, 123, 126,
  127
osteoporosis, 8–9, 161
out-of-network provider, 230
ovarian cancer, 8
Overactive Let-down Syndrome,
  214
overfeeding, avoiding, 248, 299
overheating
  avoiding, 174
  as SIDS risk factor, 172
  as sleeping hazard, 173
overhydration, 70
overlying
  as bed-sharing hazard, 173
  risk, eliminating of, 173
over-the-counter drugs, check-
  ing safety of, 176
over-the-counter pain relievers,
  65, 156
oxygen levels in car seat, 63, 64
oxytocin
  headache during let-down
    related to, 196
  milk release role of, 18
  natural and artificial com-
    pared, 22
oyster shell, 162

paced bottle feeding, 258, 296
pacifier
  for babies with colic or reflux,
    206, 209, 217
  feeding cues and, 296, 306,
    316

night wakings and, 310, 326,
  341
between nursings, 248
pre-weaning introduction,
  pitfalls of, 42, 43, 89, 143
putting aside for nursing, 317
refusal to nurse following, 95
sterilizing, 184
toddler use of, 348, 354
use guidelines, 134
pain during nursing (baby), 209
pain during nursing (mother),
  8, 187, 189, 192
painful nipples, 185–186
pain medication
  after cesarean birth, 156
  during birth process, 88
  for engorgement, 70
  during first week, 65, 70
  before nursing, 82
  during nursing, 177
  safety of, 382–383
  for sore nipples, 74
palate defects, 57, 59, 102–103,
  107, 150–151, 219, 241
Palmer, Gabrielle, 3
Pamelor, 200
panic attacks, 197
Pantley, Elizabeth, 310, 342–343
papilloma, 83
Parent Directed Feeding, 167,
  168
paroxetine (Paxil), 200
partner
  breastfeeding, attitude con-
    cerning, 336
  childcare provided by, 290
  exhaustion of, 304
  post-childbirth adjustment
    role of, 66, 87
part-time work, 289
Paxil, 200
PCB, 19
PCEA (patient-controlled epidural anesthesia), 24, 25
peanut butter, 160, 211, 213, 330
peanuts, 213, 331
Pedialyte, 178
pediatric dentists, 99
pediatrician, selecting, 30–31
pelvic floor, strengthening, 156
penicillin, 190, 191, 379
Pepcid, 215
perfume, 203
periods. See menstrual periods
personal-use pumps, 227, 234–
  235, 237, 263–275
pesticides, 19, 61
phencyclidine (PCP), 392

phenylalanine, 135–136
phenylketonuria (PKU), 135–136
phenylpropanolamine, 212
Philips Avent Comfort Double
  pump, 269, 277
Philips Avent Comfort Single
  Electric pump, 277
Philips Avent Isis Manual pump,
  280
phosphorus, 140
phototherapy
  dark stools due to, 90
  nursing during, 92, 93
  overview of, 92
pH probe, 216
physical changes, postpartum,
  155–157
physical therapist, 152
phytoestrogens, 127
pillows, nursing
  obtaining, 364
  positioning at breast with help
    of, 35–36, 147, 338
"pinch test," 26–27
Pitocin
  epidural combined with, 23
  purpose of, 22
  side effects on baby, 23, 91
PJ's Bliss pump, 268
PJ's Comfort pump, 234, 268
PJ's Manual Breast pump, 283
placental fragments in uterus
  milk supply, low due to, 70,
    223
  symptoms, 73
  underfeeding risks associated
    with, 57, 70
plastic bags for milk storage,
  251, 253, 365
plastic bottles, 251
plastic carriers, 35
Platypus Media, 359
Playtex bottle nipples, 256
pneumonia, 163, 216
Politics of Breastfeeding, The
  (Palmer), 3
Polycystic Ovary Syndrome
  (PCOS)
  milk production and, 72, 107,
    111, 223, 363
  overview of, 119
  pumping in cases of, 241
  underfeeding risks associated
    with, 57
portion sizes
  for babies, 333
  for toddlers, 351–352
positioning at breast
  cleft lip and palate, babies
    with, 150